ATLAS OF SPEECH AND HEARING ANATOMY

JOEL C. KAHANE, Ph.D.
Associate Professor
Department of Audiology and Speech Pathology
Memphis State University

JOHN F. FOLKINS, Ph.D.
Associate Professor
Department of Speech Pathology and Audiology
University of Iowa

Charles E. Merrill Publishing Company
A Bell & Howell Company
Columbus Toronto London Sydney

This book is dedicated to our families.

Published by
Charles E. Merrill Publishing Company
A Bell & Howell Company
Columbus, Ohio 43216

This book was set in Zapf.
Production Coordination and Text Design: Cherlyn B. Paul
Layout: Steve Botts

Library of Congress Catalog Card Number: 83–061497
International Standard Book Number: 0–675–20126–8
Printed in the United States of America

1 2 3 4 5 6 7 8 9 10 — 88 87 86 85 84

Preface

The *Atlas of Speech and Hearing Anatomy* is designed as a comprehensive source of anatomy for professionals in communication sciences and disorders. This *Atlas* is composed largely of material from anatomical specimens, such as photographs of human dissections and photomicrographs. This format was chosen because we feel that structural relationships are ideally illustrated with actual anatomical preparations. Drawings and illustrations have been taken from the literature to clarify and depict certain anatomical concepts; most are detailed drawings based on human dissections. We have restricted use of stylized line drawings to places in which it was necessary to present a highly schematic form.

The figures and illustrations in this *Atlas* are drawn from a variety of sources and represent a blend of classical and contemporary research. Drawings from vintage anatomy atlases have been included at the beginning of many chapters to provide a historical backdrop for the ways in which structures of speech and hearing have been studied by classical anatomists. In addition to conveying basic anatomical information, the figures in this *Atlas* are intended to acquaint the reader with various techniques used in anatomical research. These research methods enable us to illustrate different aspects of structures and provide a more comprehensive description than would be possible with a single technique. Throughout this *Atlas* are examples of gross dissection, microdissection, light microscopy, scanning and electron microscopy, and macrophotography.

The 22 chapters of the *Atlas* are divided into three parts: the speech mechanism, the auditory system, and the nervous system. Although obvious differences in anatomy dictate some differences in presentation, most chapters begin by presenting general relationships, followed by greater detail through close-up photography or microscopic anatomy. The large number of figures within chapters allow structures to be viewed from many perspectives to reinforce basic morphology, help to clarify structural detail, and illustrate three-dimensional relationships. Along with each structure of the speech and hearing mechanism, we have endeavored to present as much pertinent regional anatomy as possible. This has been done to preserve relationships which might be obscured by taking structures out of their anatomical contexts. In most figures, numbers or letters have been used to identify the parts of a structure. The anatomical name of a part of a structure is contained in the accompanying legend.

We have designed the *Atlas* to accompany existing textbooks and to supplement a variety of courses in speech and hearing sciences, communicative disorders, and allied disciplines. We hope it helps to focus attention on some of the intricacies of structure that make the processes of speech and hearing possible.

ACKNOWLEDGMENTS

We wish to thank the many people who contributed to this book. Without their substantial input it would not have been completed. First, we would like to express our appreciation to all the authors and publishers who allowed us to use their published materials. We feel that the quality of this book is greatly increased by supplementing the original material with the best figures available in the literature.

There are a number of people whom we would especially like to recognize for their contributions: Dr. Nikolajas Cauna for his generous permission to photograph dissections from the Anatomy Museum of the Department of Anatomy and Cell Biology, School of Medicine, University of Pittsburgh; Bob Moore and Jan Hart for the kindness shown and assistance given to us while working in the University of Pittsburgh Anatomy Museum; Terence Williams for allowing us access to and use of many of the resources of the Department of Anatomy, University of Iowa; many members of the Department of Otolaryngology and Maxillofacial Surgery, University of Iowa, for offering help, advice, and the use of equipment; Alfred S. Lavorato for the dissections he made for this book; Gary van Hoesen for providing the photographs of brain sections from the Yakovlev Collection, and Vernon Armbrustmachter for giving permission to use them.

Appreciation is also extended to the scientists who contributed specific unpublished material or who helped with procurement of material. They include: Richard Babin, Ysae Barnwell, Diane Bless, Keith Clark, Ivan Hunter-Duvar, Berit Engström, Hans Engström, Edward Friedman, Lori Galey, Nedzad Gluhbegovic, Edward Harris, Alice Kahn, Jesse Kennedy III, Robert Kimura, Herbert Langdon, David Lim, Raymond Linville, Biagio J. Melloni, Robert Purdy, Christopher Squier, and Gary van Hoesen. There are many other scientists around the world who offered us advice and encouragement in our search for unpublished material.

Our appreciation and admiration is extended to several photographers whose efforts resulted in many of the figures. They include Dan Dixon, University of Pittsburgh; Thurman Hobson, University of Tennessee, Center for the Health Sciences; Paul Riemann, University of Iowa; and Ruben Barreras, University of Iowa. We would also like to thank Larry Perkins and the staff at the Medical Photography Center, University of Iowa, for reproducing a number of photographs.

We express our gratitude to the librarians who assisted in our research. Richard Eimas, Miriam Morgan, and Edwin Holtum of the University of Iowa Health Sciences Library were especially helpful. The historical figures are from the John Martin Rare Book Room, University of Iowa Health Sciences Library.

We would also like to thank our research assistants — Edna Dixon, Mary Hardin, Alice Kahn, Raymond Linville, Linda Newman, Carol Zeenhov, and Cathy Zimmerman — for their assistance during various phases of this project. We thank Georgia Folkins for her help with the index, and Marcia Elam, Madonna Gaume, and Shirley Rias for typing the manuscript, the permission forms, and the index.

Many thanks are extended to colleagues in our respective faculties at the Department of Audiology and Speech Pathology, Memphis State University, and the Department of Speech Pathology and Audiology, University of Iowa, for the interest and encouragement shown during the preparation of this book.

Finally, our sincerest appreciation goes to Charles E. Merrill Publishing Company and to the editorial staff with whom we have worked: Marianne Taflinger, Vicki Knight, and Cherlyn Paul. We have greatly valued their unqualified support, encouragement, and guidance.

The figures in this *Atlas* are the products of various anatomical methods, each of which allows structural relationships to be illustrated in unique ways. No one method is best for all purposes — each has its own advantages and disadvantages. The principal techniques used in this book include viewing surface anatomy, dissection, and histological techniques. Material prepared using these techniques is presented either through conventional photography, photomicrographs, or detailed drawings. A number of electron-micrographs, which require special tissue preparation techniques, are also presented. Each of these methods is briefly described below.

SURFACE ANATOMY

Some anatomical relationships can be observed from the surface of the body. Surface anatomy has one advantage over all the other anatomical techniques used here: it can be done with live human subjects. We have used photographs of surface anatomy to illustrate the face (Chapter 11), intraoral anatomy (Chapter 7), and the auricle (Chapter 14). The endoscopic views of the velopharynx (Figure 16–4) might also be considered surface anatomy.

GROSS DISSECTION

Gross dissection is the process of cutting into a cadaver or an isolated organ. Gross dissection is done with the unaided eye (in contrast to microdissection, in which a microscope is used). It is the method of choice for describing general anatomical relationships of the body and of particular organs or regions of the body. More specific structural information is obtained by separating layers of tissues, cutting through structures, and removing or reflecting portions of structures to expose more deeply situated components. Gross dissection is used to determine the size and shape of structures, boundaries between them, points of attachment and orientation of muscle fibers, and the course and general patterns of blood vessels and nerves. Studying the architecture and anatomy of bones (osteology) may also be done during dissection by removing soft tissue from the underlying bone.

Gross dissection of the nervous system employs special techniques because tissues of the nervous system are fragile and subject to distortion and damage. Most dissection of the brain is done by blunt dissection, that is, with blunt instruments such as an orangewood manicure stick or blunt tissue forceps with a smooth edge. Scalpels or knives are rarely used except to slice the brain into thick sections to illustrate overall morophologic features. Fiber tracts, nuclear masses, and surface topography are studied by scrapping and teasing tissues and stripping away small bundles of fibers. Frequently a stream of water is run over a part of a specimen to remove tissue gently from the surface of a structure.

MICRODISSECTION

Microdissection is dissection done with the aid of a specially designed microscope. Dissecting microscopes have relatively low power (from 4× to 100×) with a large depth of field. Unlike with the light microscope, it is not necessary to stain, section, or mount specimens to study them with the dissecting microscope. Microdissection is frequently used with small structures or when detail is desired for a particular aspect of a structure, such as a nerve supply, blood supply, or muscle fiber architec-

Anatomical Methods

ture. The dissection microscope affords better views of three-dimensional relationships than the conventional light microscope.

HISTOLOGIC TECHNIQUES

Histology is the microscopic study of tissues and includes the study of cells and organ systems. Histology compliments gross anatomy by providing details of structures which cannot be seen with the unaided eye. Most techniques in histology have been developed to prepare tissues for study by the light microscope, as this has been the most common form of microscopy used.

Tissue is distorted to some degree as a result of histologic processing; however, precautions are taken to minimize these effects and preserve as much as possible the physical properties, chemical characteristics, and staining characteristics.

Specimens are first placed in solutions called *fixatives* which preserve and harden tissue. The specimens are dehydrated, then embedded in paraffin or plastic so that they may be sliced (sectioned) into thin sections (usually 5–10 μm) by a microtome. The sections are mounted on glass slides and stained with agents that selectively color or label different parts of tissue or cells which are naturally transparent. The stained section is placed on the stage of the microscope and light is passed through it from below; the image is resolved and magnified by the lens system of the microscope.

Large sections of the brain such as those found in Chapter 19 require special handling during sectioning and mounting. Sections thicker than those routinely used in transmission light microscopy require longer periods of time for fixation and staining.

Photographs made through the microscope are called *photomicrographs;* those taken with close-up or other specialized photographic lenses are called *photomacrographs.*

The invention of the electron microscope and specialized optical and acoustic microscopes has necessitated the development of specialized histologic techniques which are described in conjunction with the electron microscope in the next section.

MICROSCOPY

Photographs from light microscopy and transmission and scanning electron microscopy are presented throughout this *Atlas.* Although each type of microscope provides a different kind of information, and each requires special preparation of tissue, the usefulness of all microscopes depends on their ability to magnify and, more importantly, to resolve detail.

Light Microscopy

The light microscope is the most commonly used microscope. It operates by passing light of specific temperature and spectral characteristics through a thin (approximately 5–10 μm) and usually stained specimen. The dispersion of light passing through the specimen is gathered by the first of a series of lenses and passed on to other lenses which refine the optical properties of the image.

The final image that reaches the viewer's eye or photographic film is highly corrected and resolved. The light microscope has resolution up to 0.02 μm and is capable of magnifications up to 1500$\times$ to 2000$\times$.

Electron Microscopy

Electron microscopy permits observation of tissues and cells at levels beyond the resolution of the light microscope. One form of electron microscopy is *transmission electron microscopy*. It provides enormous levels of magnification (up to 200,000$\times$) and great resolution of detail (as small as 2Å, but usually about 30Å). This is accomplished by beams of electrons (instead of light beams) which pass through specially prepared tissues and then through electromagnetic fields (instead of optical lenses). Here electrons expose a photographic plate and create a highly resolved image.

Another form of electron microscopy is *scanning electron microscopy*. This technique provides highly magnified images of surface structure. It provides photographs with a striking three-dimensional quality. Scanning electron microscopy involves coating specimens with heavy metals such as gold or platinum alloys. The metal-coated surfaces are bombarded with a narrow beam of electrons. The reflections from the surfaces expose a photographic plate producing images with extraordinary detail and a unique display of depth.

Examples of both transmission and scanning electron microscopy are found in Part II. Electron microscopy is especially useful for showing the detail of the tiny structures within the cochlear duct in Chapter 17.

Contents

Part I covers The Speech Mechanism. The speech mechanism is not composed of a single structure or system, but rather is a functional composite of many structures. Although we have presented the various components of the speech mechanism as separate chapters, we realize that any division of a functionally integrated system is somewhat artificial. Accordingly, with the exception of Chapter 1 on the skull and skeleton, we have presented the anatomy of the structures of the head, neck, and thorax in a sequence that reflects the aerodynamic–acoustic progression of events during speech: we start with the respiratory system and work upwards to the lips. Although the auditory and nervous systems are, strictly speaking, part of the speech mechanism, they are presented separately as Parts II and III, respectively.

Part I consists of eleven chapters: skeleton and skull, thorax and abdomen, neck, larynx, pharynx, velopharynx, oral cavity, nasal cavity, tongue, craniofacial complex, and face. These chapters contain figures from diverse sources—original dissections, research literature, and textbooks. This heterogeneity, which we believe to be a strength, also creates some problems. A number of figures are photographs of cadaver dissections which contained permanent labels. These labels could not be changed to conform with the style of the rest of the Atlas without distorting anatomical features or compromising the aesthetics of the figure. In these figures the reader is directed to only certain numbers on the specimens that are defined in the legend; the other numbers refer to structures that are not described.

Chapter 1, "The Skeleton and Skull," provides an overview of the boney architecture of the thorax, vertebral column, and craniofacial skeleton. Attention is given to important structures and regions of the skull such as the hard palate and contiguous areas, the nasal cavity and paranasal sinuses, and the sphenoid bone.

Chapter 2 covers "The Thorax and Abdomen." The musculature of the trunk is reviewed, emphasizing muscles thought to be active during speech production. The presentation of muscles is followed by descriptions of the viscera of the thorax and anatomy of the lower respiratory tract.

Chapter 3, "The Neck," is a description of the anatomy of the hyoid bone and the supra- and infrahyoid muscles, and a detailed presentation on the muscles of the neck. General anatomy of the neck is illustrated to highlight structural relationships.

Presentation in Chapter 4, "The Larynx," begins with the laryngeal cartilages and is followed by gross anatomical and histological demonstrations of the cricothyroid and

I

THE
SPEECH
MECHANISM

cricoarytenoid joints. The soft tissues of the larynx are shown through dissections and micrographs of the laryngeal cavity, vocal folds, and intrinsic and extrinsic laryngeal muscles.

Chapter 5, "The Pharynx," illustrates the anatomy of the pharynx through unique views of the vocal tract during speech and via dissections and illustrations of major morphological relationships relevant to speech.

Chapter 6, "The Velopharynx," describes the morphology of this region from several perspectives. General morphological relationships are presented first. This is followed by a histological description of the soft palate which illustrates important structural relationships among the various tissues composing the region. The relationships among the muscles of the soft palate are shown through human dissections. The relationship of muscles of the soft palate to the auditory tube are shown through gross and microscopic anatomy. The functional significance of the anatomical relationships presented in this chapter are graphically illustrated in a series of nasendoscopic photographs of the velopharyngeal mechanism.

Chapter 7 presents "The Oral Cavity." Its structure is presented through micrographs of important histological relationships and through intraoral photographs. These photographs illustrate structural relationships relevant for the clinician and the basic scientist.

Chapter 8, "The Nasal Cavity," reviews the anatomy of the external aspect of the nose and the nasal cavity proper. The morphology of soft tissues and cartilages are shown via dissection and microscopic anatomy.

Chapter 9 describes "The Tongue." The general relationship of the tongue to the larynx and contiguous structures is presented first. This is followed by descriptions of the surface anatomy of the tongue and its extrinsic and intrinsic musculature.

Chapter 10 covers "The Craniofacial Complex." This presentation consists of an overview of the anatomy of the mandible, the muscles of mastication, and temporomandibular joint.

Chapter 11, "The Face," is the final chapter in Part I. In this chapter the external features of the face and the anatomy of the facial muscles are presented. The morphology of the lips including the circumoral region is presented in detail. The reader is provided with many examples of the typical variations in facial muscle morphology.

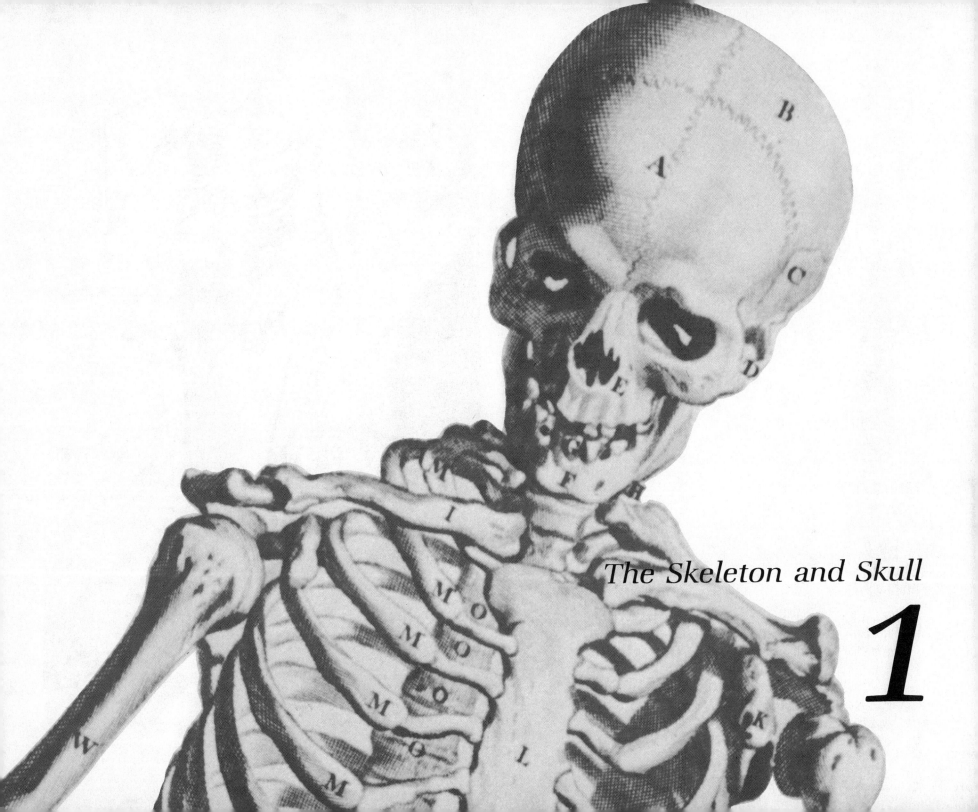

The Skeleton and Skull

1

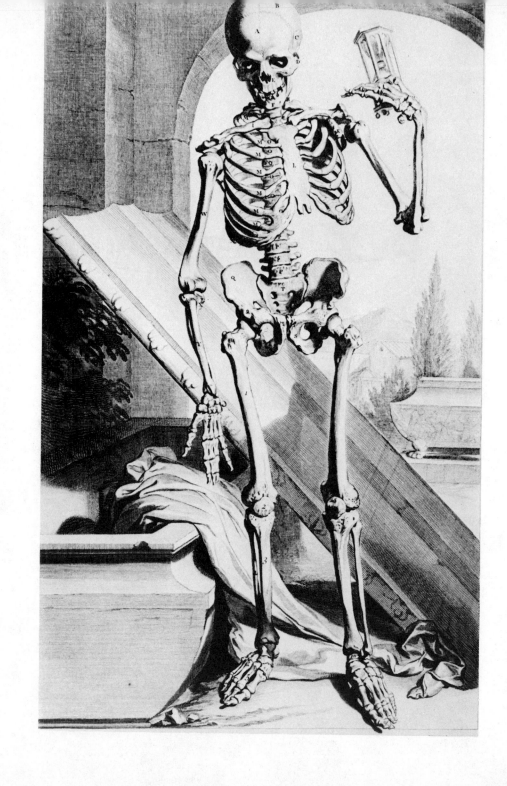

FIGURE 1–1 (From Govard Bidlvo, *Anatoma Humani Corporis*. Amsterdam: Johannis A. Someren, 1685.)

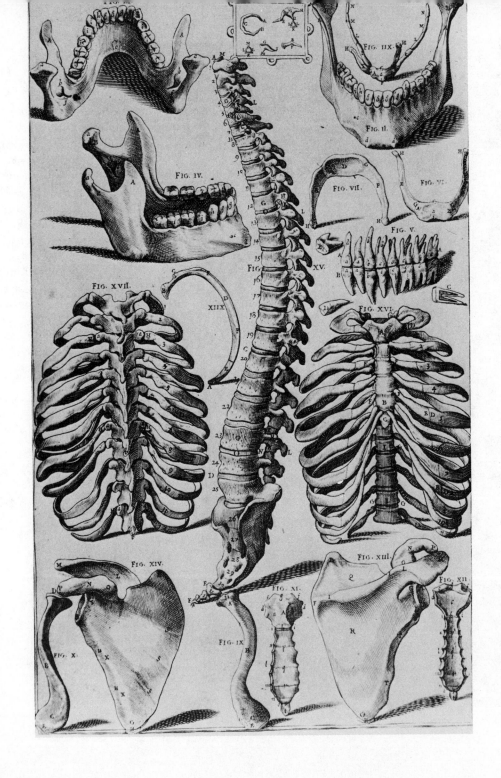

FIGURE 1–2 (From Giulio Casserio, "Tabulae Anatomica," in Adriaan van de Spiegel (Ed.), *Opera quae extant omnia*. Amsterdam: Johannem Blaeu, 1645.)

FIGURE 1–3 Frontal (A) and dorsal (B) views of skeleton. In (A): (1) skull, (2) mandible, (3) hyoid bone, (4) cervical vertebrae (3rd–7th visible), (5) clavicle, (6) acromion, (7) coracoid process and (8) part of subscapular fossa of scapula, (9) osseus portions of 1st–10th ribs, (10) cartilagenous portions of 1st–10th ribs, (11) 12th rib (lower of two pairs of floating ribs), (12) manubrium, (13) body and (14) xiphoid process of sternum, (15) lower thoracic vertebrae (9th–12th visible), (16) lumbar vertebrae (1st–4th visible), (17) intervertebral disc, (18) sacrum, (19) coccyx, (20) iliac crest, (21) ischium and (22) pubis symphasis of pelvis, (23) femur (note (*) head articulating with acentabulum of pelvis), (24) patella, (25) fibula, (26) tibia, (27) bones of foot. In (B): (28) skull, (29) 1st cervical vertebra (atlas), (30) 2nd cervical vertebra (axis), (31) clavicle, (32) superior angle, (33) acromion, (34) spine and (35) infraspinatus fossa of scapula, (36) humerous articulating at glenoid fossa of scapula, (37) radius, (38) ulna, (39) bones of hand, (40) 3rd–7th cervical vertebrae, (41) 1st–12th thoracic vertebrae, (42) 1st–5th lumbar vertebrae, (43) 1st–5th sacral vertebrae fused into sacrum, (44) 1st–4th coccygeal vertebrae fused into coccyx.

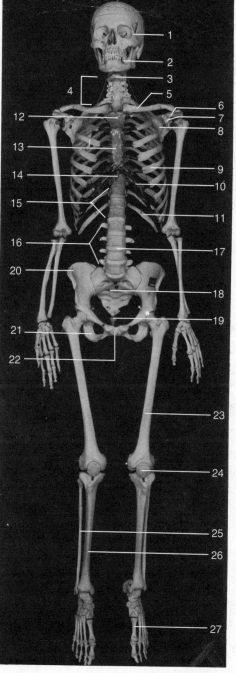

FIGURE 1–3A

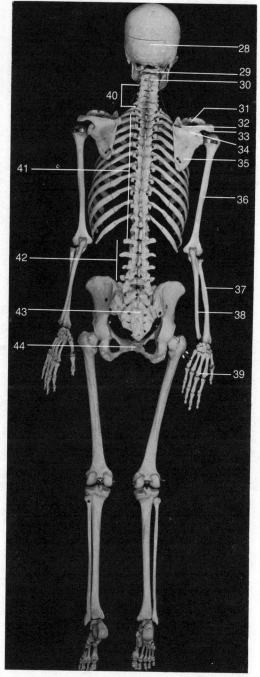

FIGURE 1–3B

FIGURE 1–4 (A) Anterosuperior view of the rib cage. (1) thoracic inlet; (2) cervical and (3) thoracic vertebrae; (4–6) sternum: (4) manubrium, (5) body, (6) xiphoid process; (7) clavical; (8) sternoclavicular joint; (9) 1st rib, containing (a) shaft, (b) neck, and (c) head; (10) osseus portion of 2nd rib; (11) cartilagenous portion (simulated) of 2nd rib; (12) costochondral joint of 2nd rib; (13) sternocostal joint of 2nd rib. Note the differences in sizes and shapes of ribs. (B) Posterior view of the rib cage, illustrating rib and vertebral relationships for 1st–10th ribs. (14) 1st thoracic vertebra; (15) portion of 1st rib; (16) clavical; (17) scapula; (18–22) morphology of a vertebra: (18) spinous process, (19) arch, (20) transverse process, (21) inferior and (22) superior articular process; (23) posterior portion of shaft of rib; (24) intercostal space; (25) nonarticular part of tubercle; (26) articular part of tubercle interconnected with costal facet of transverse process via costotransverse ligament (not shown); (27) 11th rib. (Photo by Paul Reimann, Department of Anatomy, University of Iowa.)

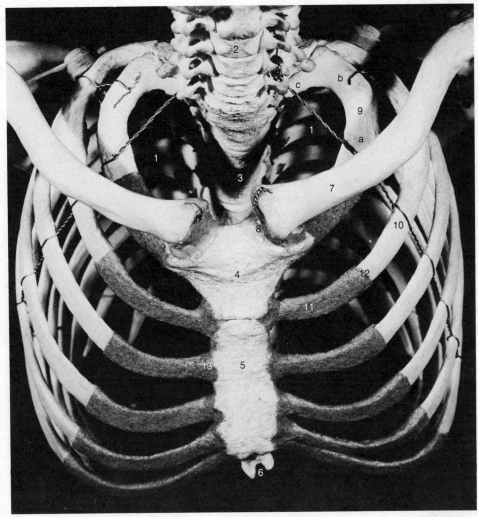

FIGURE 1–4A

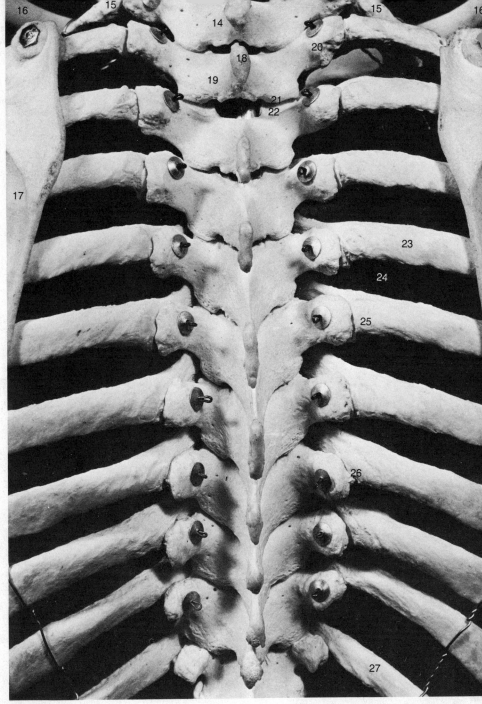

FIGURE 1–4B

THE SKELETON AND SKULL

7

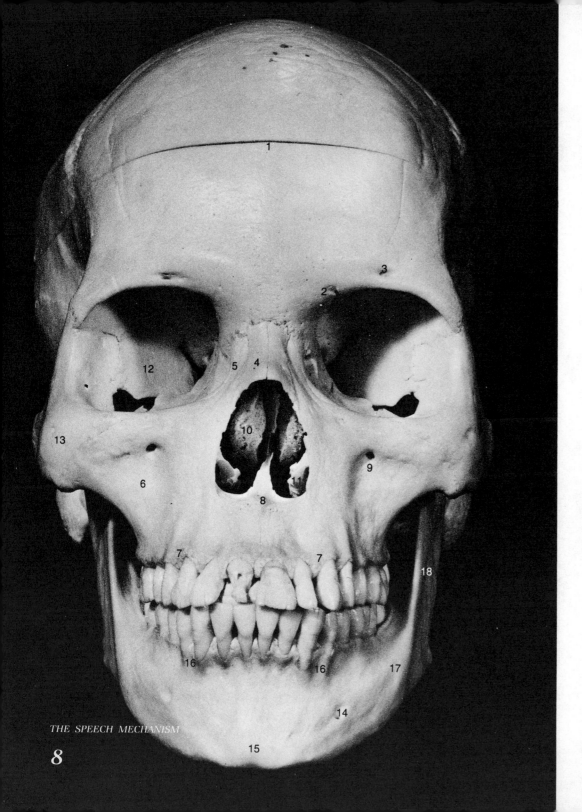

FIGURE 1–5 Frontal (anterior) view of the bones of the skull. (1) frontal bone; (2) supraorbital notch; (3) supraorbital foramen; (4) nasal bone; (5–9) parts of the maxilla: (5) frontal process, (6) maxilla, (7) alveolar process, (8) anterior nasal spine, (9) infraorbital foramen; (10) middle nasal concha; (11) inferior nasal concha; (12) orbital cavity; (13) zygomatic bone; (14–18) parts of the mandible: (14) mental foramen, (15) mental protuberance, (16) alveolar process, (17) body, (18) ramus. (Photo by Paul Reimann, Department of Anatomy, University of Iowa.)

FIGURE 1–6 Left lateral view of the bones of the skull. (1) frontal bone, (a) superior temporal line, (b) inferior temporal line; (2) nasal bone; (3–5) parts of the maxilla: (3) frontal process, (4) anterior nasal spine, (5) maxilla; (6) orbital cavity; (7) zygomatic bone; (8–11) parts of the mandible: (8) mental protuberance, (9) body, (10) ramus, (11) coronoid process; (12) condyloid process; (13) greater wing of sphenoid bone; (14) parietal bone; (15–22) parts of the temporal bone: (15) squamous portion, (16) zygomatic process, (17) articular tubercle, (18) glenoid fossa, (19) post-glenoid process, (20) external auditory meatus, (21) tympanic part, (22) mastoid process; (23) occipital bone. The styloid process has been broken off of this specimen. (Photo by Paul Reimann, Department of Anatomy, University of Iowa.)

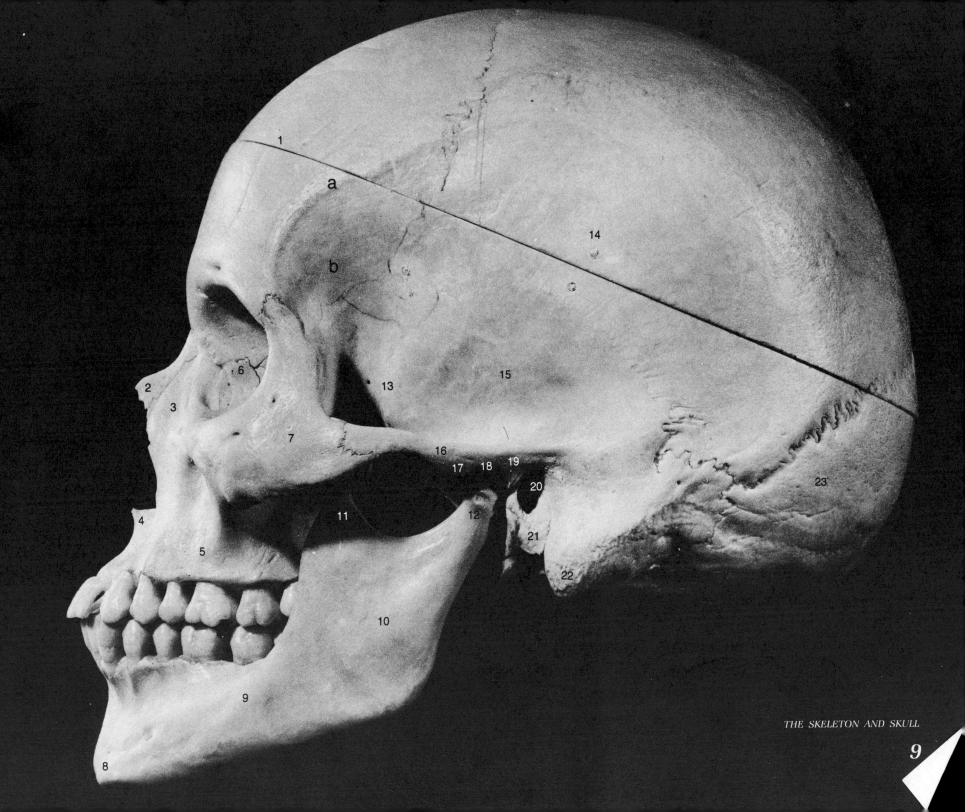

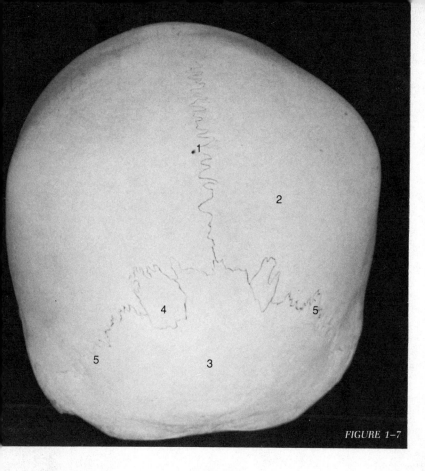

FIGURE 1–7

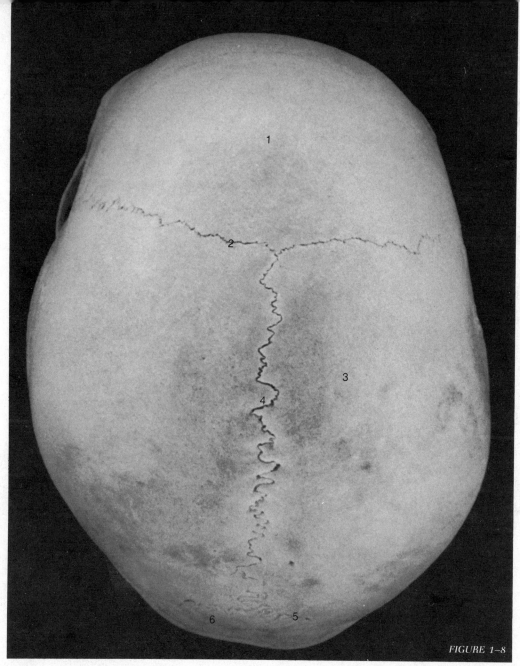

FIGURE 1–8

FIGURE 1–7 Posterior view of the calvarium. (1) sagittal suture, (2) parietal bone, (3) occipital bone, (4) interparietal bone (seen occasionally in normal skulls), (5) lambdoidal suture.

FIGURE 1–8 Superior (external) aspect of the calvarium. (1) frontal bone, (2) coronal suture, (3) parietal bone, (4) sagittal suture, (5) lambdoidal suture, (6) occipital bone.

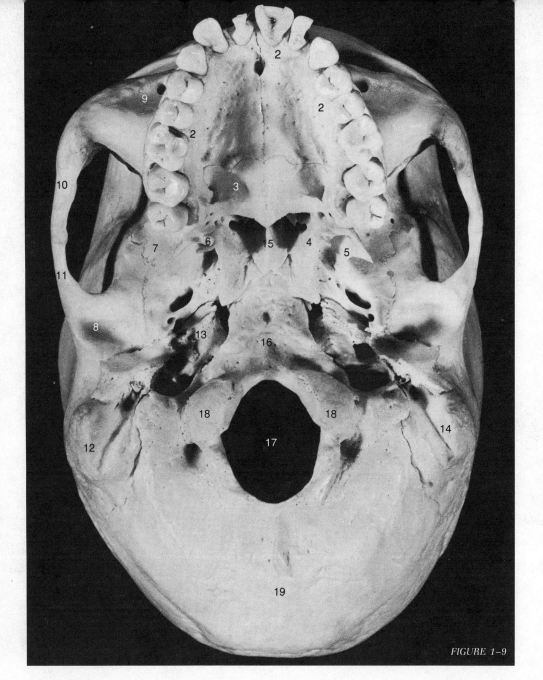

FIGURE 1-9

FIGURE 1-9 Inferior view illustrating base of the skull. (1) palatine process of maxilla, (2) alveolar process housing teeth, (3) palatine bone (horizontal plate), (4) medial and (5) lateral pterygoid plates of the sphenoid bone, (6) hamular process, (7) greater wing of sphenoid, (8) mandibular fossa, (9) zygomatic process of maxilla, (10) zygomatic bone, (11) zygomatic process of temporal bone, (12) mastoid process, (13) petrous portion of temporal bone, (14) digastric fossa, (15) vomer, (16) basioccipital of the occipital bone, (17) foramen magnum, (18) occipital condyles, (19) occipital bone (squamous portion). (Photo by Paul Reimann, Department of Anatomy, University of Iowa.)

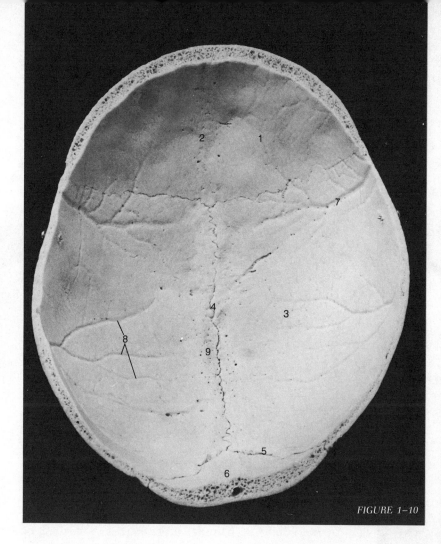

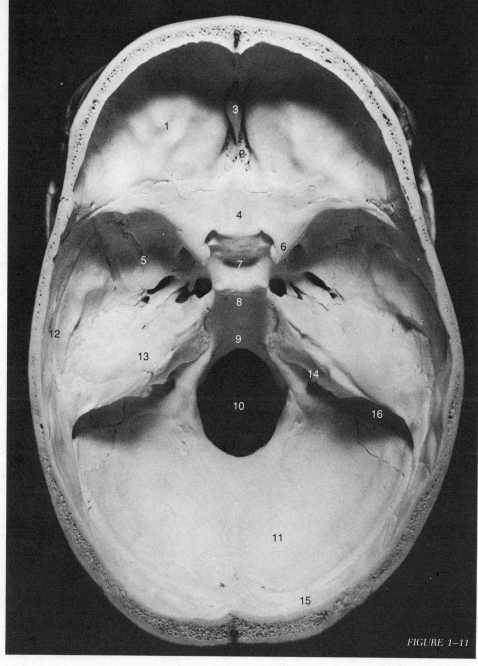

FIGURE 1–10

FIGURE 1–11

FIGURE 1–10 Internal surface of calvarium.
(1) frontal bone, (2) coronal suture, (3) parietal bone,
(4) sagittal suture, (5) lambdoidal suture, (6) squamous
part of occipital bone, (7) groove for middle meningeal
artery and (8) grooves for branches of the meningeal
artery, (9) granulae foveola.

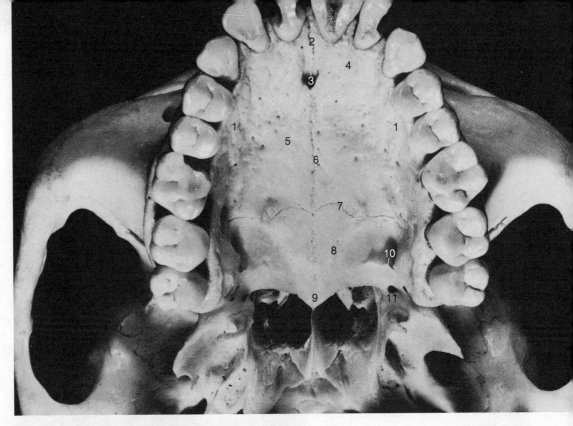

FIGURE 1–11   Internal view of the floor of the skull. (1) frontal bone, (2) cribriform plate and (3) crista galli of ethmoid bone, (4) lesser wing and (5) greater wing of sphenoid bone, (6) anterior clinoid process, (7) hypophyseal fossa, (8) dorsum sellae and posterior clinoid process, (9) basioccipital part of occipital bone, (10) foramen magnum, (11) occipital bone, (12) squamous part of temporal bone, (13) petrous part of temporal bone, (14) internal auditory meatus, (15) transverse groove, (16) sigmoid groove. See Figures 21–2 and 21–3 for details on relationships between cranial nerves and their foramena in the skull. (Photo by Paul Reimann, Department of Anatomy, University of Iowa.)

FIGURE 1–12   Hard palate. (1) alveolar ridge (encircles palatine processes), (2) premaxilla (incisive bone), (3) incisive foramen, (4) incisive suture, (5) palatine process of the maxilla, (6) median palatine suture, (7) transverse palatine suture, (8) horizontal plate of the palatine bone, (9) posterior nasal spine, (10) greater and (11) lesser palatine foramina. (Photo by Paul Reimann, Department of Anatomy, University of Iowa.)

FIGURE 1–13   Close-up of boney relationships in the posterior aspect of the hard palate and nasal cavity. (1) posterior nasal spine, (2) maxillary tuberosity, (3) hamular process, (4) medial pterygoid plate, (5) lateral pterygoid plate, (6) vomer, (7) posterior choana (one of a pair), (8) inferior turbinate.

FIGURE 1–12

FIGURE 1–13

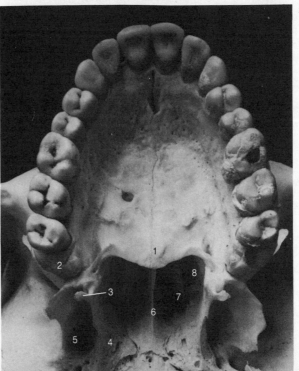

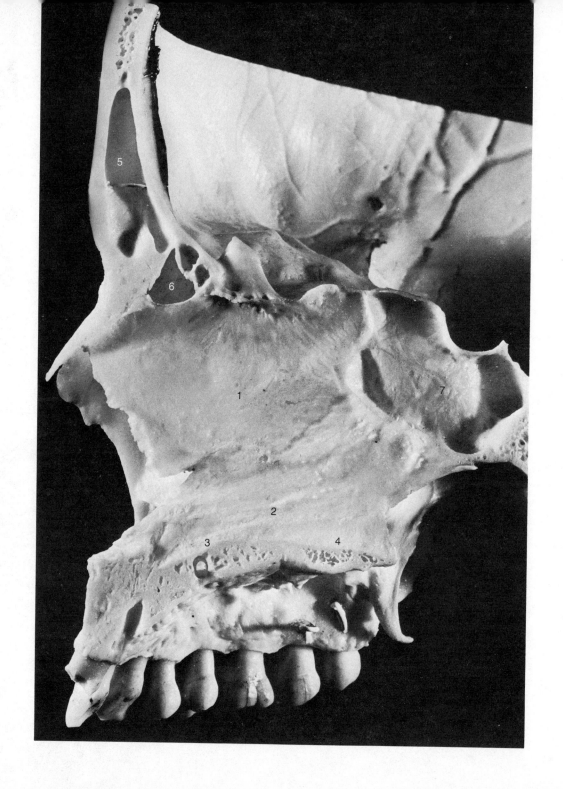

FIGURE 1–14 Boney nasal septum and related paranasal sinuses. (1) perpendicular plate of ethmoid bone;
(2) vomer; (3) nasal crests of maxilla and (4) palatine
bones; (5) frontal, (6) ethmoid, and (7) sphenoid sinuses. (Photo by Paul Reimann, Department of Anatomy, University of Iowa.)

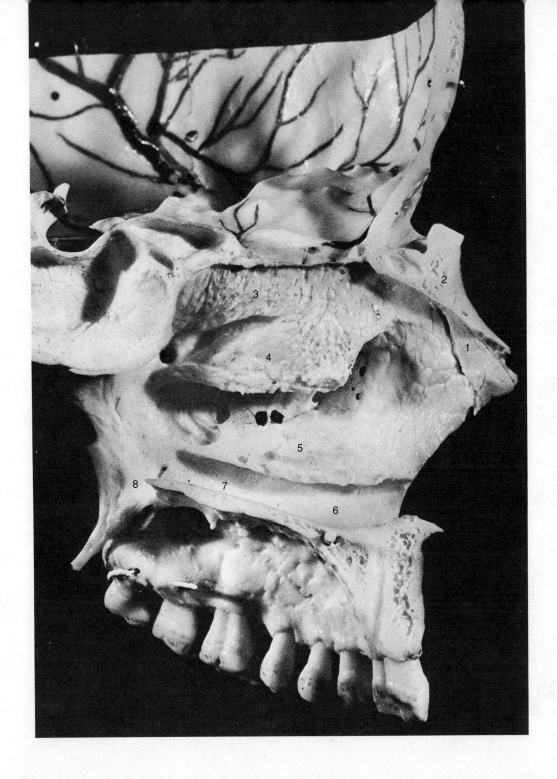

FIGURE 1–15 Lateral wall of nasal cavity. (1) frontal process of maxilla, (2) nasal bone, (3) superior concha, (4) middle concha, (5) inferior concha, (6) nasal crest of maxillary and (7) palatine bones, (8) medial pterygoid plate of sphenoid bone. (Photo by Paul Reimann, Department of Anatomy, University of Iowa.)

THE SKELETON AND SKULL

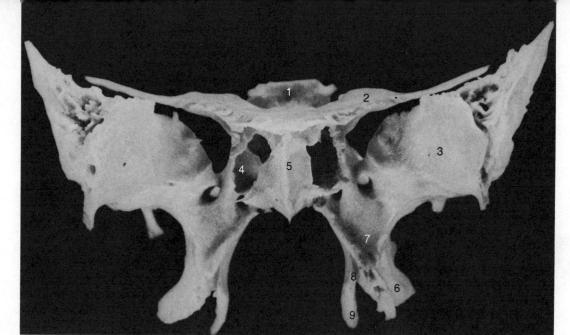

FIGURE 1–16   Anterior aspect of the sphenoid bone.
(1) posterior clinoid process, (2) lesser wing, (3) greater
wing, (4) sphenoidal sinus and (5) sphenoid crest of
the body, (6) lateral pterygoid plate, (7) pterygoid fossa,
(8) medial pterygoid plate, (9) hamular process.

FIGURE 1–17   Posterior aspect of the sphenoid bone.
(1) lesser wing, (2) posterior clinoid process, (3) greater
wing, (4) dorsum sellae and body, (5) lateral pterygoid
plate, (6) hamular process and (7) medial pterygoid
plate, (8) pterygoid fossa, (9) rostrum.

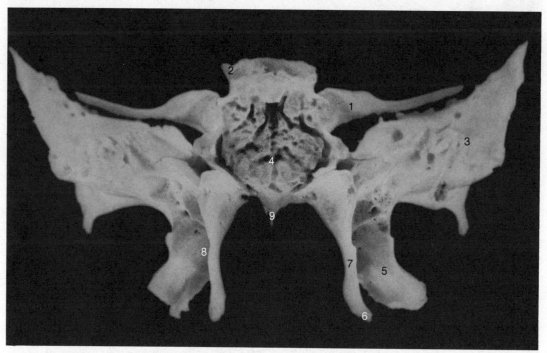

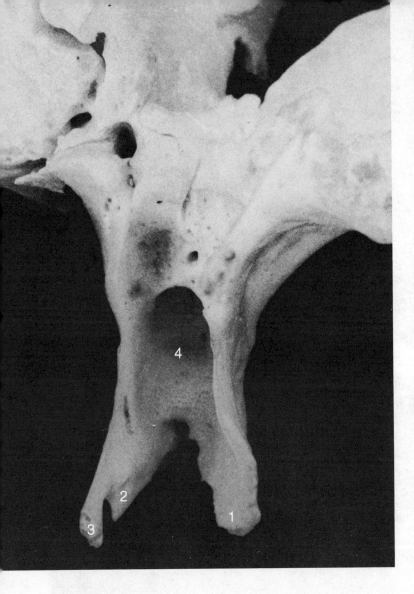

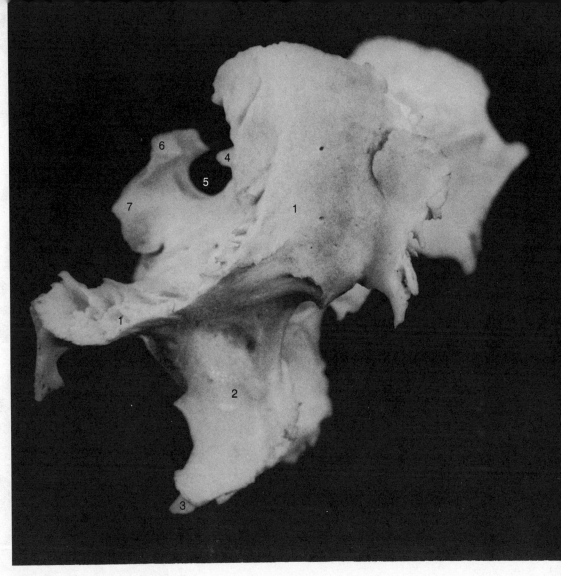

FIGURE 1–18 Close-up of pterygoid plates. (1) lateral pterygoid plate, (2) medial pterygoid plate and (3) hamular process, (4) pterygoid fossa.

FIGURE 1–19 Lateral aspect of sphenoid bone. (1) greater wing, (2) lateral pterygoid plate, (3) hamular process, (4) anterior clinoid process, (5) hypophyseal fossa, (6) posterior clinoid process, (7) dorsum sellae.

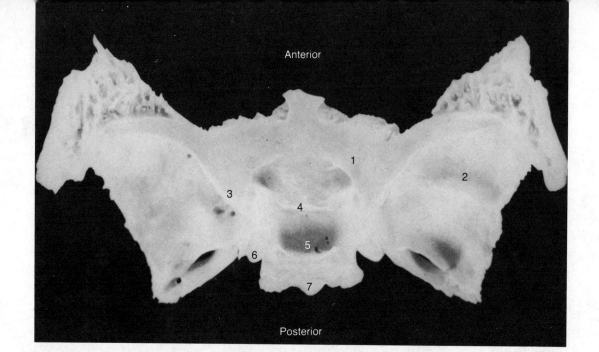

FIGURE 1–20 Superior aspect of sphenoid bone. (1) lesser wing, (2) greater wing, (3) anterior clinoid process, (4) tuberculum sellae, (5) hypophyseal fossa, (6) posterior clinoid process, (7) dorsum sellae.

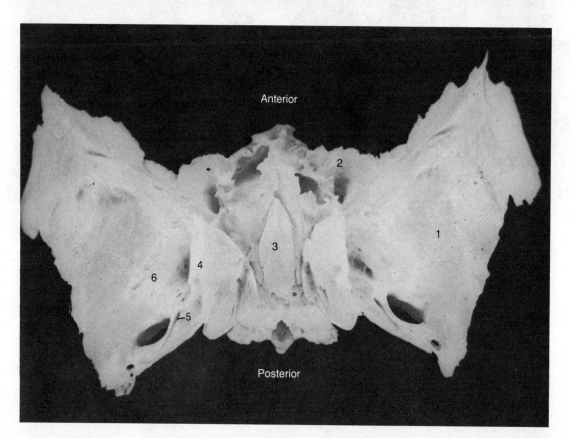

FIGURE 1–21 Inferior view of sphenoid bone. (1) greater wing, (2) lesser wing, (3) body, (4) medial pterygoid plate, (5) hamular process, (6) lateral pterygoid plate.

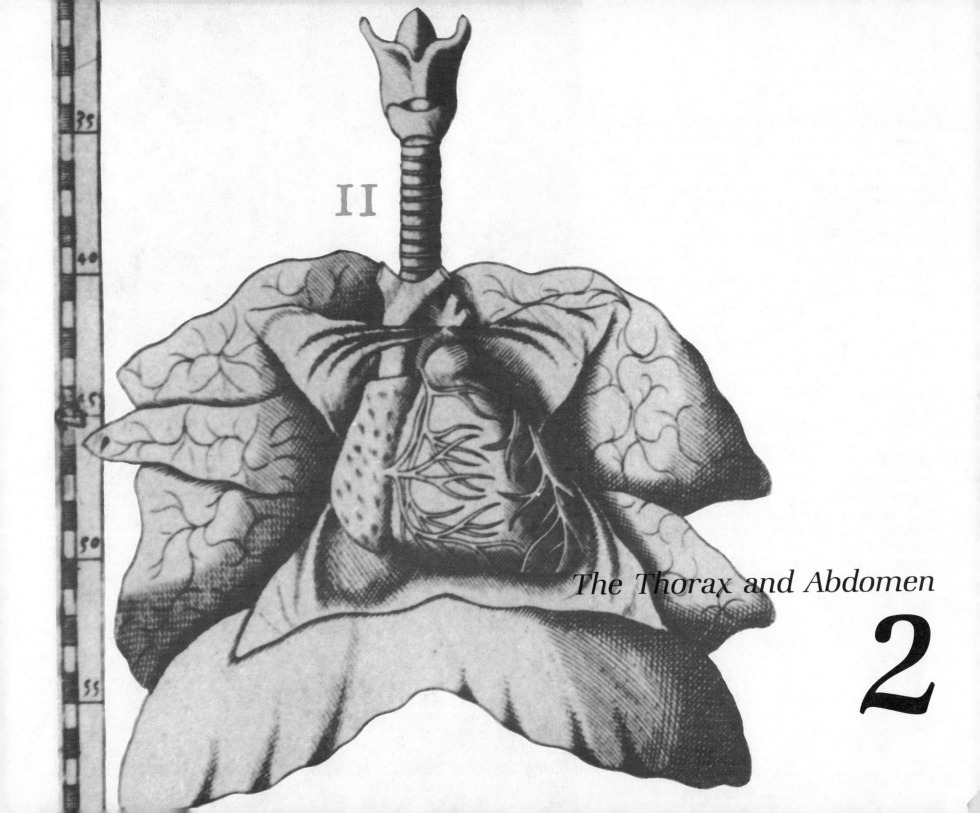

II

The Thorax and Abdomen

2

FIGURE 2–1 Anterior view of the musculature of the trunk. (24) pectoralis major muscle, (30) latissimus dorsi muscle, (37) pectoralis minor muscle (sectioned), (47) serratus anterior muscle, (53) external abdominal oblique muscle, (56) rectus abdominis muscle, (58) rectus sheath. (Courtesy of the Anatomy Museum of the Department of Anatomy and Cell Biology, University of Pittsburgh, School of Medicine, Pittsburgh.)

FIGURE 2–2 Lateral view of musculature of the trunk. (24) pectoralis major muscle, (30) latissimus dorsi muscle, (37) pectoralis minor muscle, (47) serratus anterior muscle, (53) external abdominal oblique muscle. (Courtesy of the Anatomy Museum of the Department of Anatomy and Cell Biology, University of Pittsburgh, School of Medicine, Pittsburgh.)

FIGURE 2–3 Dissection of muscles of posterior aspect of neck and trunk. (VII) spine of 7th cervical vertebra, (XII) spine of 12th thoracic vertebra, (1) external occipital protuberance, (12) sternocleidomastoid muscle, (26) trapezius muscle, (27) thoracolumbar fascia, (29) erector spinae muscle (iliocostalis portion), (30) latissimus dorsi muscle, (32) internal abdominal oblique muscle, (35) levator scapulae muscle, (36) rhomboideus minor muscle, (37) rhomboideus major muscle, (38) serratus posterior superior muscle, (39) serratus posterior inferior muscle, (40) iliocostalis muscle (sacrospinal muscle group), (41) external intercostal muscle, (42) splenius capitus muscle. (Courtesy of the Anatomy Museum of the Department of Anatomy and Cell Biology, University of Pittsburgh, School of Medicine, Pittsburgh.)

FIGURE 2–1

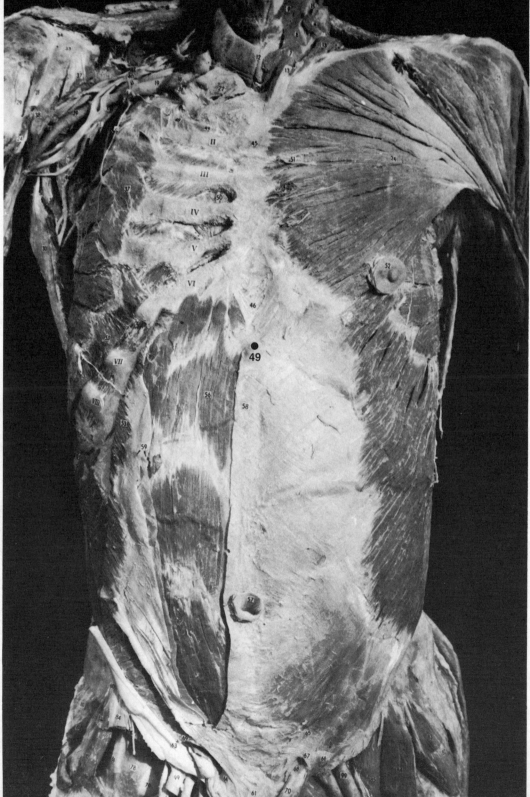

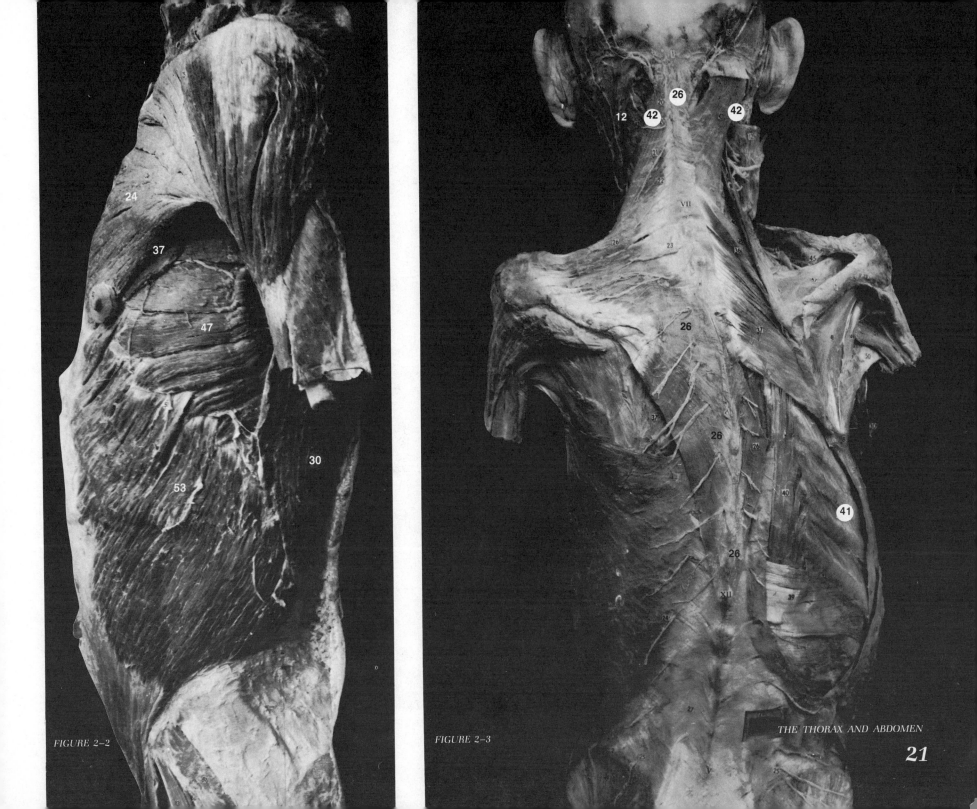

FIGURE 2–2

FIGURE 2–3

THE THORAX AND ABDOMEN

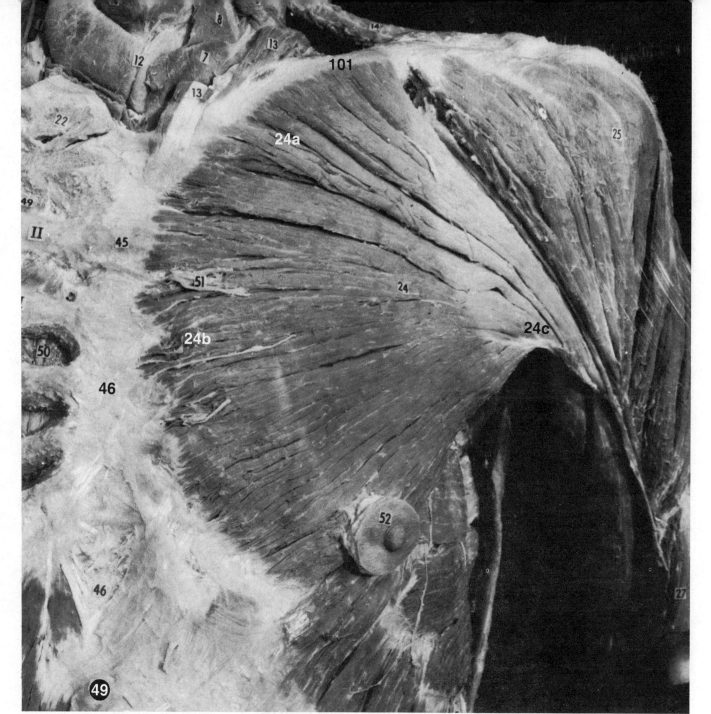

FIGURE 2–4   Pectoralis major muscle and related structures on anterior wall of thorax. (II–VI) 2nd–6th ribs; (24a) clavicular attachment and (24b) humerous attachment of pectoralis major muscle; (25) deltoid muscle; (45) manubrium; (46) body of sternum; (49) xiphoid process; (101) clavical. (Courtesy of the Anatomy Museum of the Department of Anatomy and Cell Biology, University of Pittsburgh, School of Medicine, Pittsburgh.)

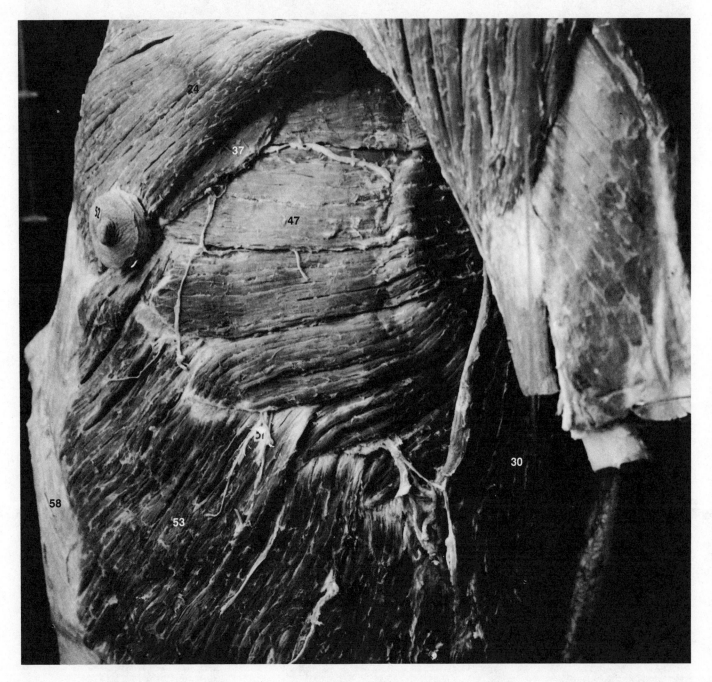

FIGURE 2–5 Lateral view of muscles of thorax on left side. (II–VIII) 2nd–8th ribs (sectioned), (24) pectoralis major muscle (sectioned near attachment), (30) latissimus dorsi muscle, (37) pectoralis minor muscle (sectioned near attachment), (47) serratus anterior muscle, (53) external abdominal oblique muscle, (58) rectus abdominis sheath. (Courtesy of the Anatomy Museum of the Department of Anatomy and Cell Biology, University of Pittsburgh, School of Medicine, Pittsburgh.)

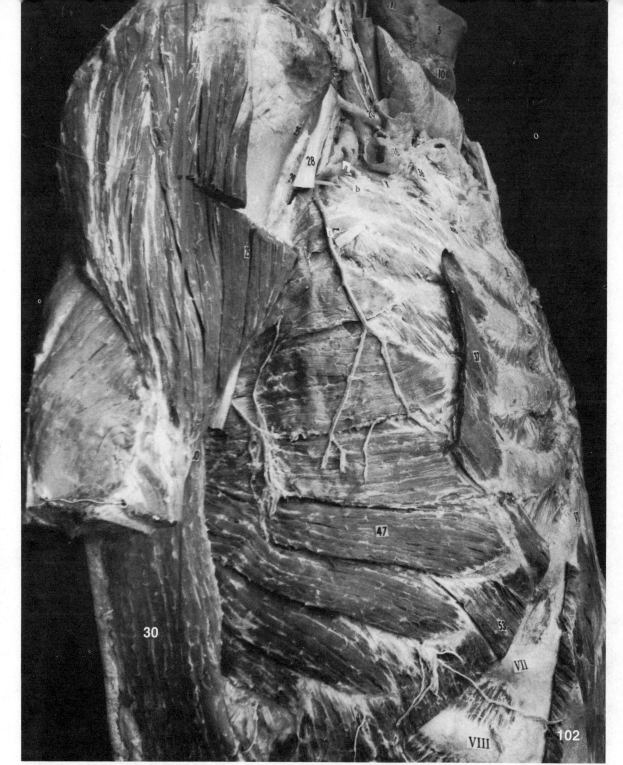

FIGURE 2–6 Lateral view of muscles of thorax on right side. (II–VIII) 2nd–8th ribs, (30) latissimus dorsi muscle, (37) pectoralis minor muscle, (47) serratus anterior muscle, (53) external abdominal oblique muscle, (102) aponeurosis of external oblique muscle. (Courtesy of the Anatomy Museum of the Department of Anatomy and Cell Biology, University of Pittsburgh, School of Medicine, Pittsburgh.)

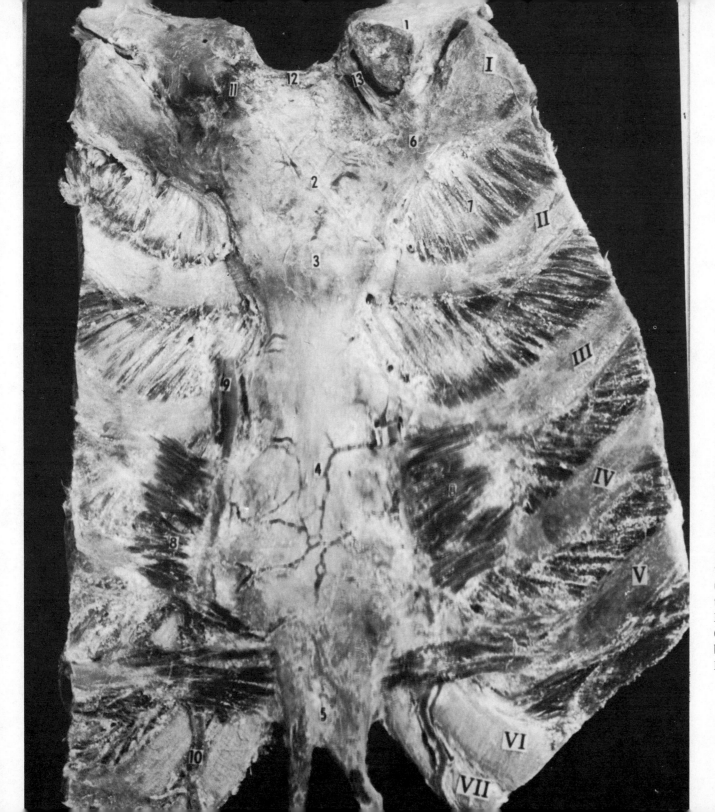

FIGURE 2–7 Deep surface of anterior portion of chest wall. (I–VII) 1st–7th ribs; (2) manubrium, (3, 4) body, and (5) xiphoid process of sternum (bifid in this specimen); (6) a costosternal joint; (7) internal intercostal muscle, (8) transverse thoracis muscle; (12) sternal notch. (Courtesy of the Anatomy Museum of the Department of Anatomy and Cell Biology, University of Pittsburgh, School of Medicine, Pittsburgh.)

THE THORAX AND ABDOMEN

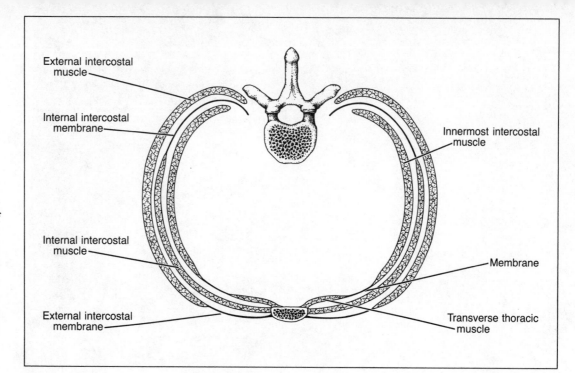

FIGURE 2–8   Cross-section illustration of the relationship of the internal, external, intercostal, and transverse thoracic muscles in the intercostal space. (Adapted from J.B. Grant, *Grant's Atlas of Anatomy*. Baltimore: The Williams & Wilkins Co., 1972.)

FIGURE 2–9   Schematic of the anatomical relationship between the internal and external intercostal muscles within the intercostal space. (Adapted from J. Langman and M.W. Woerdeman, *Atlas of Medical Anatomy*. Philadelphia: W.B. Saunders Company, 1981.)

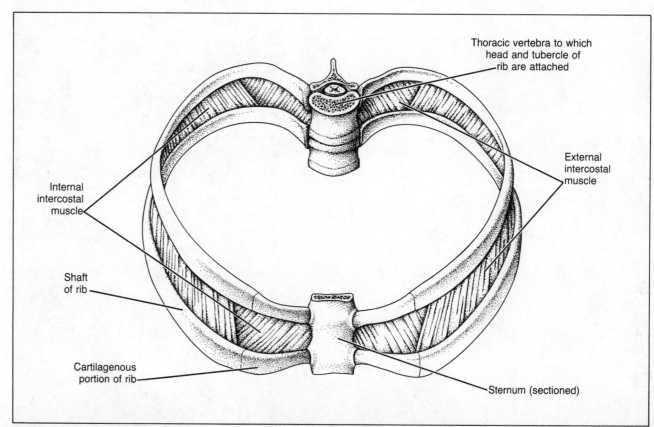

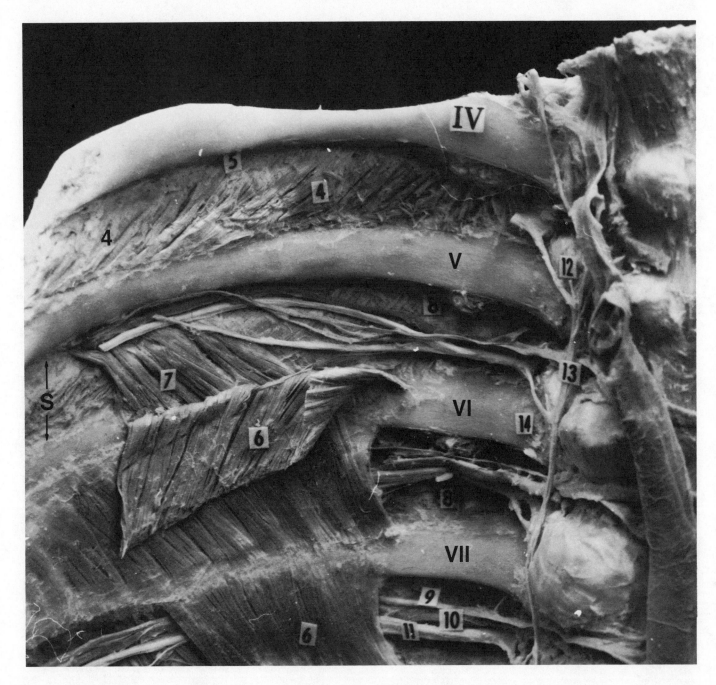

FIGURE 2–10   Posterior thoracic (chest) wall. (IV–VII) 4th–7th ribs, (S) intercostal space, (4) external intercostal muscle, (6) innermost intercostal muscle and (7) internal intercostal muscle proper separated by intercostal nerve and posterior intercostal vessels, (8) internal intercostal membrane, (12) head of rib articulating with articular facet of adjacent vertebrae. (Courtesy of the Anatomy Museum of the Department of Anatomy and Cell Biology, University of Pittsburgh, School of Medicine, Pittsburgh.)

FIGURE 2–11 Diaphragm viewed from above; solid lines indicate region of central tendon. (1) posterior wall of thorax (note that pleural membrane is intact on right but has been dissected on left), (2) external muscle of chest wall (reflected), (3) ribs and associated muscles, (4) muscle fibers of diaphragm, (4a) diaphragm covered with pleural membrane, (5) remnants of pericardial cavity, (6) sternum, (7) cartilage of rib, (8) inferior vena cava, (9) phrenic nerve, (10) esophagus, (11) aorta, (12) fat pad. (Courtesy of the Anatomy Museum of the Department of Anatomy and Cell Biology, University of Pittsburgh, School of Medicine, Pittsburgh.)

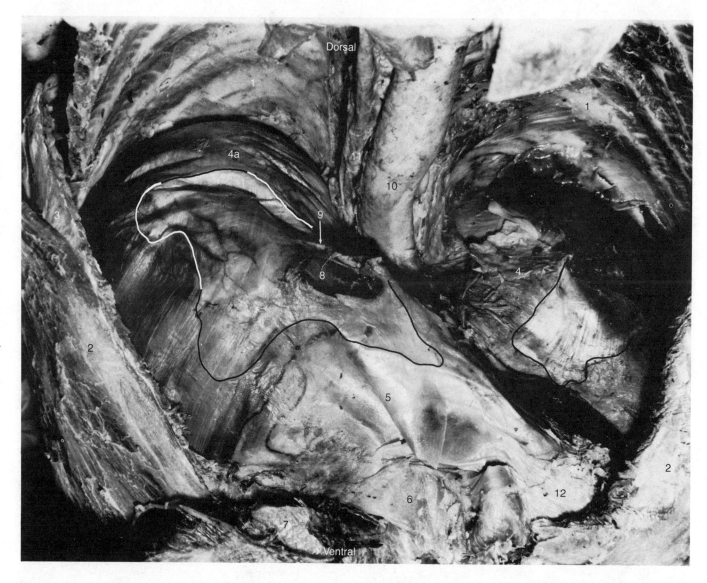

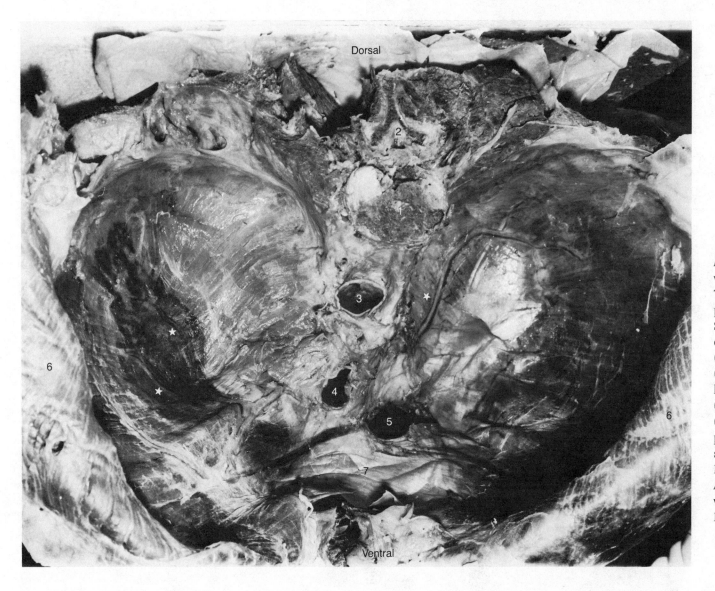

FIGURE 2–12 Diaphragm viewed from abdominal cavity. The anterior region of the diaphragm is not entirely shown. Solid lines indicate extent of central tendon. (1) body and (2) spinus process of vertebra, (3) aortic hiatus, (4) esophageal hiatus, (5) vena caval foramen, (6) abdominal wall (reflected), (7) remnants of peritoneum, (*) phrenic nerves and blood vessels. (Courtesy of the Anatomy Museum of the Department of Anatomy and Cell Biology, University of Pittsburgh, School of Medicine, Pittsburgh.)

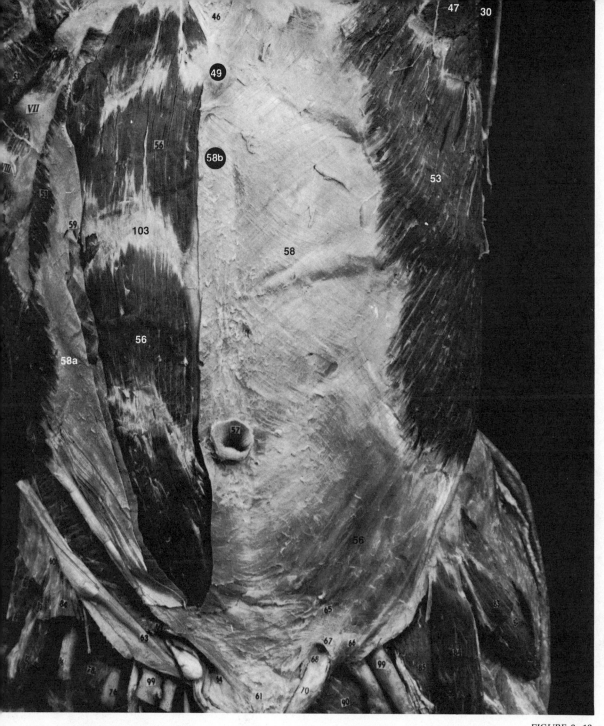

FIGURE 2–13 Anterior view of abdominal wall. (VI–VIII) 6th–8th ribs, (30) latissimus dorsi muscle, (47) serratus anterior muscle, (53) external abdominal oblique muscle, (56) rectus abdominis muscle, (57) umbilicus, (58) rectus sheath, (58a) rectus sheath reflected, (58b) linea alba, (103) tendonous intersection. (Courtesy of the Anatomy Museum of the Department of Anatomy and Cell Biology, University of Pittsburgh, School of Medicine, Pittsburgh.)

FIGURE 2–14 Right lateral view of abdominal wall. (VII–IX) 7th–9th ribs, (30) latissimus dorsi muscle, (47) serratus anterior muscle, (53) external abdominal oblique muscle, (54) internal abdominal oblique muscle, (55) transverse abdominis muscle, (56) rectus abdominis muscle, (58) rectus sheath, (104) iliac crest, (105) lumbar fascia. (Courtesy of the Anatomy Museum of the Department of Anatomy and Cell Biology, University of Pittsburgh, School of Medicine, Pittsburgh.)

FIGURE 2–15 Left lateral view of abdominal wall. (30) latissimus dorsi muscle, (47) serratus anterior muscle, (53) external abdominal oblique muscle and its (102) aponeurosis, (105) lumbar fascia, (106) linea semilunaris, (107) inguinal ligament. (Courtesy of the Anatomy Museum of the Department of Anatomy and Cell Biology, University of Pittsburgh, School of Medicine, Pittsburgh.)

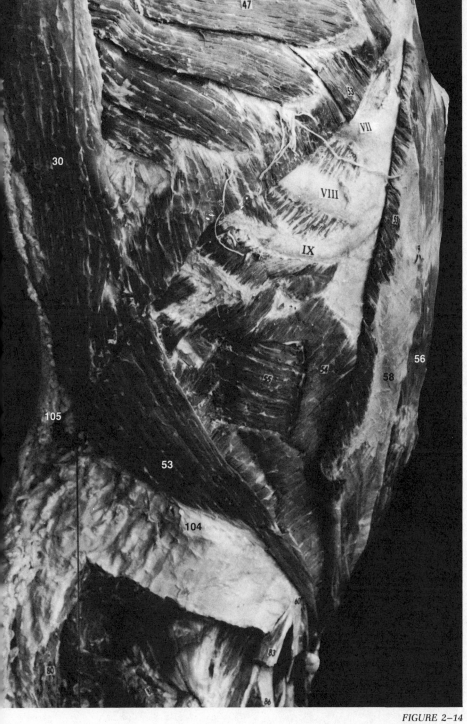

FIGURE 2-14

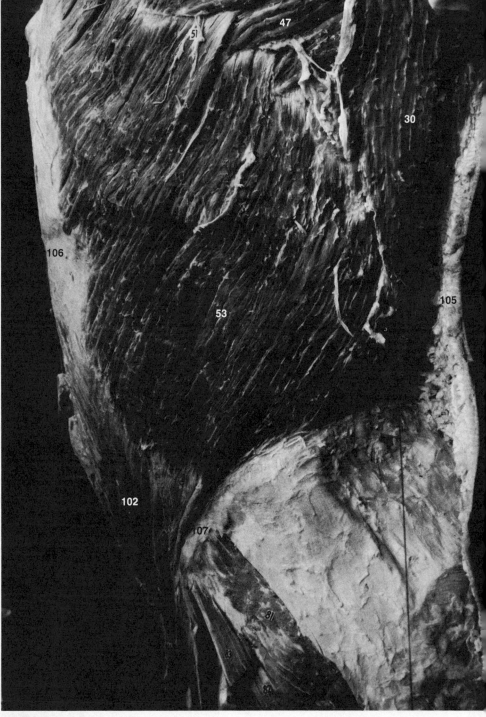

FIGURE 2-15

THE THORAX AND ABDOMEN

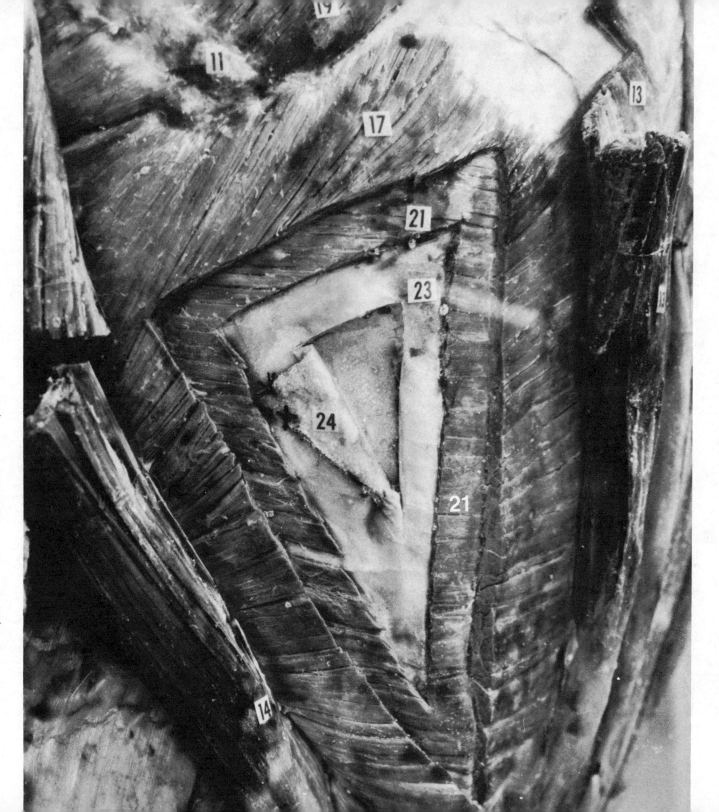

FIGURE 2–16 Close-up of musculature of lateral abdominal wall on right side. (11) costal cartilage for 7th rib, (13,14) external abdominal oblique muscle, (17) internal abdominal oblique muscle, (19) internal intercostal muscle, (21) transverse abdominis muscle, (23) transversalis fascia and its (24) parietal peritoneum, (Courtesy of the Anatomy Museum of the Department of Anatomy and Cell Biology, University of Pittsburgh, School of Medicine, Pittsburgh.)

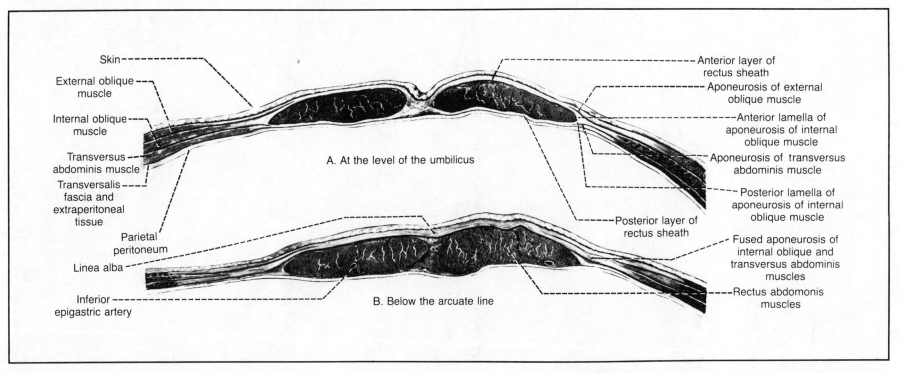

Skin

External oblique
muscle

Internal oblique
muscle

Transversus
abdominis muscle

Transversalis
fascia and
extraperitoneal
tissue

Parietal
peritoneum

Linea alba

Inferior
epigastric artery

A. At the level of the umbilicus

B. Below the arcuate line

Anterior layer of
rectus sheath

Aponeurosis of external
oblique muscle

Anterior lamella of
aponeurosis of internal
oblique muscle

Aponeurosis of transversus
abdominis muscle

Posterior lamella of
aponeurosis of internal
oblique muscle

Posterior layer of
rectus sheath

Fused aponeurosis of
internal oblique and
transversus abdominis
muscles

Rectus abdomonis
muscles

FIGURE 2–17   Horizontal sections of the anterior abdominal wall, at the level of the (A) umbilicus and below the (B) arcuate line. (Courtesy of Lord Solly Zuckerman, with Deryk Darlington and Peter Lisowski, *A New System of Anatomy*, 2nd Ed. Oxford: Oxford University Press, 1981.)

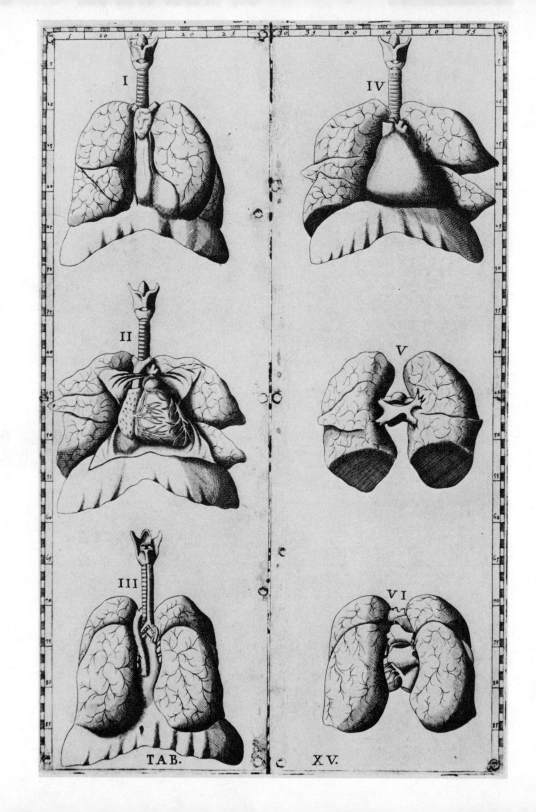

FIGURE 2–18   (From Bartolomeo Eustachi, *Tabulae Anatomicae Clarissimi*. Rome: Francisci Gonzagae, 1714.)

THE SPEECH MECHANISM

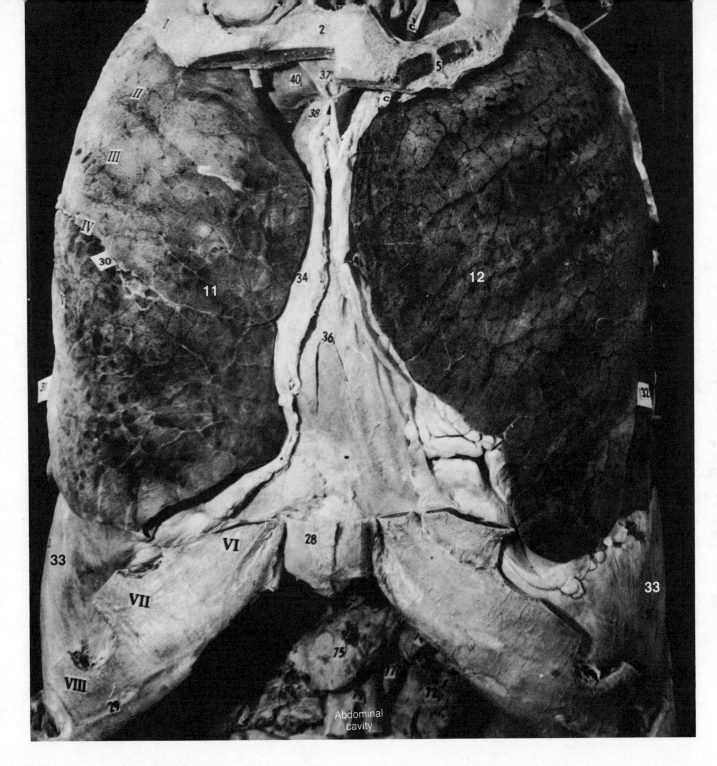

FIGURE 2–19 Viscera of thoracic cavity with chest wall removed. (I–IX) position of 1st–9th ribs, (2) manubrium of sternum, (11) right lung, (12) left lung, (28) xiphoid process of sternum, (29) interchondral articulation between ribs, (30) horizontal fissure separating superior from middle lobes, (31) oblique fissure separating middle from inferior lobes, (32) oblique fissure separating superior from inferior lobes, (33) diaphragm covered with parietal pleura, (34) mediastinal pleura, (36) pericardium with heart and great vessels beneath. (Courtesy of the Anatomy Museum of the Department of Anatomy and Cell Biology, University of Pittsburgh, School of Medicine, Pittsburgh.)

THE THORAX AND ABDOMEN

35

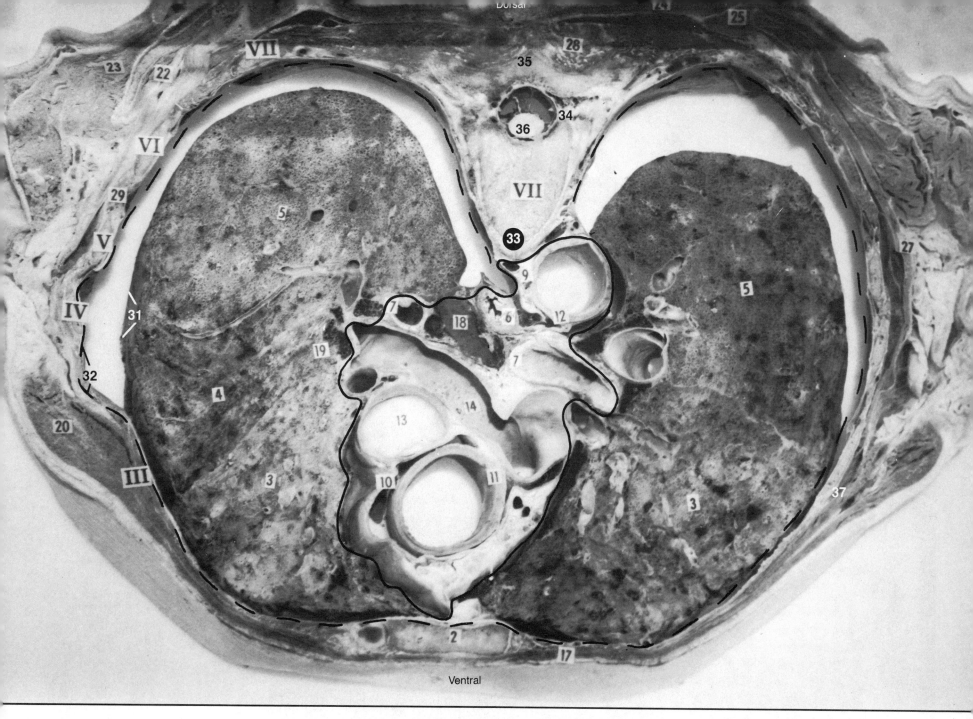

FIGURE 2–20 Transverse section through thorax at level of 7th thoracic vertebra. Solid line delimits the mediastinum, and broken line outlines the thoracic cavity. The space between the walls of the thorax and lungs is caused by postmortem shrinkage. (III–VII) portions of 3rd–7th ribs; (2) body of sternum; (3) superior, (4) middle, and (5) inferior lobes of lungs; (20) pectoralis major muscle; (26) latissimus dorsi muscle; (27) serratus anterior muscle; (31) visceral and (32) parietal pleurae; (33) body, (34) arch, and (35) spinal process of 7th vertebra; (36) vertebral canal, spinal cord; (37) pectoralis minor muscle. (Courtesy of the Anatomy Museum of the Department of Anatomy and Cell Biology, University of Pittsburgh, School of Medicine, Pittsburgh.)

FIGURE 2–21 Dissection of thorax, abdomen, and mediastinum, showing heart and great vessels. The lung has been removed to expose the posterior thoracic cavity and posterior lateral aspects of the chest wall. (I–X) 1st–10th ribs; (1) thyroid cartilage; (2) cricoid cartilage; (5) trachea; (6) thyroid gland; (14) left common carotid artery; (15) left and right subclavian arteries; (23) innominate artery; (27) right phrenic nerve; (40) right atrium and (42) left atrium of heart; (41) superior vena cava; (43) pulmonary artery; (45) aortic arch; (47) bifurcation of trachea into mainstem bronchi; (48) lobar bronchi; (49) superior, (50) middle, and (51) inferior lobes of right lung; (60, 93, 61) diaphragm: (60) left dome, (93) central tendon and attachment of pericardium to surface of diaphragm by way of pleura, (61) right dome with (*) pleural membrane removed to show underlying muscle; (91) brachial plexus (nerve supply to upper limbs); (92) pulmonary vein; (94) innominate vein; (95) left thoracic cavity. (Courtesy of the Anatomy Museum of the Department of Anatomy and Cell Biology, University of Pittsburgh, School of Medicine, Pittsburgh.)

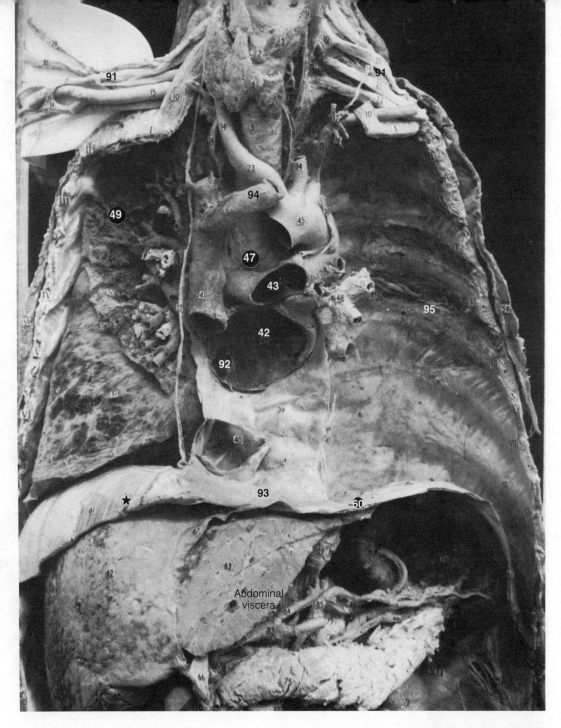

Abdominal
viscera

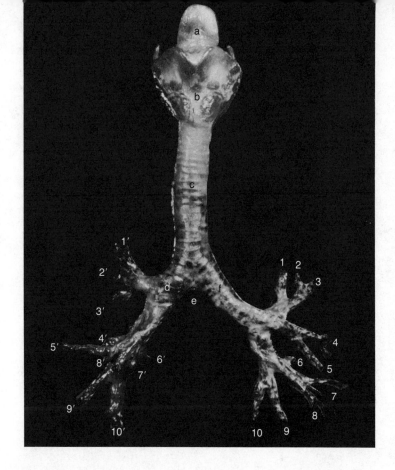

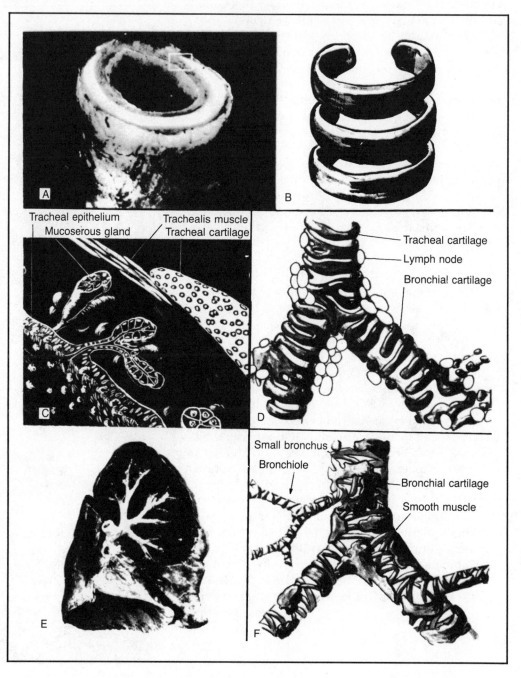

FIGURE 2–22 Anterior view of larynx, trachea, and bronchi. (a) epiglottis, (b) thyroid cartilage, (c) trachea, (d) right mainstem bronchus, (e) trachial bifurcation, (f) left mainstem bronchus. On right side, lobar and segmental bronchi for right lung: (1′–3′) to superior lobe, (4′–5′) to middle lobe, and (6′–10′) to inferior lobe. On left side, lobar and segmental bronchi for left lung: (1–5) to superior lobe and (6–10) to inferior lobe. (Courtesy of Chihiro Yokochi and Johannes W. Rohen, *Photographic Anatomy of the Human Body*, 2nd Ed. Tokyo: Igaku-Shoin, Ltd., 1978.)

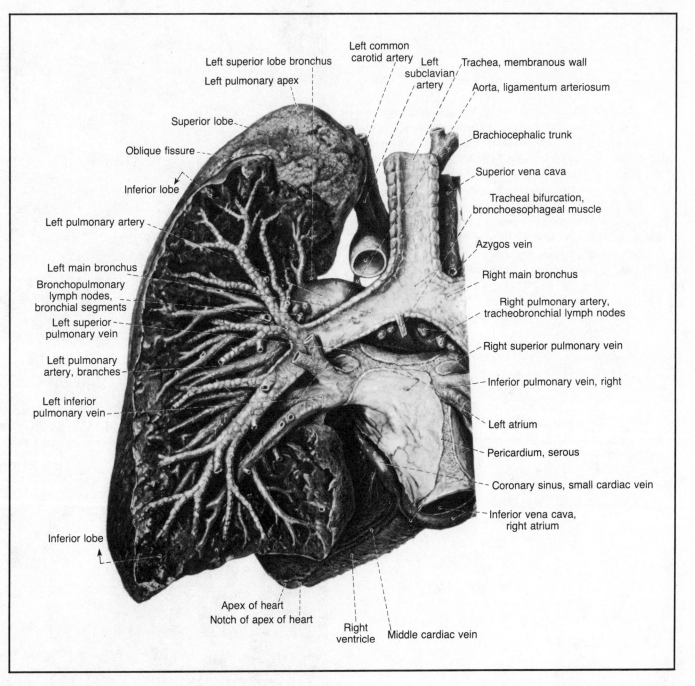

FIGURE 2–23 Trachea, bronchi, and bronchiole. (A) trachea of newborn, (B) cartilagenous open rings of trachea, (C) stereogram of wall of trachea, (D) cartilages and lymph nodes at the bifurcation of the trachea, (E) lung of 13-year-old boy, (F) small bronchi and bronchioles. (Courtesy of Hans Elias, Joun Pauly, and E. Robert Burns, *Histology and Human Microanatomy*, 4th ed. Padova, Italy: Piccin Medical Books, 1978. Originally from United States Public Health Service filmstrip by Hans Elias.)

FIGURE 2–24 Drawing of a heart-lung preparation from a dorsal view showing the bronchial tree. (From J. Sabotta and F. Figge, *Atlas of Human Anatomy*, 9th English Ed., Vol. 2. Munich and Baltimore: Urban and Schwarzenberg, 1977.)

Left superior lobe bronchus

Left common carotid artery

Left pulmonary apex

Left subclavian artery

Trachea, membranous wall

Aorta, ligamentum arteriosum

Superior lobe

Oblique fissure

Brachiocephalic trunk

Inferior lobe

Superior vena cava

Left pulmonary artery

Tracheal bifurcation, bronchoesophageal muscle

Azygos vein

Left main bronchus

Bronchopulmonary lymph nodes, bronchial segments

Right main bronchus

Left superior pulmonary vein

Right pulmonary artery, tracheobronchial lymph nodes

Left pulmonary artery, branches

Right superior pulmonary vein

Inferior pulmonary vein, right

Left inferior pulmonary vein

Left atrium

Pericardium, serous

Coronary sinus, small cardiac vein

Inferior vena cava, right atrium

Inferior lobe

Apex of heart

Notch of apex of heart

Right ventricle

Middle cardiac vein

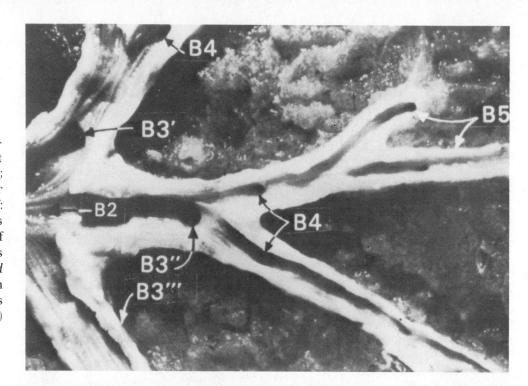

FIGURE 2–25   Anatomy of some broncho-pulmonary segments and their subdivisions (wet specimen from 13-year-old boy). (B) bronchus; (B2) bronchus of 2nd order, bronchus lobaris superior sinister; (B3) bronchus of 3rd order, consisting of: (B3'–B) segmentalis apicoposterior, (B3"–B) segmentalis anterior, (B3'''–B) segmentalis lingurais; (B4) bronchi of 4th order; (B5) bronchi of 5th order. (Courtesy of Hans Elias, Joun Pauly, and E. Robert Burns, *Histology and Human Microanatomy*, 4th ed. Padova, Italy: Piccin Medical Books, 1978. (Originally from United States Public Health Service filmstrip by Hans Elias.)

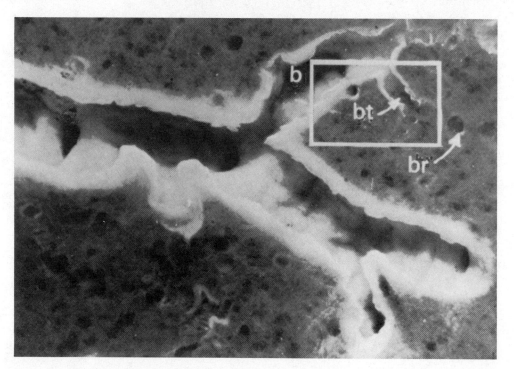

FIGURE 2–26   Terminal and respiratory bronchi (wet specimen from dog). (b) bronchiolus, (bt) bronchiolus terminalis, (br) bronchiolus respiratorius. (Courtesy of Hans Elias, Joun Pauly, and E. Robert Burns, *Histology and Human Microanatomy*, 4th ed. Padova, Italy: Piccin Medical Books, 1978. Originally from United States Public Health Service filmstrip by Hans Elias.)

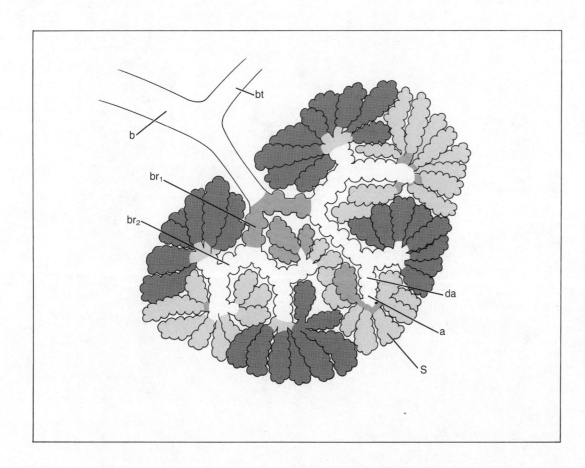

FIGURE 2–27 Diagram of lobule of lung. (b) bronchiolus, (br₁) bronchiolus respiratorius of 1st order, (br₂) bronchiolus respiratorius of 2nd order, (bt) bronchiolus terminalis, (da) ductulus alveolaris, (a) atrium, (S) sacculus alveolaris. (Courtesy of Hans Elias, Joun Pauly, and E. Robert Burns, *Histology and Human Microanatomy*, 4th ed. Padova, Italy: Piccin Medical Books, 1978. Originally from United States Public Health Service filmstrip by Hans Elias.)

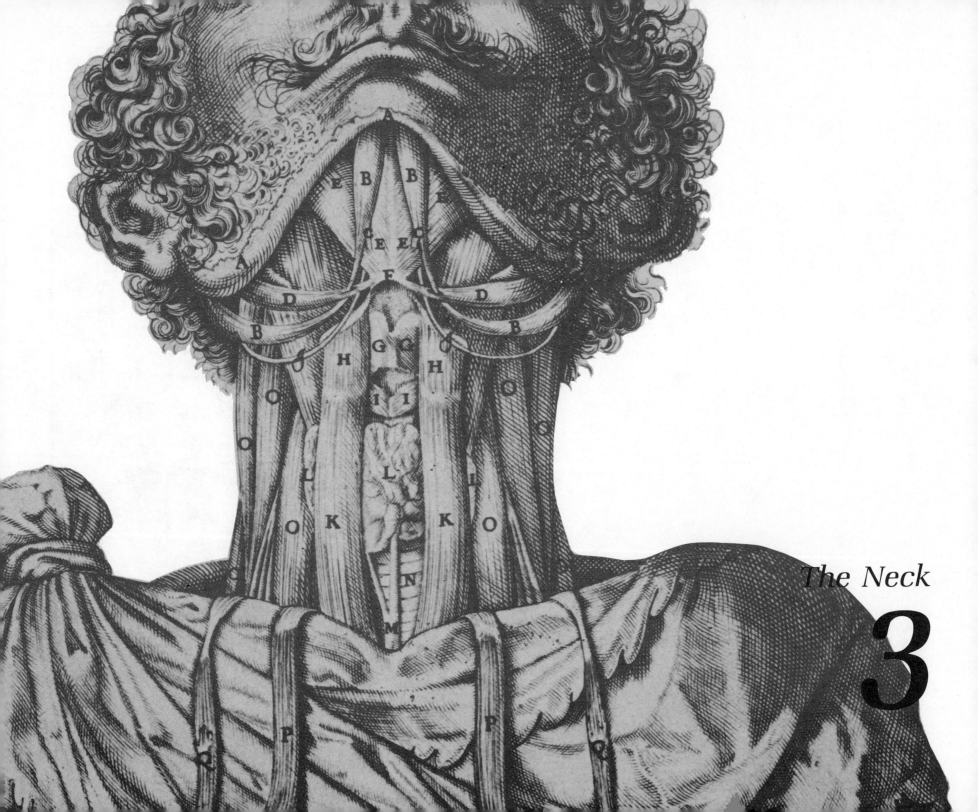

The Neck

3

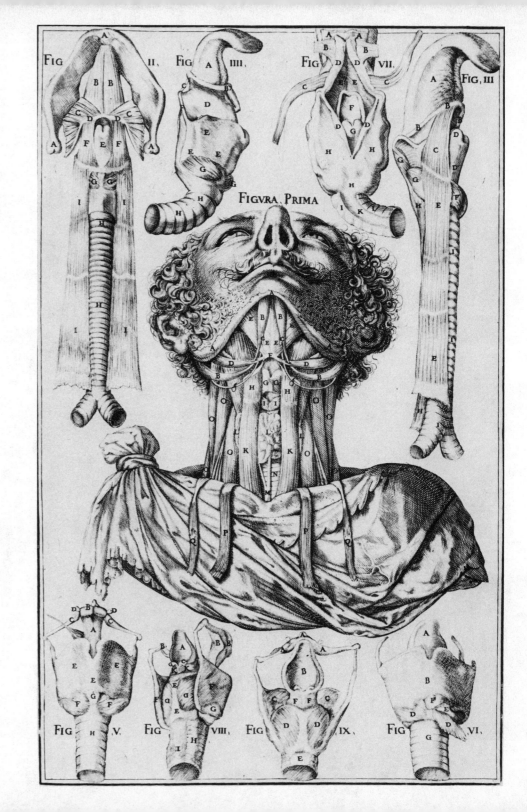

FIGURE 3–1 (From Giulio Casserio, *De Vocis Auditusque Organis Historia Anatomica*. Ferrare: Victorius Baldimus, 1600–1601.)

THE SPEECH MECHANISM

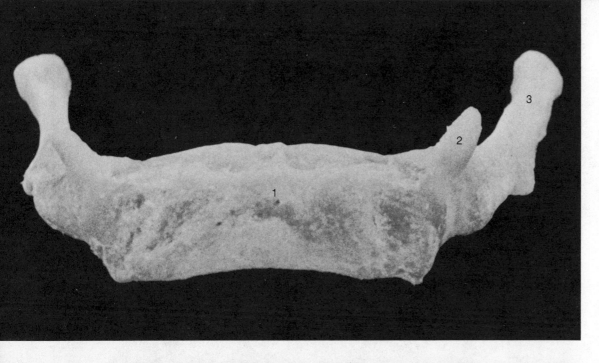

FIGURE 3–2   Anterior view of the hyoid bone. (1) body, (2) lesser horn, (3) greater horn.

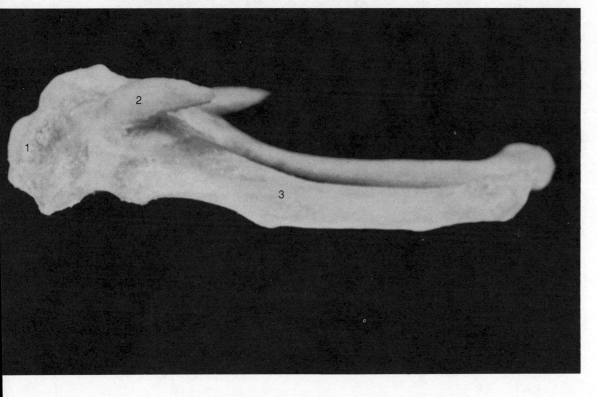

FIGURE 3–3   Lateral view of hyoid bone. (1) body, (2) lesser horn, (3) greater horn.

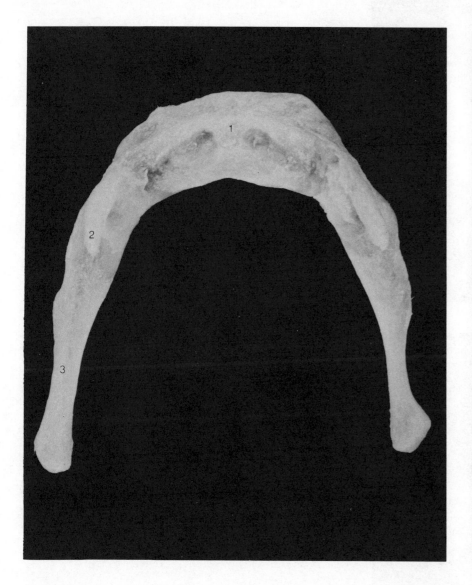

FIGURE 3–4   Superior view of hyoid bone. (1) body, (2) lesser horn, (3) greater horn.

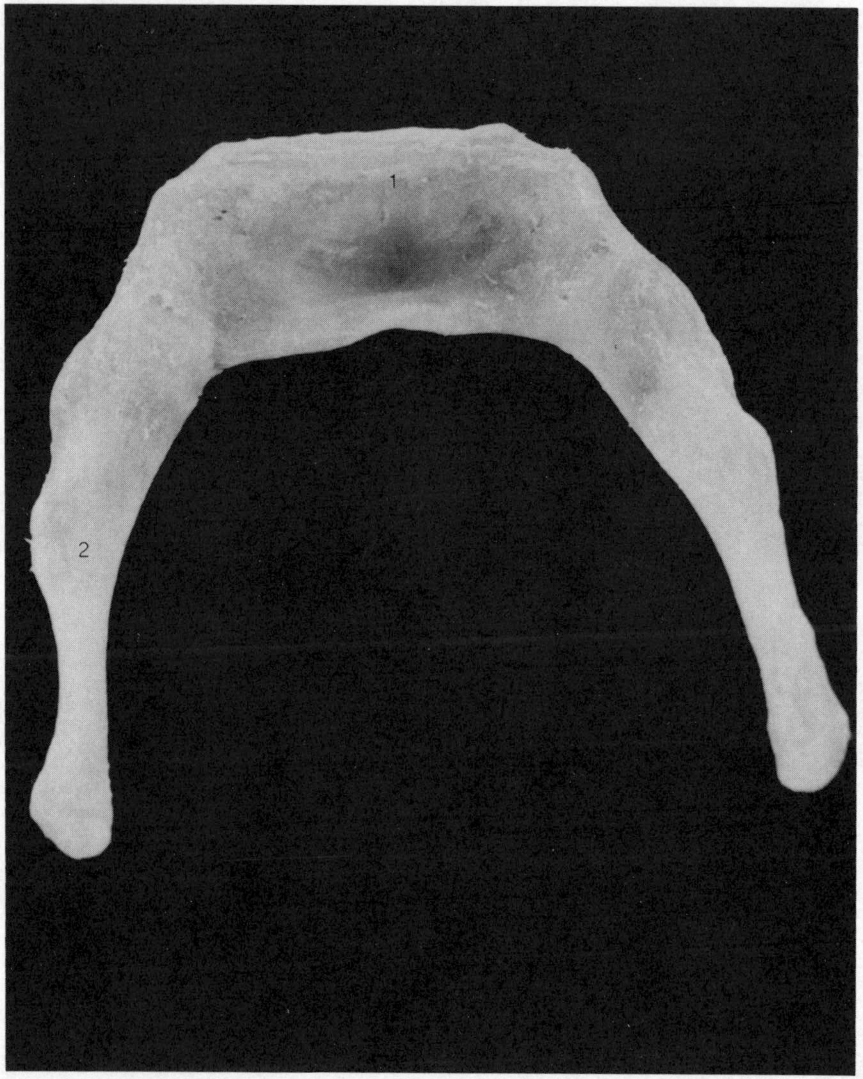

FIGURE 3–5   Inferior view of hyoid bone. (1) body, (2) greater horn.

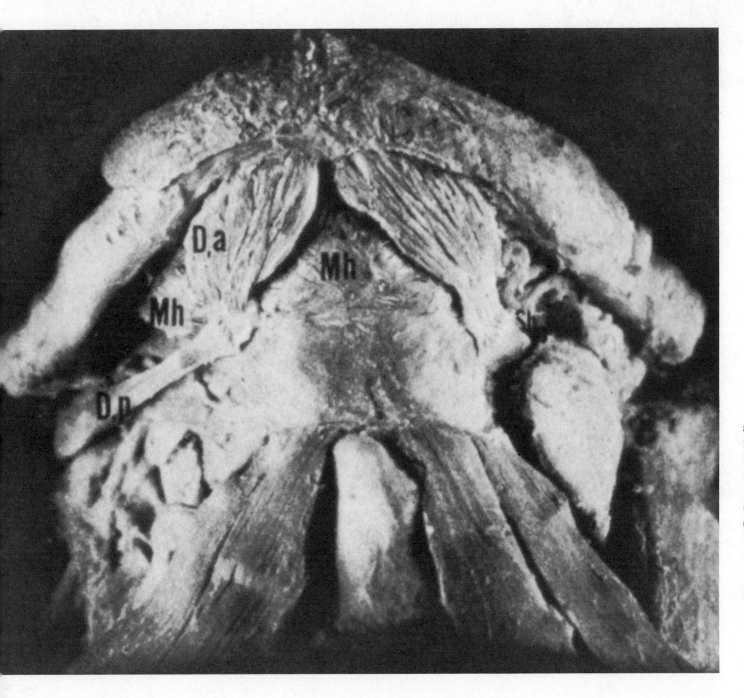

FIGURE 3–6 Dissection of the suprahyoid muscles viewed from front. (D,a) anterior belly of digastric muscle, (D,p) posterior belly of digastric muscle, (Sh) stylohyoid muscle, (Mh) mylohyoid muscle. (Courtesy of A.L. Martone and L.F. Edwards, "Anatomy of the Mouth and Related Structures: Part II, Musculature of Expression," in *Journal of Prosthetic Dentistry* 12, No. 1, 1962, p. 19.)

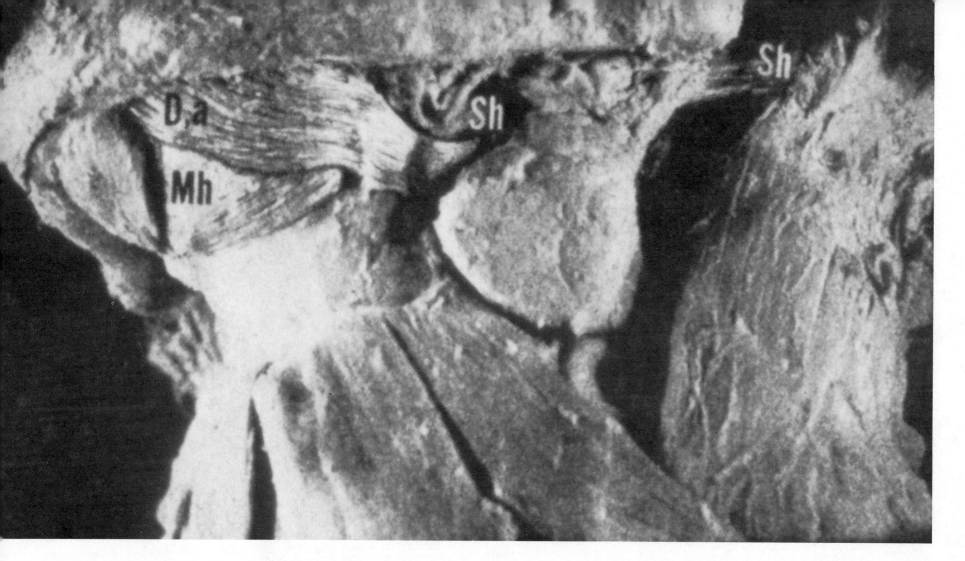

FIGURE 3–7 Dissection of suprahyoid muscles viewed laterally from left. (D,a) anterior belly of digastric muscle, (Sh) stylohyoid muscle, (Mh) mylohyoid muscle. (Courtesy of A.L. Martone and L.F. Edwards, "Anatomy of the Mouth and Related Structures: Part II, Musculature of Expression," in *Journal of Prosthetic Dentistry*, 12, No. 1, 1962, p. 19.)

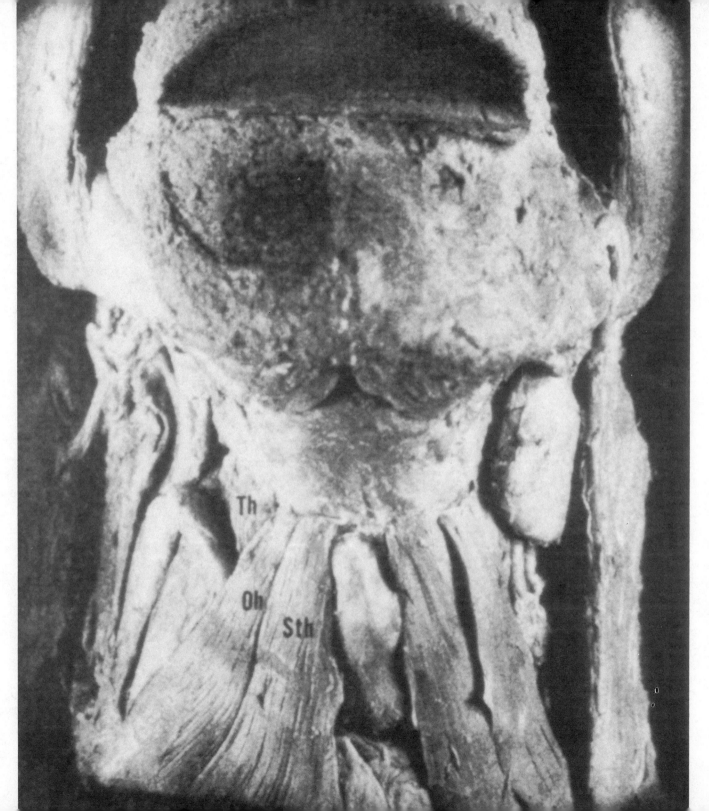

FIGURE 3–8 Dissection of infrahyoid muscles viewed from front. (Th) thyrohyoid muscle, (Oh) omohyoid muscle, (Sth) sternohyoid muscle. (Courtesy of A.L. Martone and L.F. Edwards, "Anatomy of the Mouth and Related Structures: Part II, Musculature of Expression," in *Journal of Prosthetic Dentistry*, 12, No. 1, 1962, p. 21.)

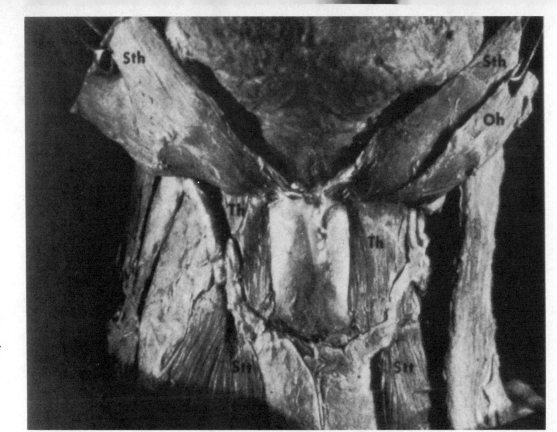

FIGURE 3–9   Dissection of neck, viewed from front, to show extrinsic laryngeal muscles. The (Sth) sternohyoid and (Oh) omohyoid muscles have been retracted. Both left and right (Th) thyrohyoid and (Stt) sternothyroid muscles are evident. (Courtesy of A.L. Martone and J.W. Black, "An Approach to Prosthetics Through Speech Science: Part IV, Physiology of Speech," in *Journal of Prosthetic Dentistry* 12, No. 3, 1962, p. 413.)

FIGURE 3–10   Superficial dissection of neck viewed anteriorly to show platysma muscles. (Courtesy of Lord Solly Zucherman, with Deryk Darlington and Peter Lisowski, *A New System of Anatomy*, 2nd Ed. Oxford: Oxford University Press, 1981.)

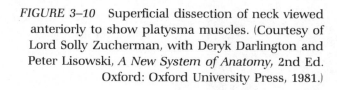

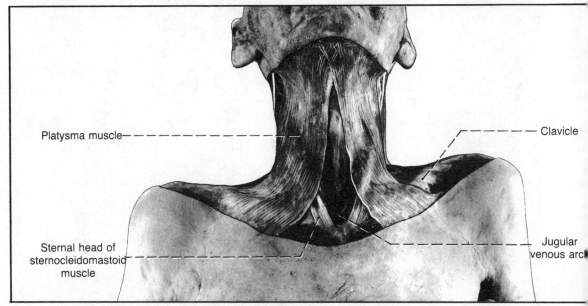

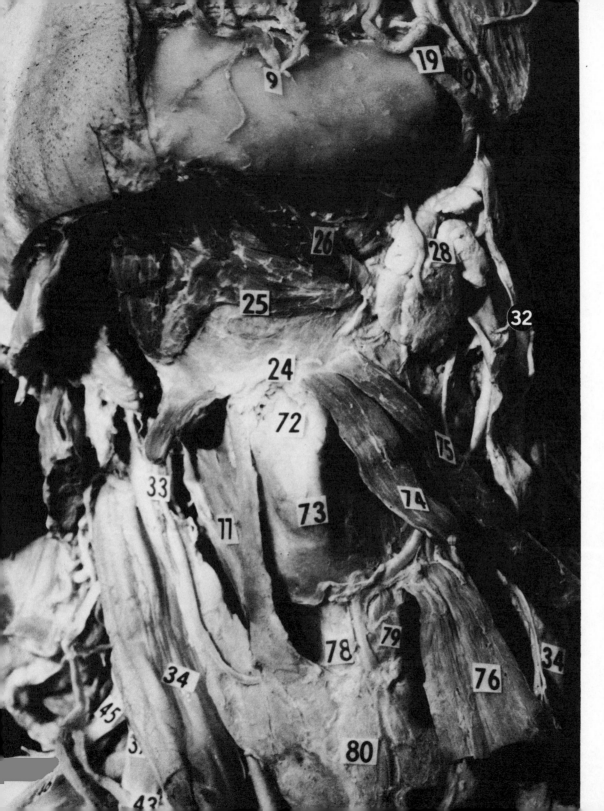

FIGURE 3–11 Dissection of anterior and lateral aspects of neck and submandibular regions. (9) mandible, (24) body of hyoid bone, (25) mylohyoid muscle, (26) anterior digastric muscle (note that its anterior attachment has been laid onto mandible surface), (28) submandibular gland, (32) carotid sinus at bifurcation of carotid artery into internal and external divisions, (34) internal jugular vein (opened on subject's right side but intact on left), (72) thyrohyoid membrane, (73) laryngeal prominence of thyroid cartilage, (74) sternohyoid muscle, (75) omohyoid muscle (on subject's right side, this muscle is removed except for its attachment to hyoid bone), (76) sternothyroid muscle, (78) cricoid cartilage, (79) cricothyroid muscle, (80) thyroid gland. (Courtesy of the Anatomy Museum of the Department of Anatomy and Cell Biology, University of Pittsburgh, School of Medicine, Pittsburgh.)

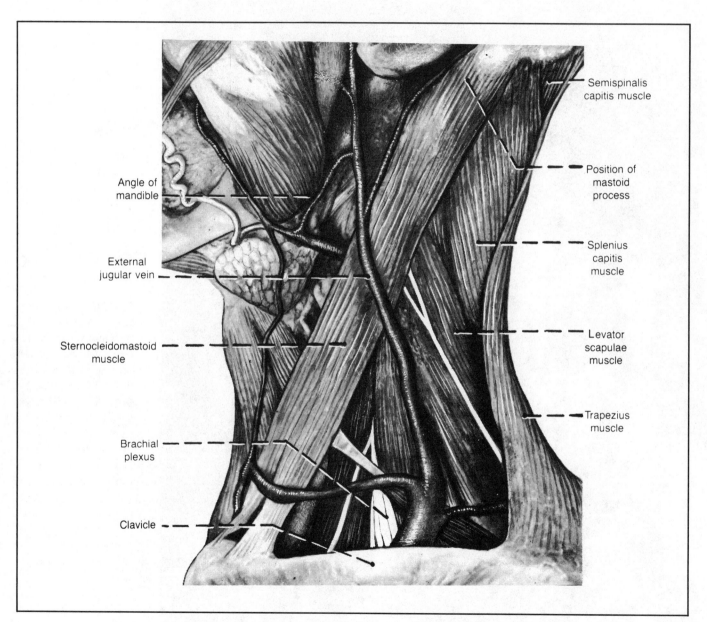

Semispinalis
capitis muscle

Position of
mastoid
process

Angle of
mandible

Splenius
capitis
muscle

External
jugular vein

Sternocleidomastoid
muscle

Levator
scapulae
muscle

Trapezius
muscle

Brachial
plexus

Clavicle

FIGURE 3–12 Dissection of left posterior triangle of neck. (Courtesy of Lord Solly Zuckerman, with Deryk Darlington and Pete Lisowski, *A New System of Anatomy*, 2nd Ed. Oxford: Oxford University Press, 1981.)

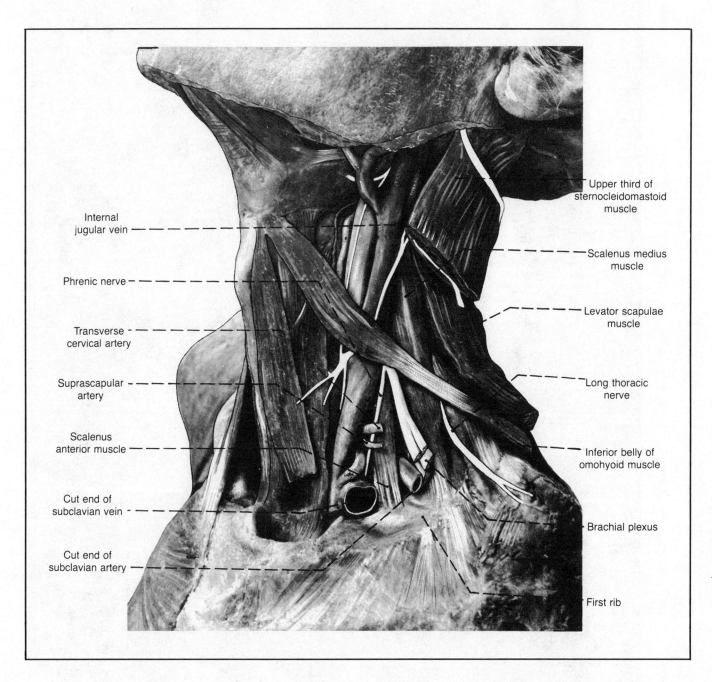

Internal
jugular vein

Phrenic nerve

Transverse
cervical artery

Suprascapular
artery

Scalenus
anterior muscle

Cut end of
subclavian vein

Cut end of
subclavian artery

Upper third of
sternocleidomastoid
muscle

Scalenus medius
muscle

Levator scapulae
muscle

Long thoracic
nerve

Inferior belly of
omohyoid muscle

Brachial plexus

First rib

FIGURE 3–13 Dissection of root of the neck viewed from left side. (Courtesy of Lord Solly Zuckerman, with Deryk Darlington and Peter Lisowski, *A New System of Anatomy*, 2nd Ed. Oxford: Oxford University Press, 1981.)

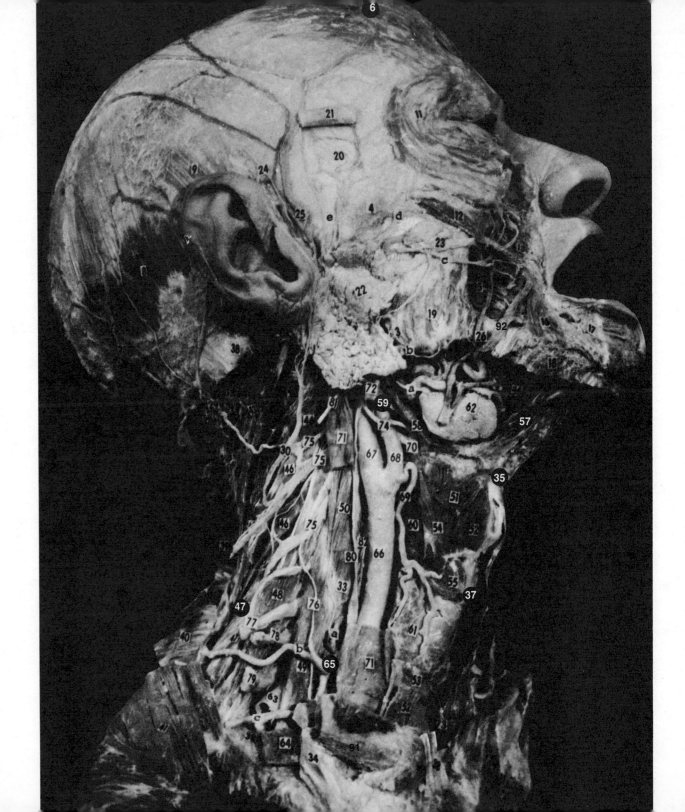

FIGURE 3–14 Lateral view of dissection of head and neck. (4) zygomatic arch; (6) frontal belly and (8) occipital belly of occipito-frontalis muscle; (9) superior and posterior auricularis muscles; (11) orbicularis oculi muscle; (12) zygomatic major muscle; (13) levator anguli muscle; (15) buccinator muscle; (16) depressor anguli oris muscle; (18) platysma muscle; (19) masseter muscle; (20) temporalis muscle; (21) temporal fascia; (22) parotid gland; (a) cervical, (b) mandibular, (c) buccal, (d) zygomatic, and (e) temporofrontal branches of the facial nerve; (23) parotid duct; (24) auriculotemporal nerve; (25) superficial temporal nerve and artery; (26) facial vein; (28) greater occipital nerve and occipital artery; (29) lesser occipital nerve; (30) greater auricular nerve; (34) subclavius muscle; (35) body of hyoid bone; (37) cricoid cartilage (anterior arch); (38) sternocleidomastoid muscle; (39) trapezius muscle; (40) rhomboid muscle; (41) serratus anterior muscle; (43) splenius capitus muscle; (46) levator scapulae muscle; (47) posterior, (48) medial, and (49) anterior scalene muscles; (50) longus capitus muscle; (51) omohyoid muscle; (52) sternohyoid muscle; (53) sternothyroid muscle; (54) thryohyoid muscle; (55) cricothyroid muscle; (56) mylohyoid muscle; (57) anterior and (58) posterior digastric muscles; (59) stylohyoid muscle; (60) inferior constrictor muscle; (61) thyroid gland; (62) submandibular gland; (63) subclavian artery; (65) thyrocervical trunk; (66) common carotid artery; (67) internal and (68) external carotid arteries; (69) superior thyroid artery; (70) lingual artery; (71) internal jugular vein; (74) hypoglossal nerve; (75) cervical plexus; (76) phrenic nerve; (77) upper, (78) middle, and (79) lower trunks of brachial plexus; (80) vagus nerve; (81) spinal accessory nerve; (91) clavical; (92) facial artery. (Courtesy of the Anatomy Museum of the Department of Anatomy and Cell Biology, University of Pittsburgh, School of Medicine, Pittsburgh.)

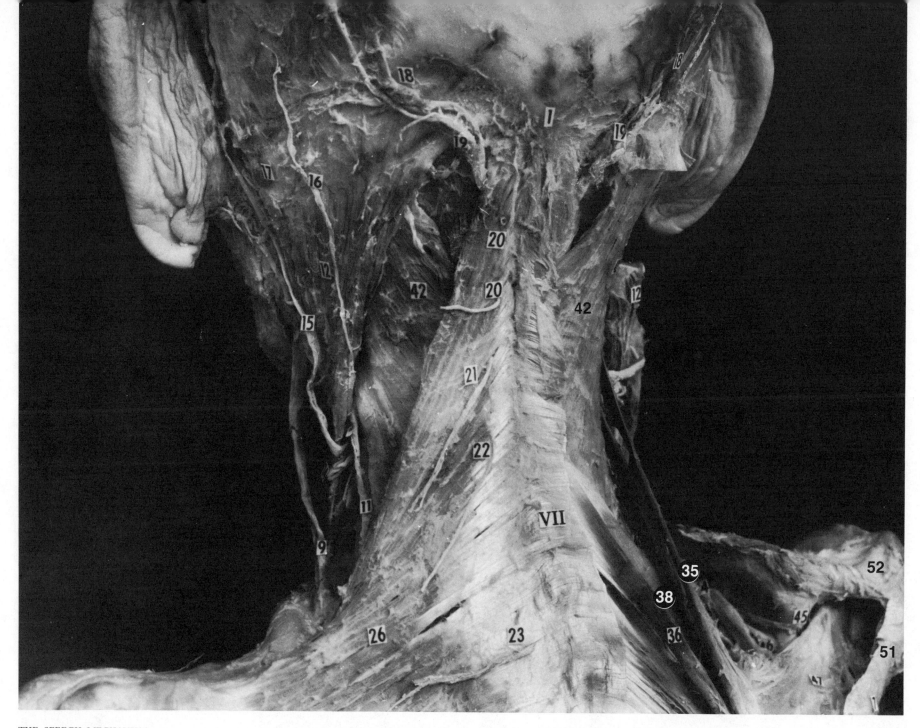

FIGURE 3–15 Dissection of posterior aspect of neck, back, and shoulder. (VII) spine of 7th cervical vertebra, (1) external occipital protuberance, (9) external jugular vein, (12) sternocleidomastoid muscle, (15) greater auricular nerve, (16) lesser occipital nerve, (19) occipital artery and nerve, (20–23) spinal nerves piercing the (26) trapezius muscle, (35) levator scapulae muscle, (36) rhomboidius major muscle, (38) serratus posterior superior muscle, (42) splenius capitus muscle, (51) spine and (52) acromion of scapula. (Courtesy of the Anatomy Museum of the Department of Anatomy and Cell Biology, University of Pittsburgh, School of Medicine, Pittsburgh.)

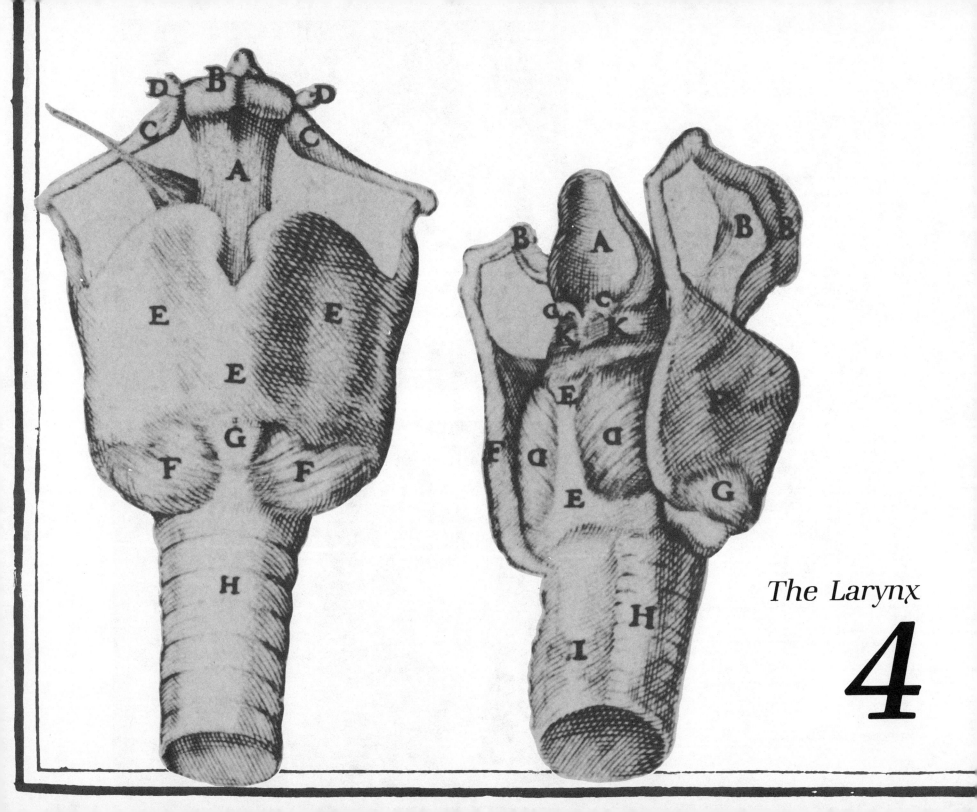

The Larynx

4

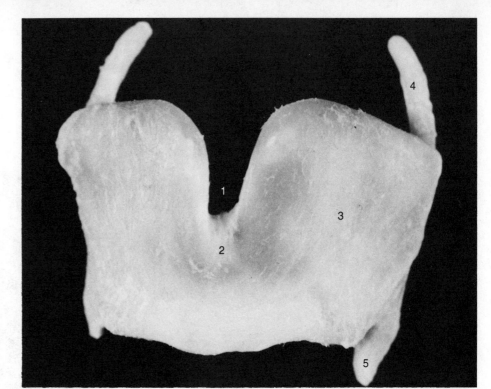

FIGURE 4–1   Anterior view of thyroid cartilage. (1) thyroid notch, (2) thyroid prominence (eminence), (3) lamina, (4) superior horn (cornu), (5) inferior horn. (Dissection by Joel C. Kahane.)

FIGURE 4–2   Anterior-inferior view of thyroid cartilage. (1) inferior thyroid horn, (2) cricothyroid articular facet, (3) inferior tubercle, (4) thyroid notch, (5) lamina. (Dissection by Joel C. Kahane.)

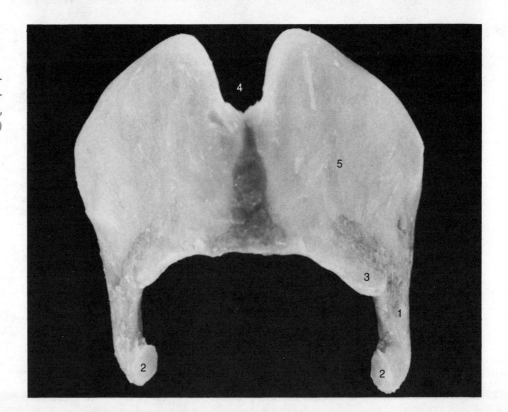

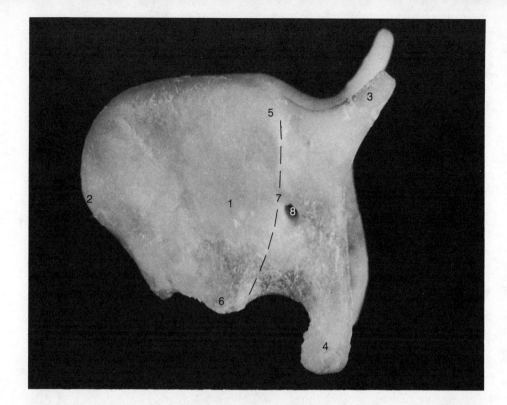

FIGURE 4–3 Left lateral view of thyroid cartilage. (1) lamina, (2) laryngeal prominence, (3) superior thyroid horn, (4) inferior thyroid horn, (5) superior and (6) inferior tubercle, (7) oblique line, (8) foramen occasionally found in lamina of thyroid cartilage. (Dissection by Joel C. Kahane.)

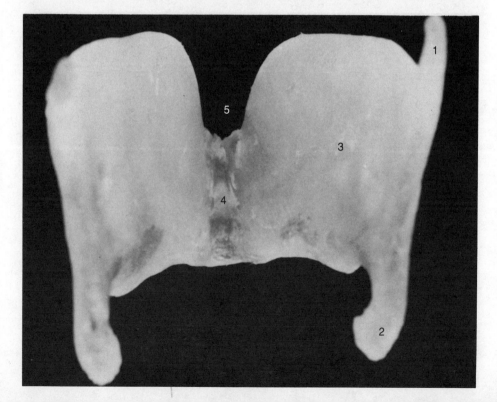

FIGURE 4–4 Posterior view of thyroid cartilage. (1) superior and (2) inferior thyroid horns; (3) lamina; (4) points of attachment for vestibular folds, vocal folds, and thyroepiglottic ligament; (5) thyroid notch. (Dissection by Joel C. Kahane.)

THE LARYNX

61

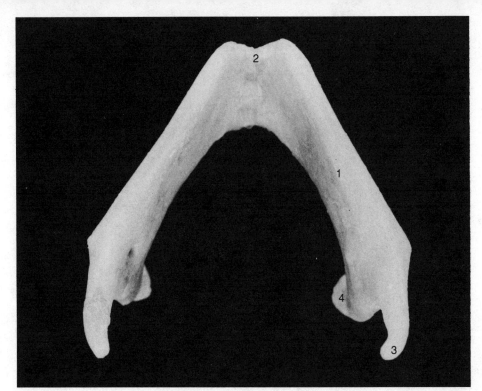

FIGURE 4–5 Superior view of thyroid cartilage. (1) lamina, (2) thyroid notch, (3) superior horn, (4) inferior horn. (Dissection by Joel C. Kahane.)

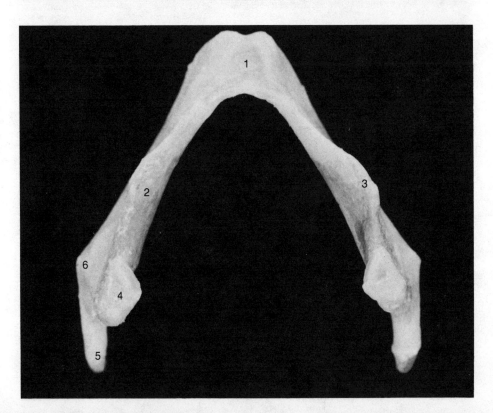

FIGURE 4–6 Inferior view of thyroid cartilage. (1) thyroid prominence, (2) lamina, (3) inferior tubercle, (4) inferior thyroid horn and articular facets, (5) superior thyroid horn, (6) superior tubercle. (Dissection by Joel C. Kahane.)

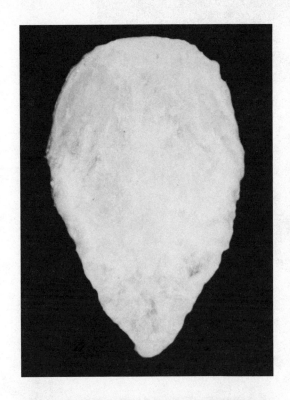

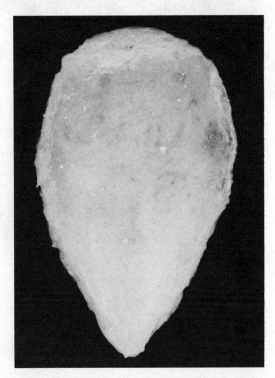

FIGURE 4–7   Lingual surface of epiglottis with mucosa intact. (Dissection by Joel C. Kahane.)

FIGURE 4–8   Laryngeal surface of epiglottis with mucosa intact. (Dissection by Joel C. Kahane.)

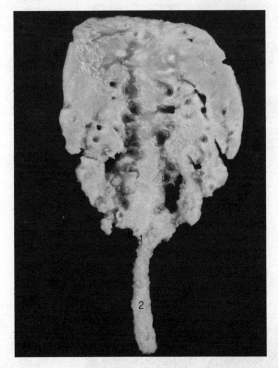

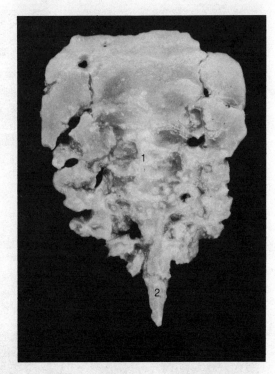

FIGURE 4–9   Epiglottic cartilage with numerous pits for mucous glands contained therein. (1) petiole, (2) thyroepiglottic ligament. (Dissection courtesy of Alice R. Kahn, Memphis, Tennessee.)

FIGURE 4–10   Epiglottic cartilage from child of unknown age. Note similarities to adult. (1) region of epiglottic tubercle, (2) petiole. (Dissection courtesy of Alice R. Kahn, Memphis, Tennessee.)

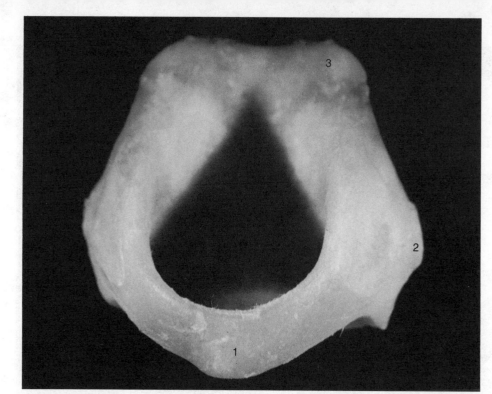

FIGURE 4–11   Anterior view of cricoid cartilage. (1) arch at midline, (2) cricothyroid articular facets, (3) cricoarytenoid articular facets. (Dissection by Joel C. Kahane.)

FIGURE 4–12   Right lateral view of cricoid cartilage. (1) anterior portion and (2) lateral portion of arch, (3) cricothyroid articular facet, (4) cricoarytenoid articular facet, (5) lamina. (Dissection by Joel C. Kahane.)

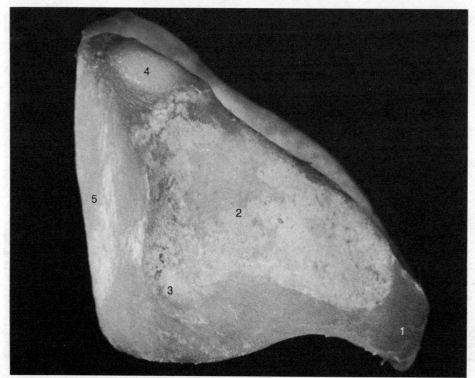

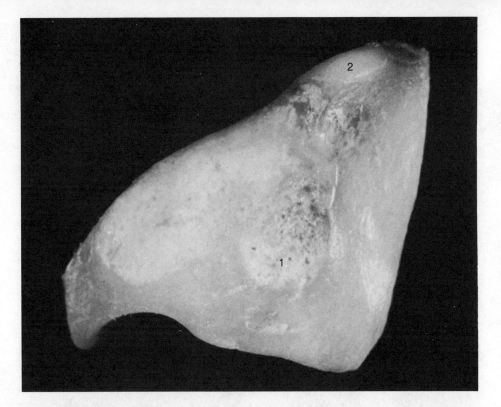

FIGURE 4–13 Left lateral view of cricoid cartilage. Note asymmetry between (1) cricothyroid articular facet on left side and its counterpart on right side. Compare this with the bilateral symmetry of the (2) cricoarytenoid articular facet on left and right sides. (Dissection by Joel C. Kahane.)

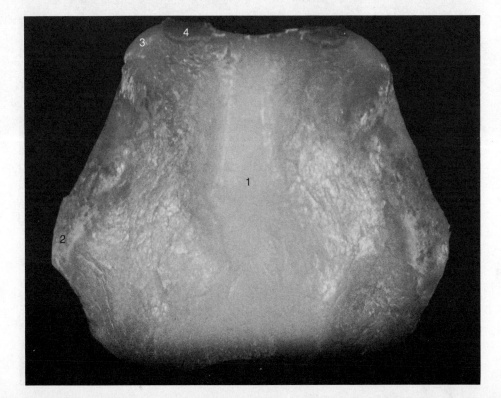

FIGURE 4–14 Posterior view of cricoid cartilage. (1) dorsal ridge dividing lamina, (2) cricothyroid articular facets, (3) cricoarytenoid articular facets, (4) ossified points of attachment of posterior cricoarytenoid ligaments. (Dissection by Joel C. Kahane.)

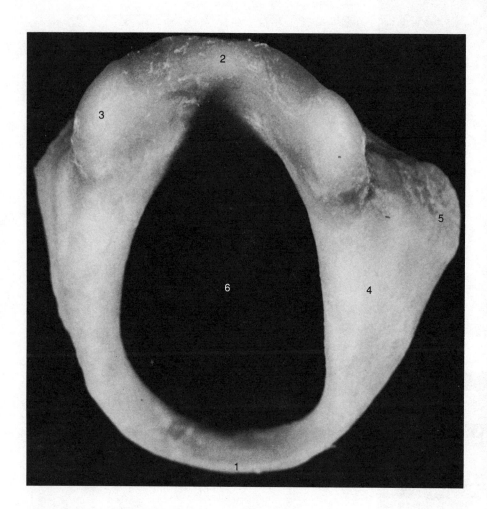

FIGURE 4-15 Superior view of cricoid cartilage.
(1) superior border of arch, anteriorly, (2) superior border of lamina, (3) cricoarytenoid articular facets, (4) arch, laterally, (5) cricothyroid articular facets, (6) cricoid lumen. (Dissection by Joel C. Kahane.)

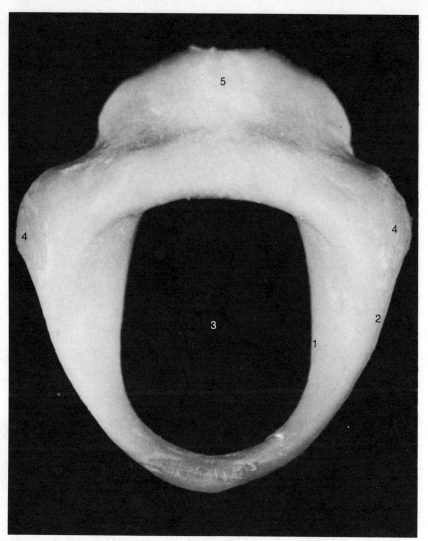

FIGURE 4-16 Inferior view of cricoid cartilage. (1) superior and (2) inferior borders of cricoid arch, (3) lumen of cricoid cartilage, (4) cricothyroid articular facets, (5) lamina. (Dissection by Joel C. Kahane.)

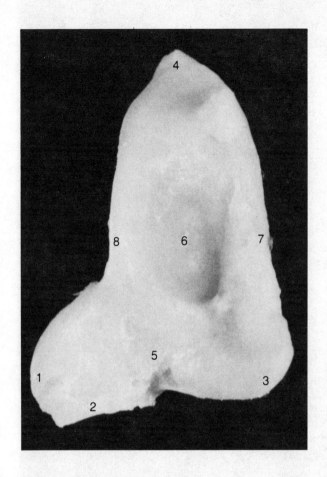

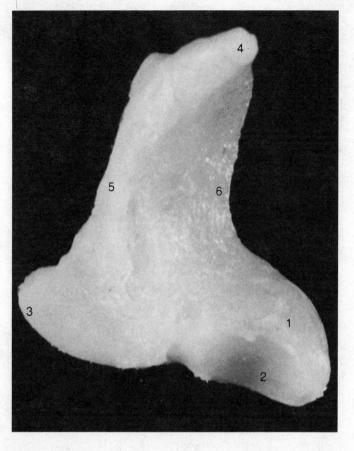

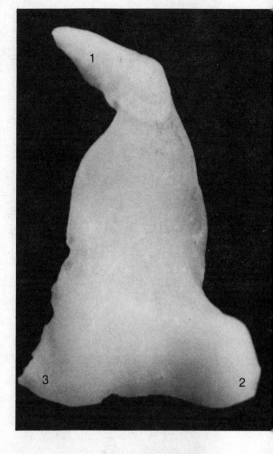

FIGURE 4–17 Anterolateral view of left arytenoid cartilage. (1) muscular process, (2) articular facet, (3) vocal process, (4) apex, (5) fovea oblonga, (6) fovea triangularis, (7) anterior and (8) dorsolateral ridges. (Dissection by Joel C. Kahane.)

FIGURE 4–18 Medial view of right arytenoid cartilage. (1) muscular process, (2) articular facet, (3) vocal process, (4) apex, (5) anterior ridge, (6) dorsolateral ridge. (Dissection by Joel C. Kahane.)

FIGURE 4–19 Right arytenoid cartilage with corniculate cartilage attached. (1) corniculate cartilage on top of apex, (2) muscular process, (3) vocal process. (Dissection by Joel C. Kahane.)

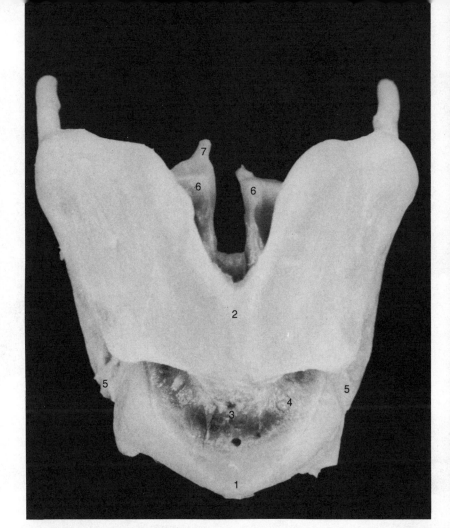

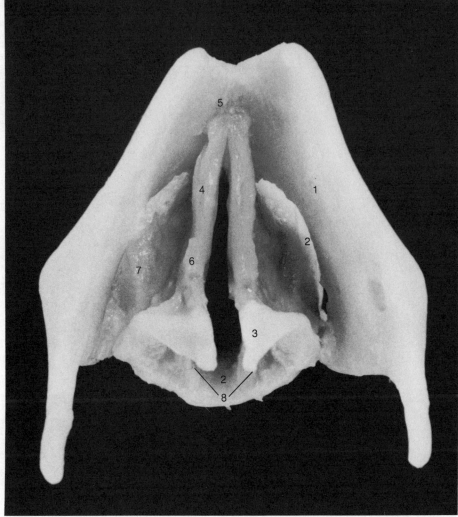

FIGURE 4–20 Anterior view of articulated laryngeal cartilages. (1) cricoid cartilage (arch), (2) thyroid cartilage, (3) cricothyroid membrane and (4) part of conus elasticus, (5) cricothyroid joint, (6) arytenoid cartilages with (7) corniculate cartilages. (Dissection by Joel C. Kahane.)

FIGURE 4–21 Superior view of articulated laryngeal cartilages and attached connective tissues. (1) thyroid cartilage, (2) cricoid cartilage, (3) arytenoid cartilage, (4) vocal ligament with attachment at (5) anterior commissure and (6) vocal process of arytenoid cartilage, (7) conus elasticus, (8) posterior cricoarytenoid ligaments. (Dissection by Joel C. Kahane.)

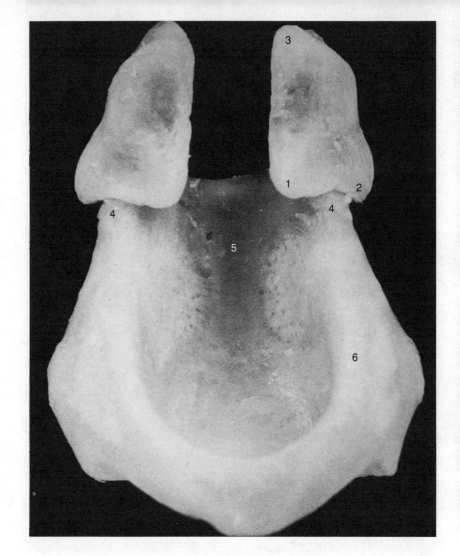

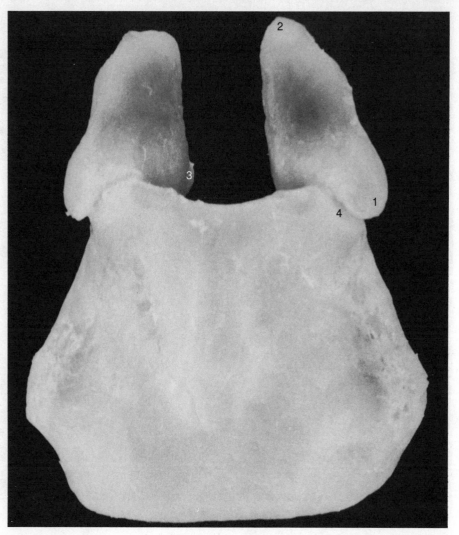

FIGURE 4–22 Articulation of arytenoid and cricoid cartilages at cricoarytenoid joint, viewed anteriorly. (1) vocal process, (2) muscular process and (3) apex of arytenoid cartilage, (4) cricoarytenoid articular facets of cricoid, (5) lamina and (6) arch of cricoid cartilage. (Dissection by Joel C. Kahane.)

FIGURE 4–23 Articulation of arytenoid and cricoid cartilages at cricoarytenoid joint, viewed posteriorly. (1) muscular process, (2) apex, (3) vocal process of arytenoid cartilage, (4) cricoarytenoid facet. (Dissection by Joel C. Kahane.)

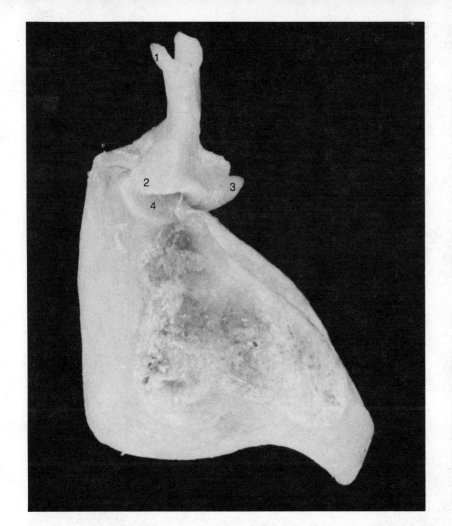

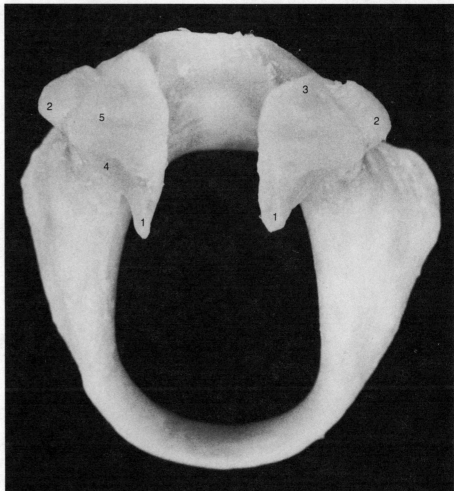

FIGURE 4–24   Articulation of arytenoid and cricoid cartilages at cricoarytenoid joint, viewed laterally. (1) corniculate cartilage attached to apex, (2) muscular process, (3) vocal process, (4) cricoarytenoid articular facet of cricoid exposed by separating corresponding articular surface of arytenoid cartilage, which is located on the undersurface of muscular process. (Dissection by Joel C. Kahane.)

FIGURE 4–25   Articulation of arytenoid and cricoid cartilages at cricoarytenoid joint, viewed superiorly. (1) vocal process (2) muscular process, (3) apex, (4) fovea oblonga, (5) fovea triangularis. (Dissection by Joel C. Kahane.)

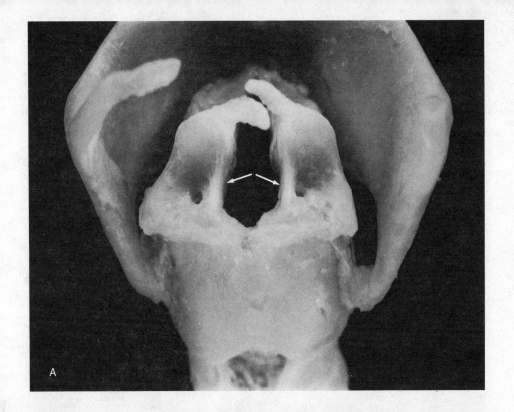

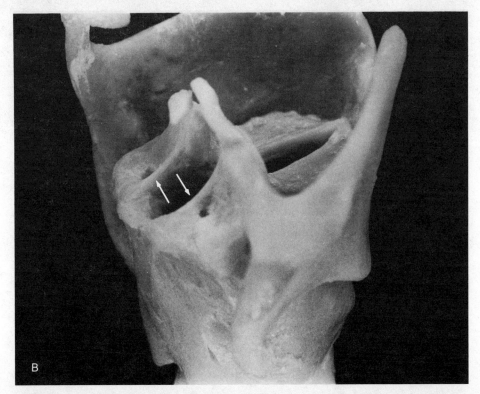

FIGURE 4–26   Posterior cricoarytenoid ligaments
(shown by arrows). (A) posterior attachment,
(B) attachment to medial surface of arytenoid cartilage.
(Dissection by Joel C. Kahane.)

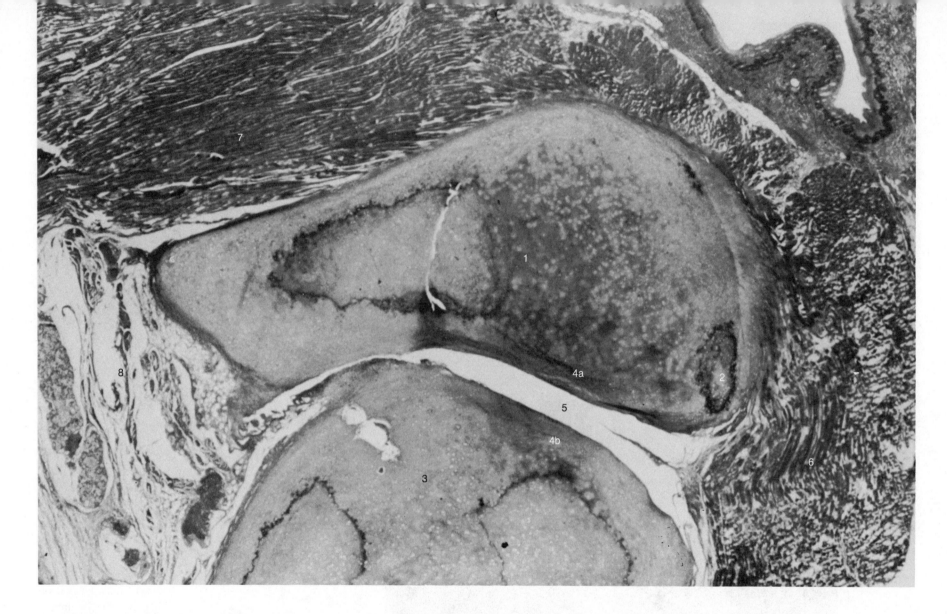

FIGURE 4–27 Photomicrograph of a coronal section through adult left cricoarytenoid joint. (1) body and (2) muscular process of arytenoid cartilage, (3) cricoid cartilage, (4a) articular facet of arytenoid cartilage, (4b) articular facet of cricoid cartilage, (5) joint cavity of cricoarytenoid cartilage with portion of synovial membrane shown at right, (6) posterior cricoarytenoid muscle, (7) interarytenoid muscle, (8) loose connective tissue and glands in contiguous tissues. (Photomicrographs by Joel C. Kahane.

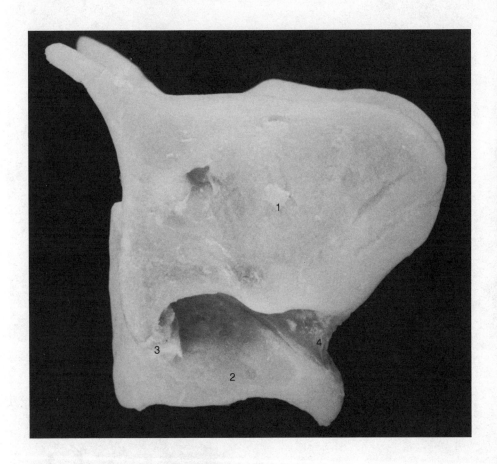

FIGURE 4–28   Lateral view of thyroid and cricoid cartilages. (1) thyroid cartilage, (2) cricoid cartilage, (3) cricothyroid joint, (4) cricothyroid membrane. (Dissection by Joel C. Kahane.)

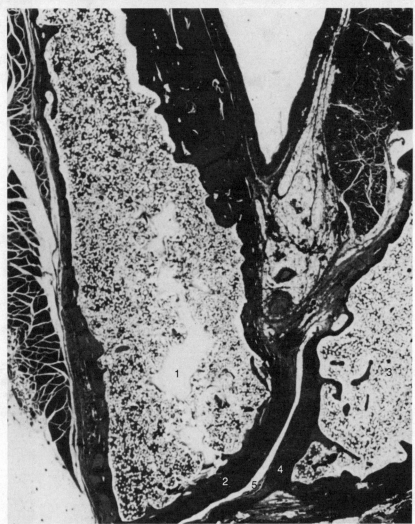

FIGURE 4–29   Photomicrograph of coronal section through adult cricothyroid joint. (1) inferior horn of thyroid cartilage and (2) surface of articular facet, (3) cricoid cartilage and (4) surface of articular facet, (5) joint space, (6) pars oblique portion of cricothyroid muscle. (Photomicrograph by Joel C. Kahane.)

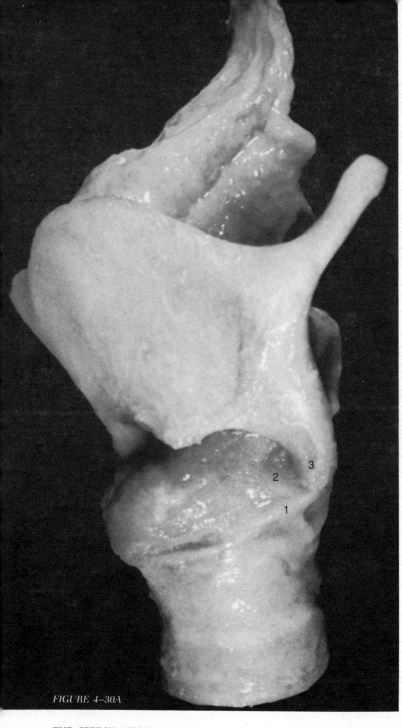

FIGURE 4-30A

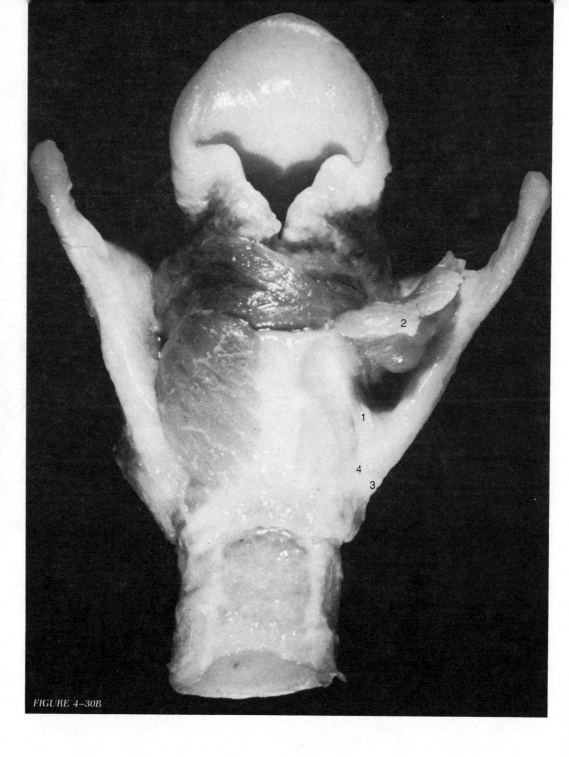

FIGURE 4-30B

THE SPEECH MECHANISM

FIGURE 4–30 Ligaments of cricothyroid joint. In lateral view (A): (1) lateral and (2) anterior cricothyroid (ceratocricoid) ligaments composing part of joint capsule of (3) cricothyroid joint formed through joining articular facets on inferior thyroid horn and arch of cricoid cartilage, respectively. In posterior view (B): (1) posterior cricothyroid (ceratocricoid) ligament lays deep to (2) posterior cricoarytenoid muscle. Note attachment of ligament to (3) inferior thyroid horn through (4) joint capsule. (Dissection by Joel C. Kahane.)

FIGURE 4–31 Superior-lateral view of larynx and hyoid bone. (1) body, (2) lesser, and (3) greater horn of hyoid bone; (4) epiglottis; (5) aryepiglottic fold; (6) cuneiform and (7) corniculate tubercles; (8) piriform recess; (9) inferior pharyngeal constrictor muscle; (10) thyrohyoid muscle; (11) omohyoid muscle; (12) sternohyoid muscle. (Dissection by Joel C. Kahane.)

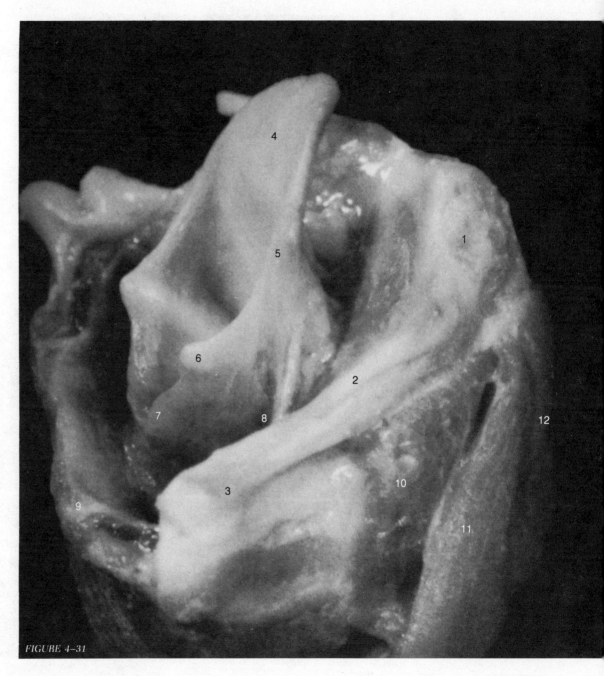

FIGURE 4–31

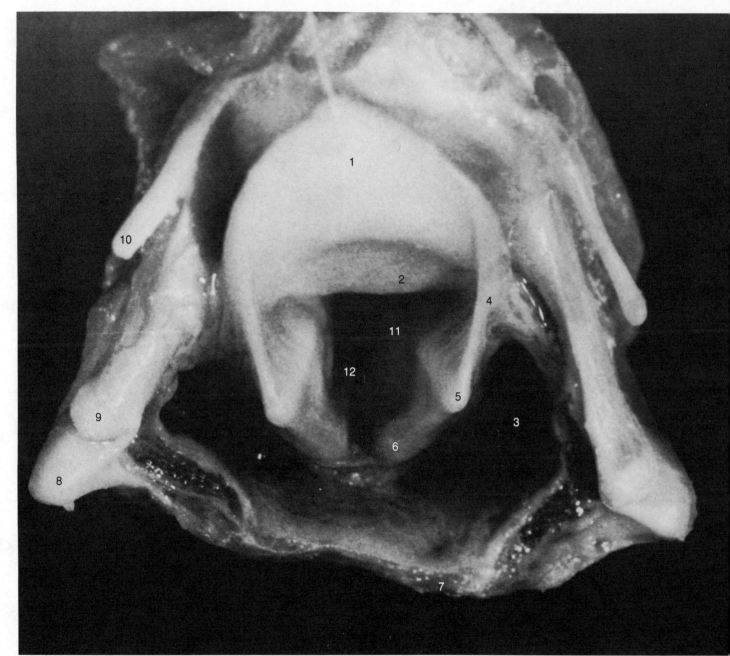

FIGURE 4–32 Superior view of larynx. (1) epiglottis, (2) epiglottic tubercle, (3) piriform recess, (4) aryepiglottic fold, (5) cuneiform and (6) corniculate tubercles, (7) inferior pharyngeal constrictor muscle, (8) tip of superior thyroid horn, (9) greater and (10) lesser horns of hyoid bone, (11) vestibular (ventricular) fold, (12) rima glottidis. (Dissection by Joel C. Kahane.)

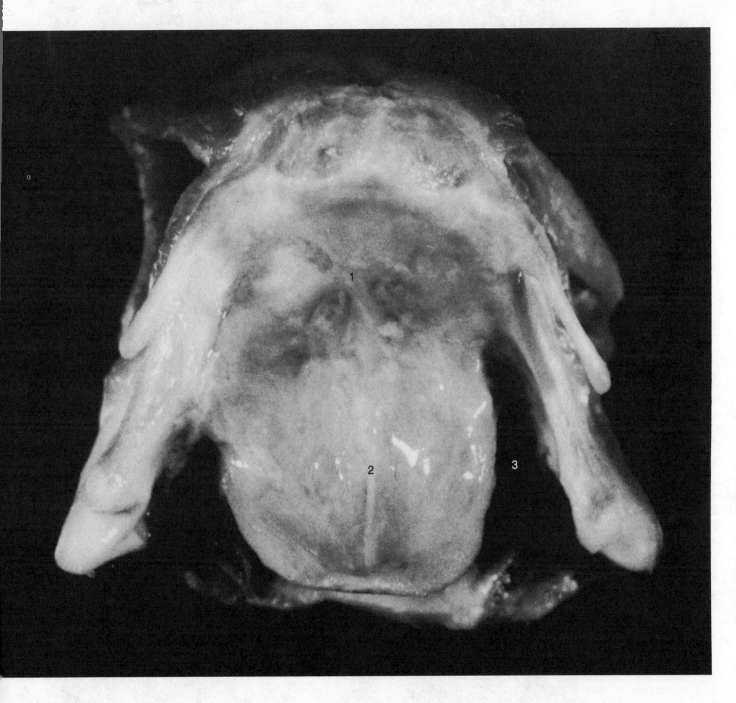

FIGURE 4–33 Superior view of larynx, identical to Figure 4–32 except that epiglottis is covering entrance into larynx. (1) remnants of hyoepiglottic ligament, (2) median glosso-epiglottic fold, (3) piriform recess. (Dissection by Joel C. Kahane.)

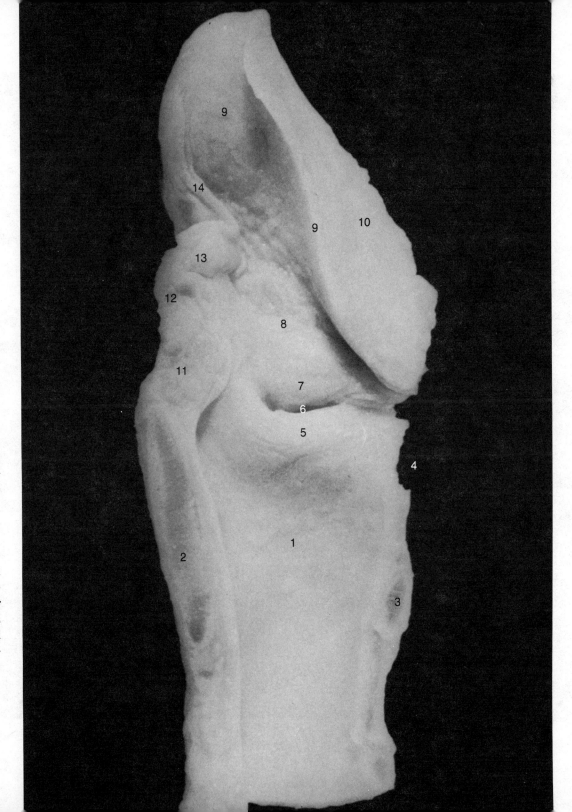

FIGURE 4–34 Midsagittal section of laryngeal cavity. The laryngeal cavity is divided into 3 parts: the *vestibule* extends from the aditus laryngeus to the vestibular (ventricular) folds; the *glottal region* is bounded by the vestibular (ventricular) and true vocal folds; (3) the *infraglottal region* (or *subglottal cavity*) extends from the vocal folds to the lower border of the cricoid cartilage. (1) conus elasticus and mucosa of subglottal cavity, (2) lamina and (3) arch of cricoid cartilage, (4) area from which thyroid cartilage has been removed, (5) vocal fold, (6) laryngeal ventricle (of Morgagni), (7) vestibular (ventricular) fold, (8) quadrangular membrane, (9) epiglottis, (10) pre-epiglottic fat pad, (11) interarytenoid muscle, (12) corniculate and (13) cuneiform tubercles, (14) aryepiglottic folds. (Dissection by Joel C. Kahane.)

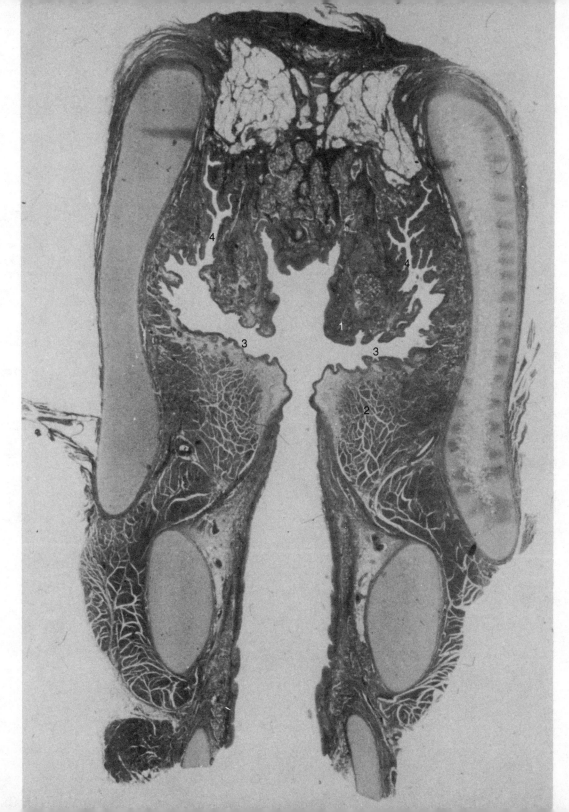

FIGURE 4–35 Photomicrograph of coronal section of an infant larynx to illustrate the anatomy of the laryngeal ventricle (of Morgagni) and sacculus. (1) vestibular fold, (2) true vocal fold, (3) laryngeal ventricle, (4) sacculus. (Photomicrograph by Joel C. Kahane.)

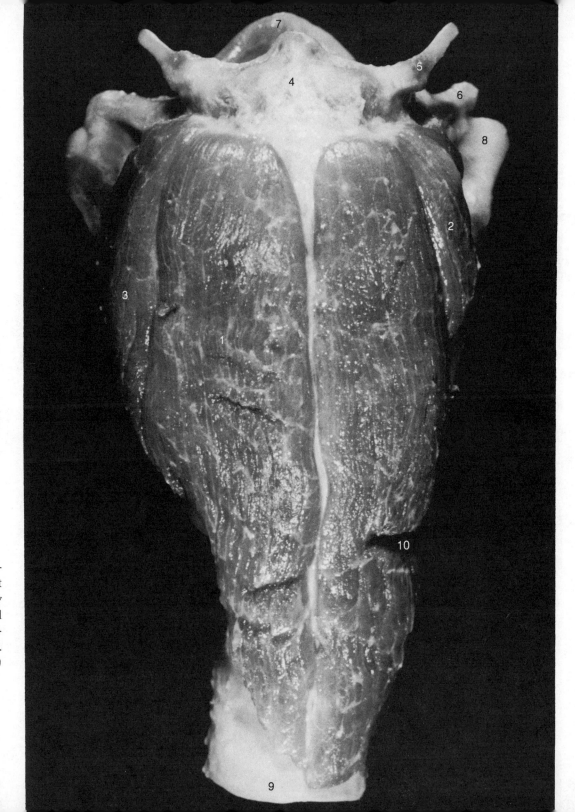

FIGURE 4–36 Anterior view of larynx showing extrinsic laryngeal muscles. (1) sternohyoid muscle, (2) left omohyoid muscle, (3) right omohyoid muscle (4) body of hyoid bone, (5) lesser and (6) greater horns of hyoid bone, (7) epiglottis, (8) superior horn of thyroid cartilage, (9) trachea, (10) artifact. (Dissection by Joel C. Kahane.)

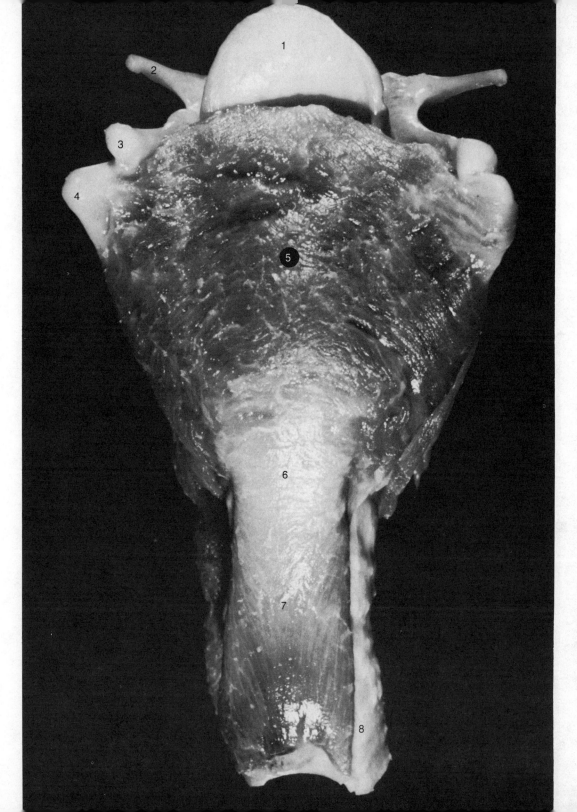

FIGURE 4–37 Posterior view of larynx. (1) epiglottis, (2) lesser and (3) greater horns of hyoid bone, (4) tip of superior thyroid horn, (5) inferior constrictor muscle, (6) cricopharyngeal fibers of inferior pharyngeal constrictor muscle, (7) esophagus, (8) trachea. (Dissection by Joel C. Kahane.)

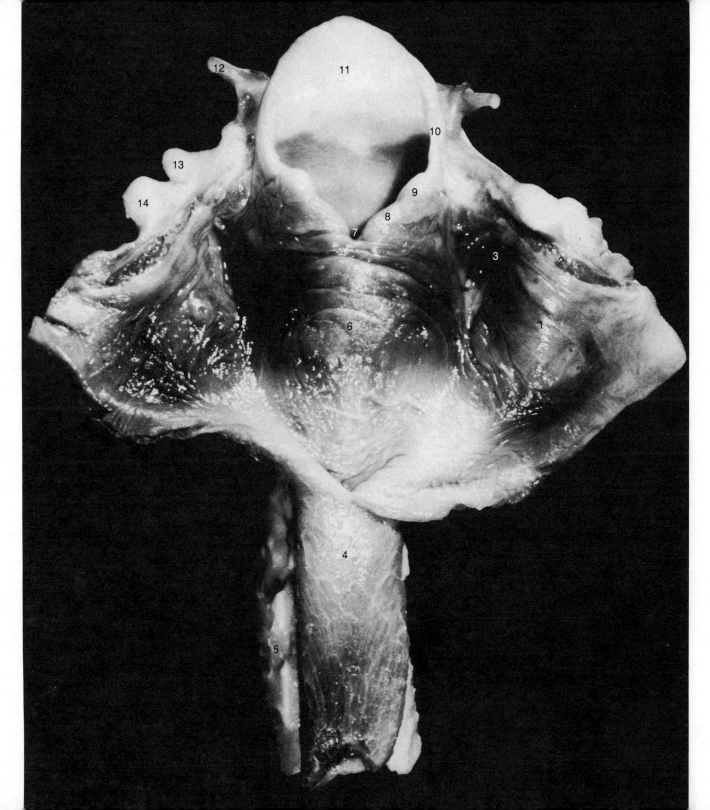

FIGURE 4–38 Posterior view of larynx with inferior pharyngeal constrictor muscle sectioned medially and reflected. (1) pharyngeal mucosa and (2) musculature, (3) piriform recess, (4) esophagus, (5) trachea, (6) mucosa overlying cricoid and arytenoid cartilages, (7) interarytenoid notch, (8) corniculate and (9) cuneiform tubercles, (10) aryepiglottic fold, (11) epiglottis, (12) lesser and (13) greater horns of hyoid bone, (14) tip of superior thyroid horn. (Dissection by Joel C. Kahane.)

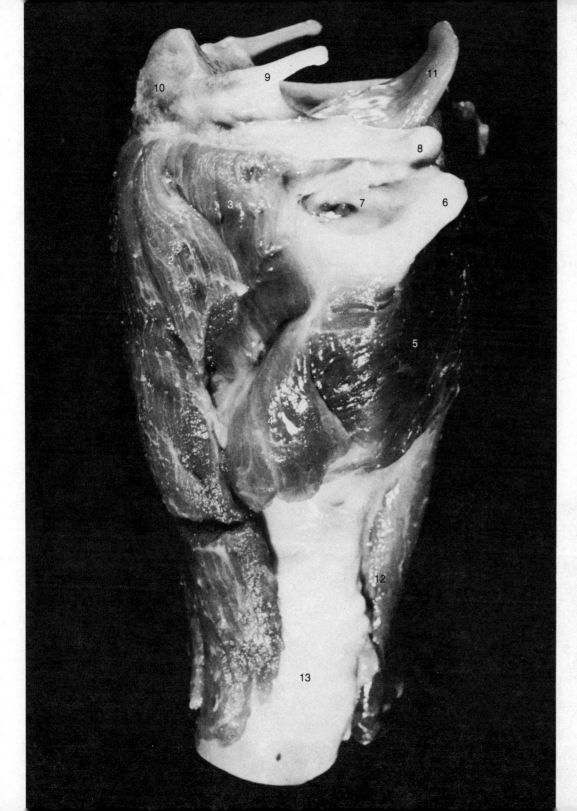

FIGURE 4–39 Left lateral view of larynx. (1) sternohyoid muscle, (2) omohyoid muscle (sectioned), (3) thyrohyoid muscle, (4) sternothyroid muscle (sectioned) attached to oblique line, (5) inferior pharyngeal constrictor muscle, (6) superior horn of thyroid cartilage, (7) thyrohyoid membrane pierced by vessels and nerve, (8) greater and (9) lesser horns and (10) body of hyoid bone, (11) epiglottis, (12) esophagus, (13) trachea. (Dissection by Joel C. Kahane.)

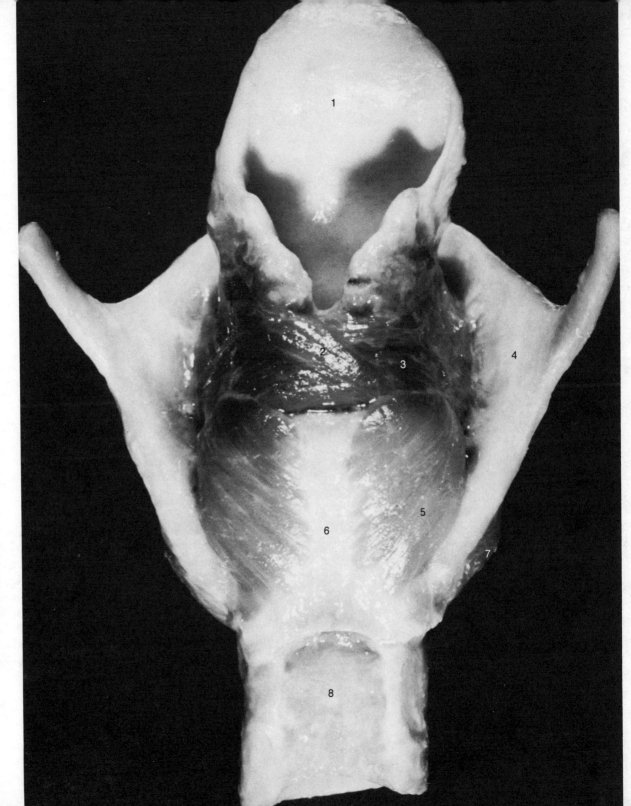

FIGURE 4–40   Posterior view of larynx and intrinsic laryngeal muscles. (1) epiglottis, (2) oblique interarytenoid muscle, (3) transverse interarytenoid muscle, (4) lamina of thyroid cartilage, (5) posterior cricoarytenoid muscle, (6) lamina of cricoid cartilage, (7) pars oblique portion of cricothyroid muscle, (8) trachea with trachealis muscle connecting the sides of the cartilage. (Dissection by Joel C. Kahane.)

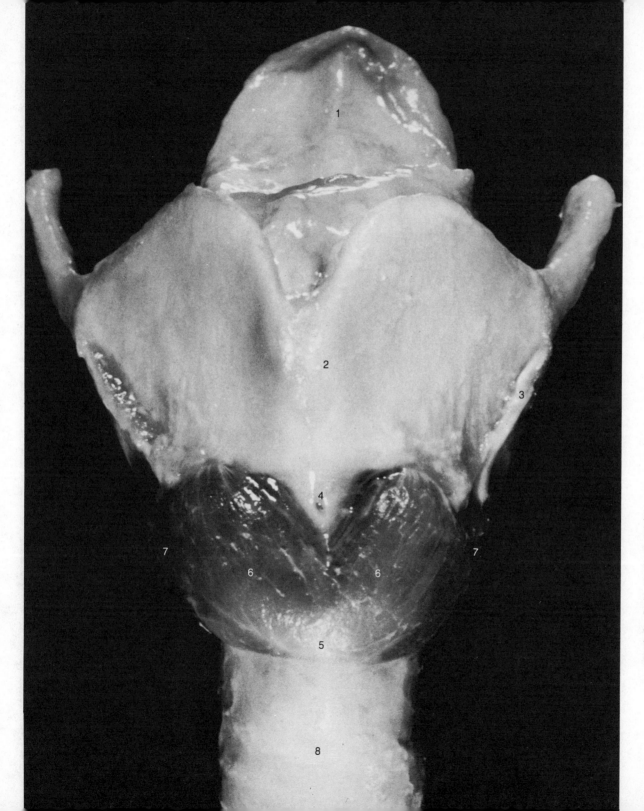

FIGURE 4–41 Anterior view of
larynx and cricothyroid muscle. (1) epiglottis, (2) thyroid
cartilage, (3) oblique line,
(4) portion of median cricothyroid ligament, (5) arch of cricoid cartilage, (6) pars recta
and (7) pars oblique of cricothyroid muscle, (8) trachea.
(Dissection by Joel C. Kahane.)

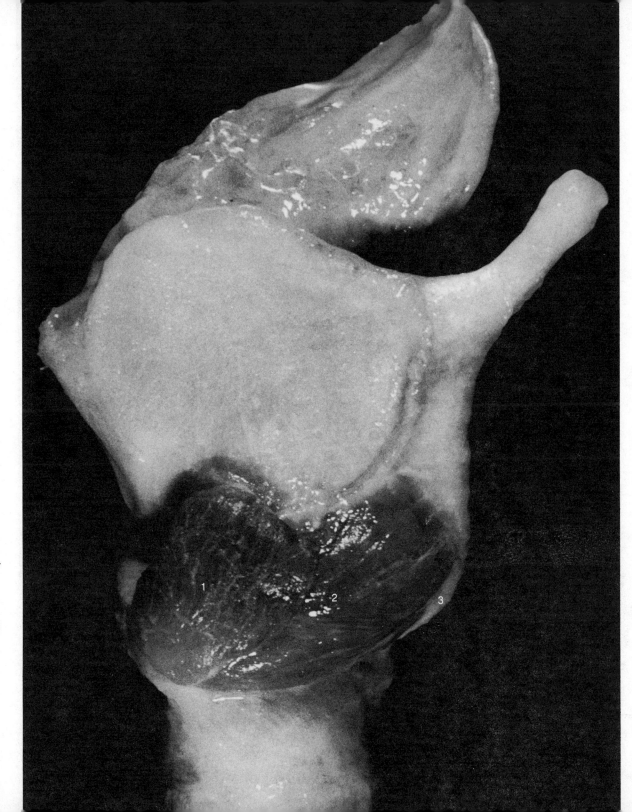

FIGURE 4–42   Lateral view of larynx and cricothyroid muscle. (1) pars recta and (2) pars oblique of cricothyroid muscle, (3) inferior horn of thyroid cartilage. (Dissection by Joel C. Kahane.)

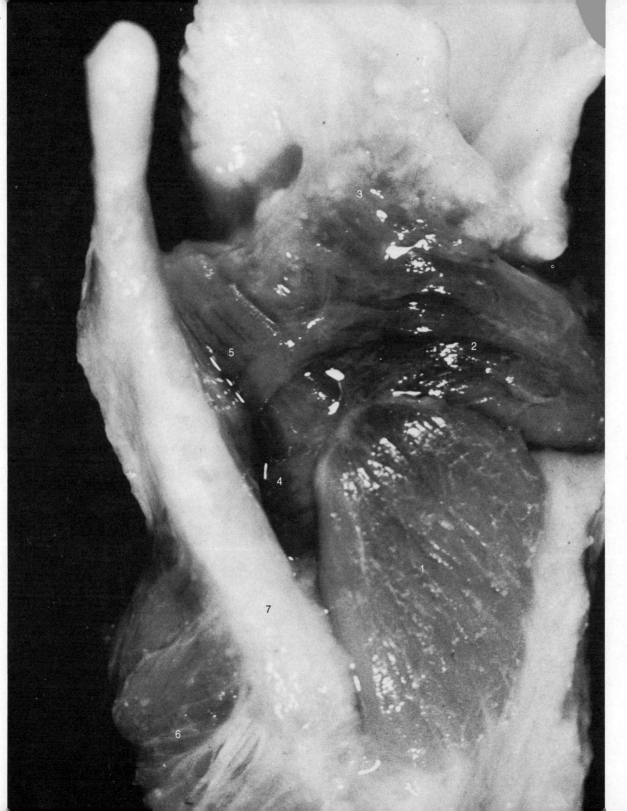

FIGURE 4–43 Oblique view of larynx and intrinsic laryngeal muscles. (1) posterior cricoarytenoid muscle, (2) interarytenoid muscle with oblique fibers prominent, (3) fibers of aryepiglottic muscle, (4) lateral cricoarytenoid muscle, (5) portion of lateral part of thyroarytenoid muscle, (6) pars oblique of cricothyroid muscle, (7) inferior horn of thyroid cartilage. (Dissection by Joel C. Kahane.)

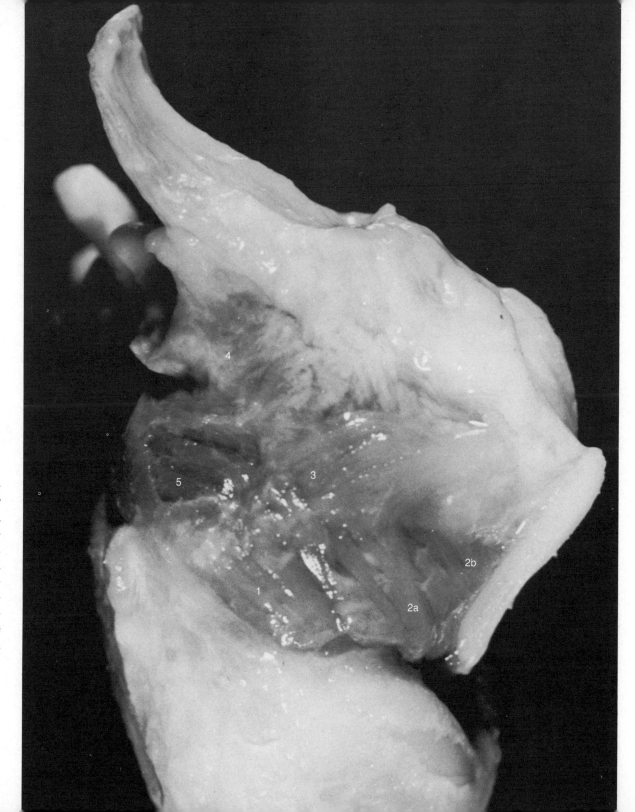

FIGURE 4–44 Intrinsic laryngeal muscles seen laterally
(thyroid cartilage removed).
(1) lateral cricoarytenoid muscle; (2) thyroarytenoid muscle,
(2a) oblique and (2b) horizontal
fibers; (3) fibers from thyro-
muscularis portion of thyroarytenoid muscle; (4) aryepiglottic muscle; (5) transverse
arytenoid muscle. (Dissection
by Joel C. Kahane.)

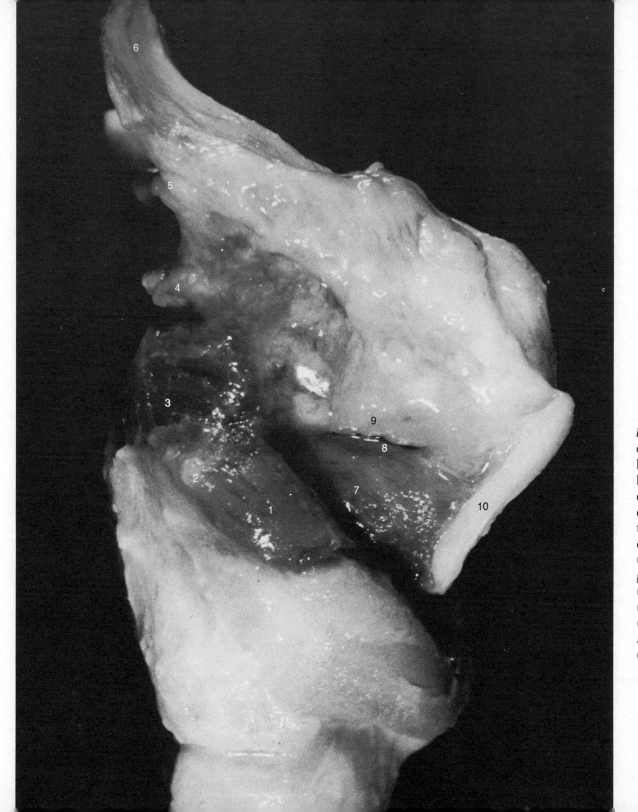

FIGURE 4–45 Lateral cricoarytenoid muscle seen in lateral view, with thyroid cartilage removed. (1) lateral cricoarytenoid muscle, (2) muscular process of arytenoid cartilage, (3) interarytenoid muscle, (4) corniculate cartilages, (5) cuneiform cartilage, (6) epiglottis, (7) conus elasticus, (8) ventricle of Morgagni, (9) vestibular (ventricular) fold, (10) thyroid cartilage sectioned at midline. (Dissection by Joel C. Kahane.)

THE LARYNX

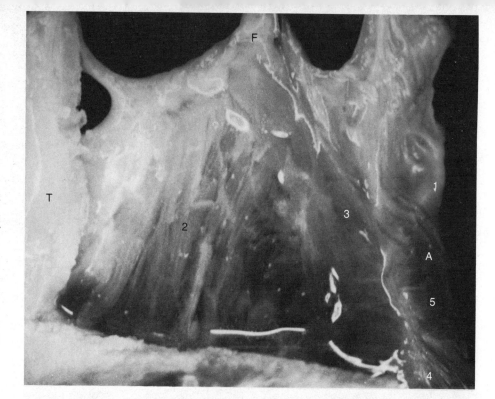

FIGURE 4–46 Lateral view of vestibule of larynx showing some muscle fibers which invest this region. Anterior (T, thyroid cartilage) is left, and posterior (A, arytenoid cartilage) is to right, covered by interarytenoid musculature. The (F) aryepiglottic fold has been stretched along the upper portion of the photograph. (1) apex of arytenoid cartilage, (2) thyroepiglottic muscle, (3) aryepiglottic muscle, (4) posterior cricoarytenoid muscle, (5) interarytenoid muscle. (Dissection by Joel C. Kahane.)

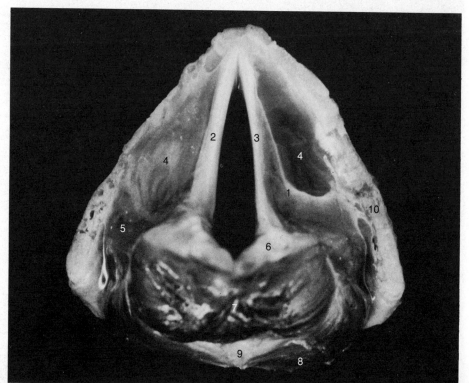

FIGURE 4–47 Superior view of larynx illustrating vocal folds and other intrinsic laryngeal muscles. (1) right vocal fold with some fascia removed to illustrate muscle fibers, (2) vocal ligament with mucosa attached (see Figure 4–48 for detailed morphology), (3) vocal ligament with mucosa removed, (4) thyroarytenoid muscle, (5) lateral cricoarytenoid muscle, (6) arytenoid cartilage, (7) transverse and oblique interarytenoid muscles, (8) posterior cricoarytenoid muscle, (9) cricoid cartilage (lamina), (10) thyroid cartilage sectioned above level of cricothyroid joint. (Dissection by Joel C. Kahane.)

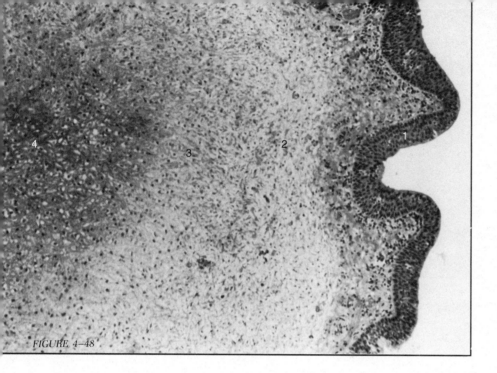

FIGURE 4–48

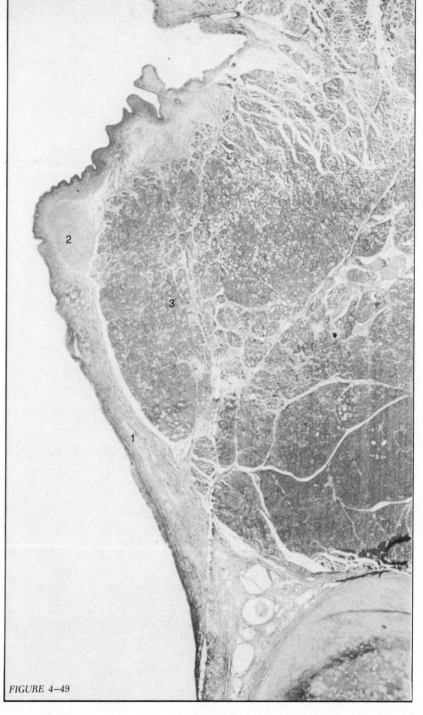

FIGURE 4–49

FIGURE 4–48 Photomicrograph of mucosa and lamina propria of vocal fold sectioned in the coronal plane. Vibrating surface is to the right. (1) stratified squamous epithelium and subepithelial connective tissue, (2) superficial (Reinke's space), (3) middle and (4) deep layers of the lamina propria. Note that connective tissue fiber denseness is progressively greater in regions more distant from the epithelial surface. (Photomicrograph by Joel C. Kahane.)

FIGURE 4–49 Photomicrograph of coronal section of adult vocal fold to illustrate relationships of dense connective tissue to thyroarytenoid muscle. (1) conus elasticus, (2) vocal ligament, (3) thyroarytenoid muscle. Compare with Figures 4–30 and 4–47. (Photomicrograph by Joel C. Kahane.)

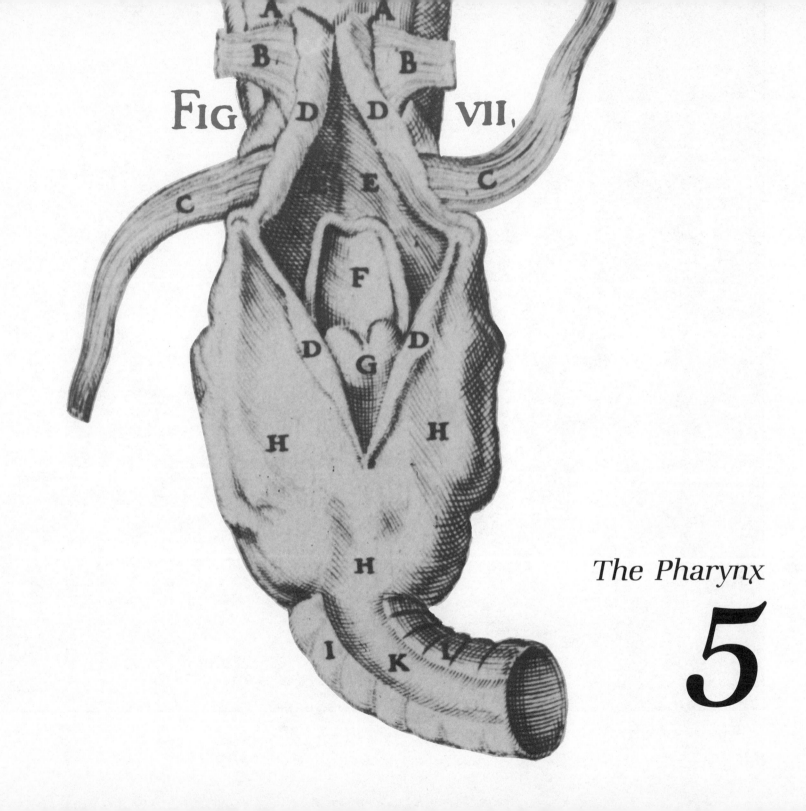

FIG VII,

The Pharynx

5

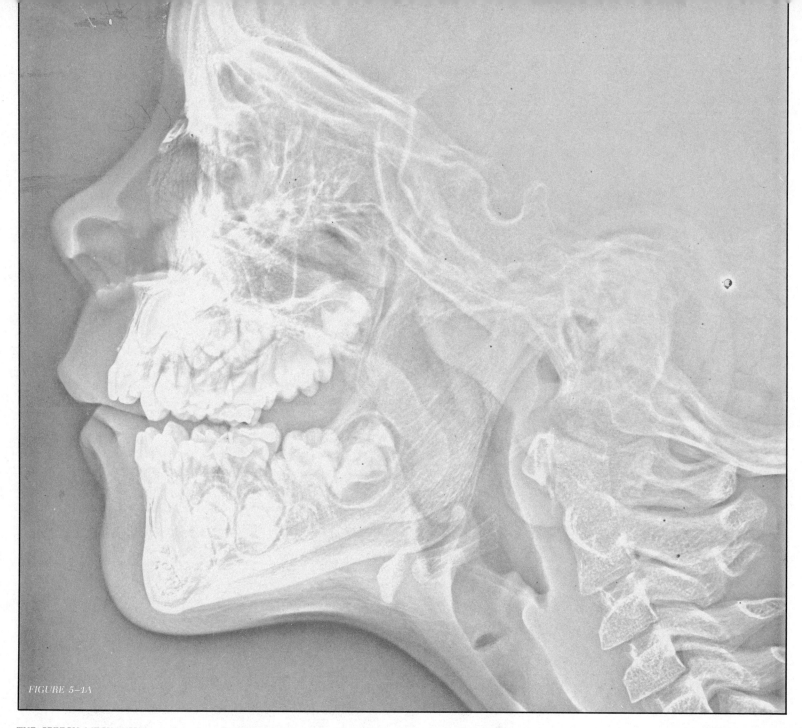

THE SPEECH MECHANISM

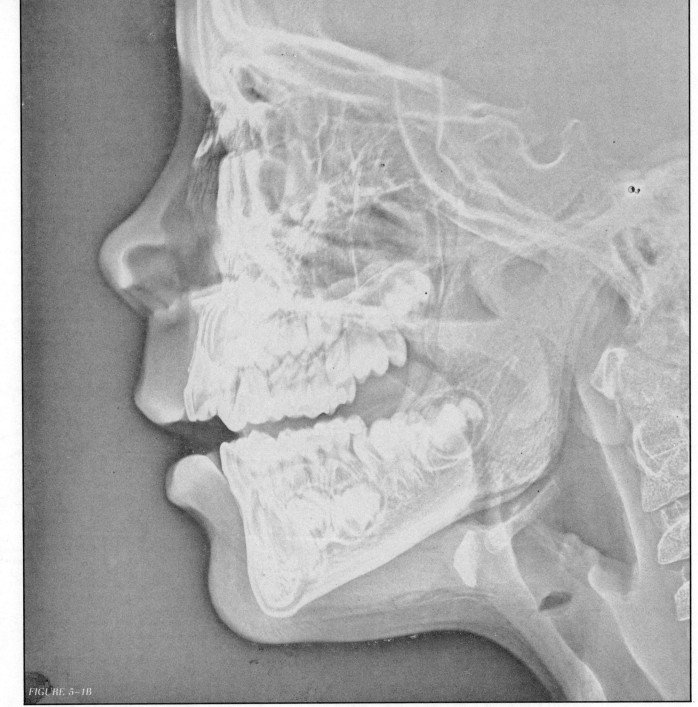

FIGURE 5–1 Lateral xeroradiograms of 8-year-old child. (A) shows the velum lowered during rest breathing. In (B) the velum is raised; the subject is producing a sustained [s]. (C) is a composite tracing of the rest and [s] xeroradiograms. For [s] the subject demonstrates only a small contact between the elevated velum and the posterior pharyngeal wall. If the posterior nasopharyngeal adenoidal tissue were removed, this subject might have difficulty making a complete velopharyngeal closure. Xeroradiography is a relatively new technique which provides greater contrasts at areas of changes in density and thereby better detail of both hard and soft tissue than conventional radiograms. (Courtesy of Diane M. Bless, Department of Communicative Disorders, University of Wisconsin, Madison.)

FIGURE 5–1B

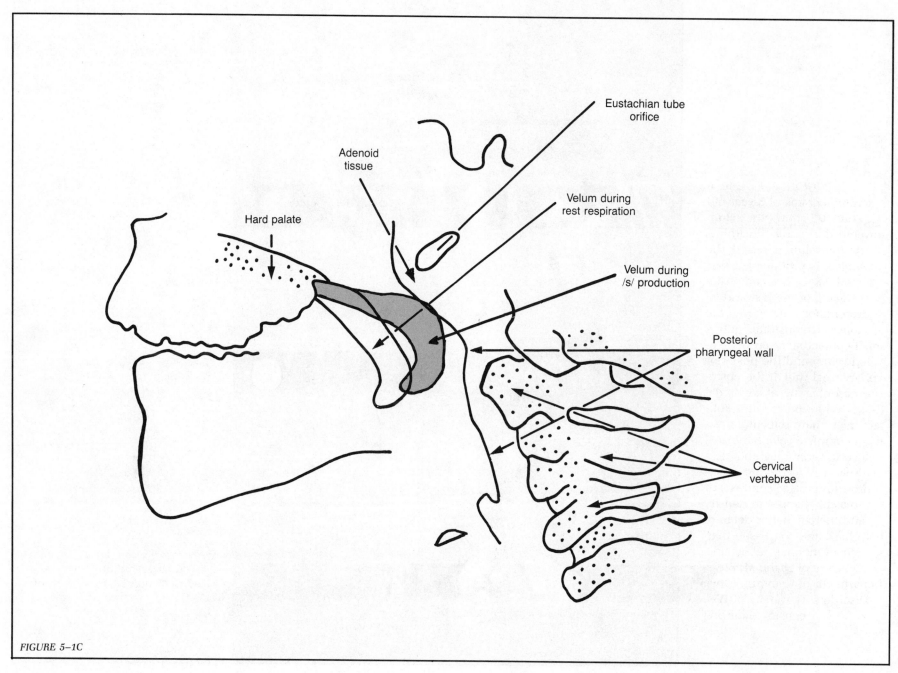

FIGURE 5-1C

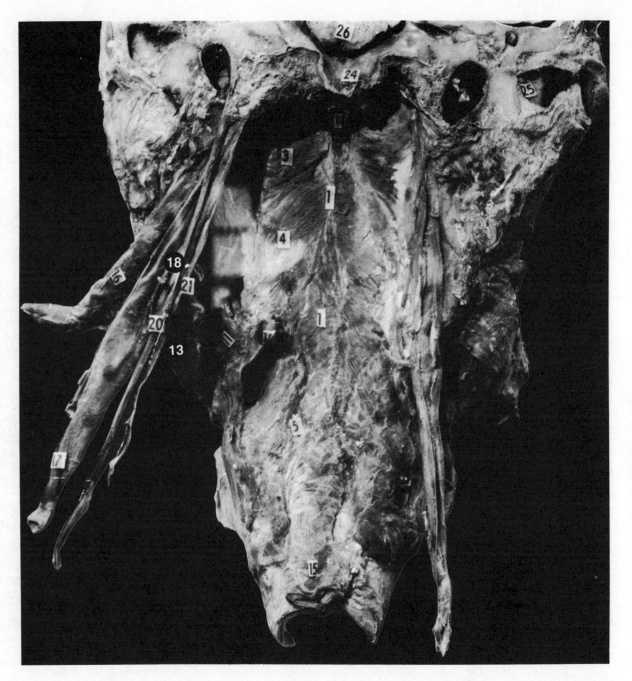

FIGURE 5–2   Dorsal view of pharynx. (1) pharyngeal raphe; (3) superior, (4) middle, and (5) inferior pharyngeal constrictor muscles; (8) spinal accessory nerve; (11) submaxillary gland; (12) greater horn of hyoid bone; (15) esophagus; (16) internal jugular vein; (17) common carotid artery; (20) vagus nerve; (21) superior laryngeal nerve; (24) dura mater; (26) pons varoli. (Courtesy of the Anatomy Museum of the Department of Anatomy and Cell Biology, University of Pittsburgh, School of Medicine, Pittsburgh.)

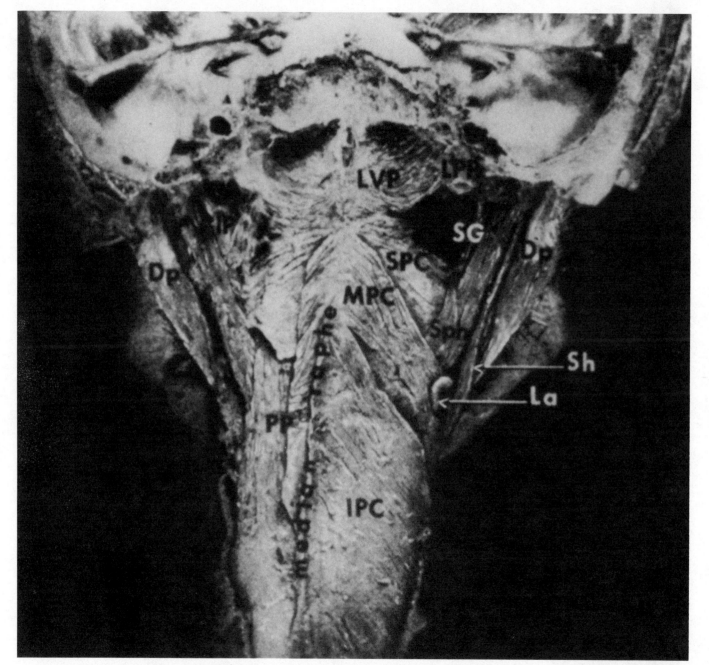

FIGURE 5–3 Dorsal view of posterior pharyngeal wall. (LVP) levator veli palatini muscle, (LPP) lateral pterygoid plate, (SPC) superior pharyngeal constrictor muscle, (MPC) middle pharyngeal constrictor muscle, (IPC) inferior pharyngeal constrictor muscle, (Sph) stylopharyngeus muscle, (Dp) posterior belly of digastric muscle, (PP) palatopharyngeus muscle, (Ip) medial pterygoid muscle, (SG) styloglossus muscle, (Sh) stylohyoid muscle, (La) lingual artery. (Courtesy of A.L. Martone and J.W. Black, "An Approach to Prosthetics Through Speech Science: Part IV, Physiology of Speech," in *Journal of Prosthetic Dentistry* 12, No. 3, 1962, p. 413.)

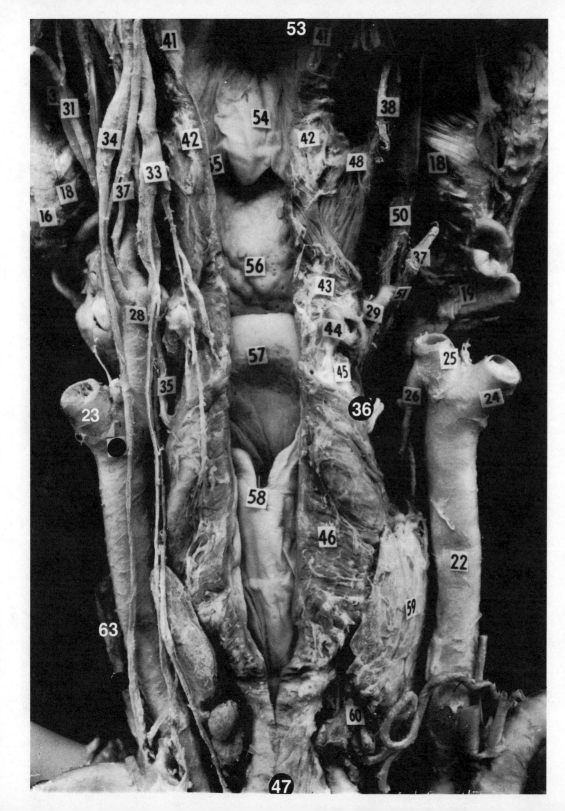

FIGURE 5–4 Posterior view of pharynx and deep neck structures. (16) angle of the mandible, (18) medial pterygoid muscle, (22) common carotid artery, (23) carotid body, (24) internal carotid artery, (25) external carotid artery, (28) left ascending pharyngeal artery, (29) right lingual artery, (31) posterior auricular artery, (33) left sympathetic trunk, (34) vagus nerve, (35) left superior laryngeal nerve, (36) internal branch of right superior laryngeal nerve, (37) hypoglossal nerve, (38) right glossopharyngeal constrictor muscle, (41) pharyngobasilar membrane, (42) superior pharyngeal constrictor muscle, (43) middle pharyngeal constrictor muscle, (44) greater horn of hyoid bone, (45) thyrohyoid membrane, (46) inferior pharyngeal constrictor muscle, (47) esophagus, (48) stylopharyngeus muscle, (50) stylohyoid muscle, (51) intermediate tendon of digastric muscle, (53) salpigopharyngeal fold, (54) soft palate, (56) dorsum of tongue, (57) epiglottis, (58) interarytenoid arch, (59) thyroid gland, (60) parathyroid glands, (63) internal jugular vein. (Courtesy of the Anatomy Museum of the Department of Anatomy and Cell Biology, University of Pittsburgh, School of Medicine, Pittsburgh.)

THE PHARYNX

99

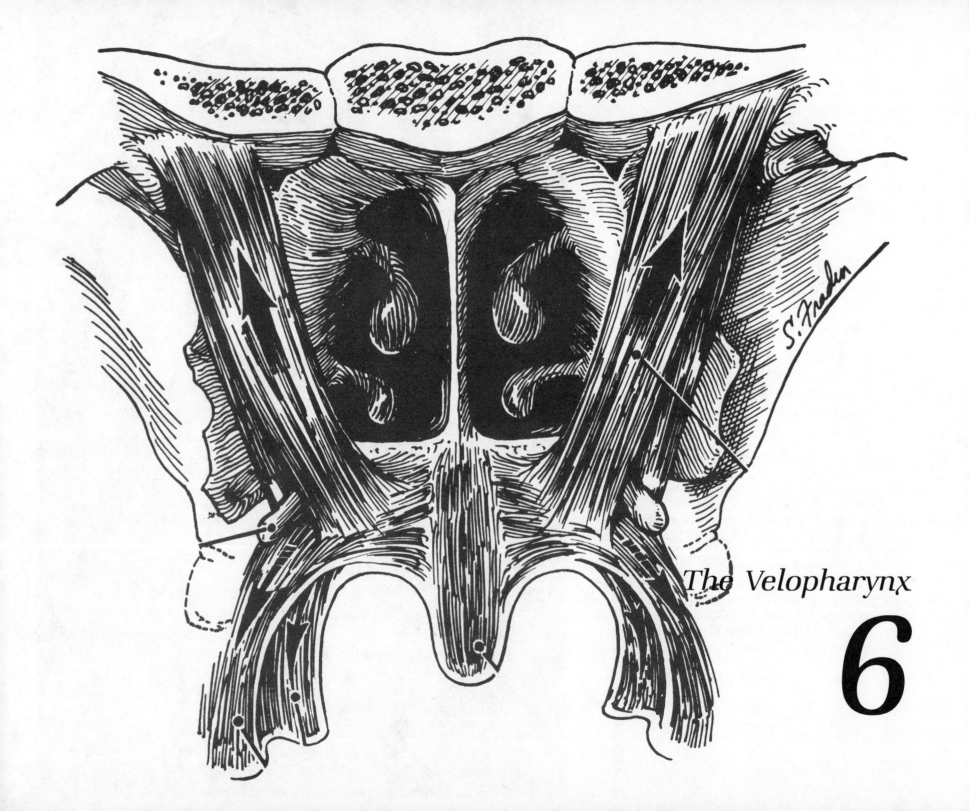

The Velopharynx

6

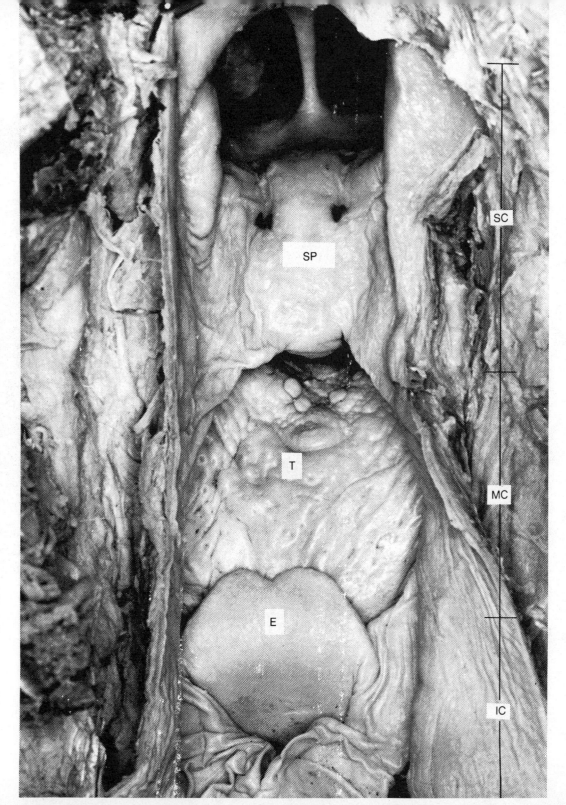

FIGURE 6–1   Posterior view of interior of pharynx illustrating position of soft palate. The pharyngeal muscles have been sectioned at midline and drawn laterally to expose underlaying structures. (SC) superior pharyngeal constrictor muscle, (MC) middle pharyngeal constrictor muscle, (IC) inferior pharyngeal constrictor muscle. The nasal surface of the (SP) soft palate, the dorsum of (T) tongue and (E) epiglottis are clearly visible. The pairs of dots on the velum mark the anterior and posterior margins of the insertion of the levator veli palatini muscle. (Courtesy of Nabil A. Azzam and David P. Kuehn, "The Morphology of Musculus Uvulae," in *Cleft Palate Journal* 14, No. 1, 1977, p. 81.)

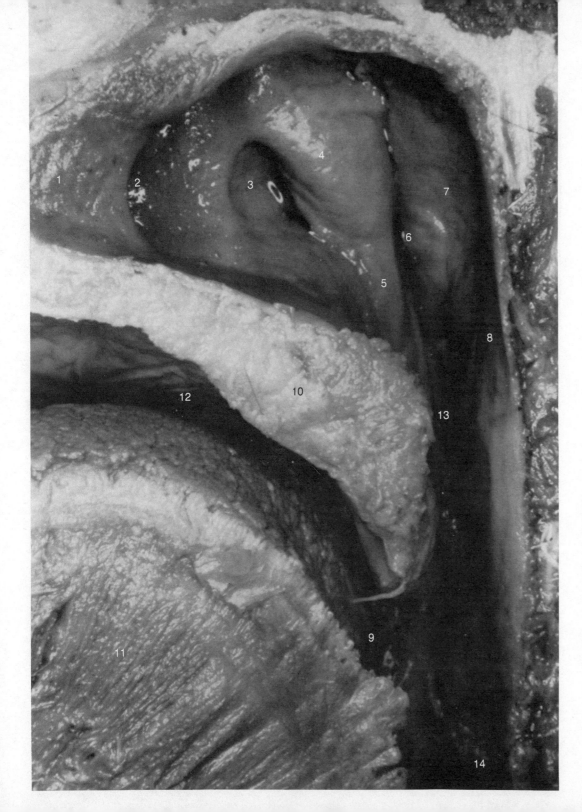

FIGURE 6–2 Close-up view of nasopharynx with mucosal surface intact. (1) nasal septum, (2) posterior choana, (3) auditory (Eustachian) tube orifice, (4) auditory tube cartilage (torus tubarius), (5) salpingopharyngeal fold, (6) pharyngeal recess (Fossa of Rosenmüller), (7) posterolateral pharyngeal wall, (8) posterior pharyngeal wall, (9) posterior faucial pillar, (10) soft palate, (11) tongue, (12) oral cavity, (13) nasopharyngeal portal, (14) oropharynx. (Dissection courtesy of Alfred S. Lavorato, Department of Speech Pathology and Audiology, School of Medicine, University of Nevada.)

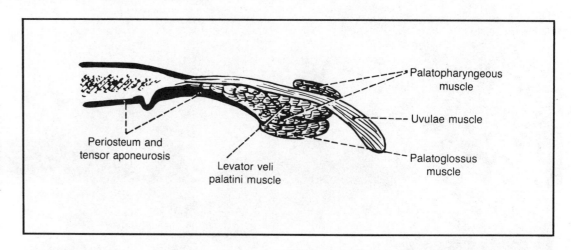

FIGURE 6–3   Schematic cross-section of soft palate illustrating relationships among velar muscles. (Courtesy of W. Henry Hollingshead, *Anatomy for Surgeons*: Vol. 1, Head and Neck, 2nd ed. New York: Harper and Row, 1968.

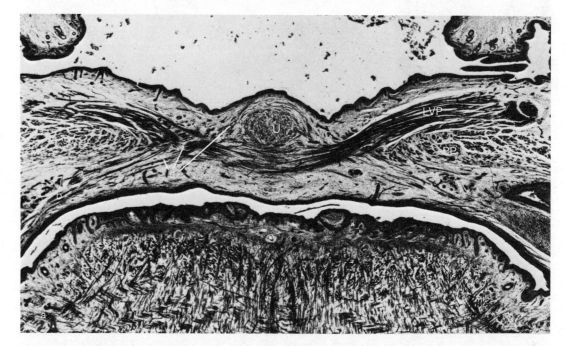

FIGURE 6–4   Coronal section through velum and upper part of tongue, illustrating course of palatoglossus muscle at level of anterior pillar. Arrows, from lower to upper, indicate: (a) fibers joining with transverse musculature of tongue, (b) muscle in anterior pillar, dividing the lateral velum into inferior and superior bundles, (c) inferior bundle terminating short of midline, (d) superior bundle running medial to (PP) palatopharyngeous muscle, penetrating (LVP) levator veli palatini muscle, and terminating in connective tissue lateral to (U) musculus uvulae. The linear streaks just left of center are artifacts caused by reproduction.

(Courtesy of H.L. Langdon, K.M. Klueber, and Y.M. Barnwell, "The Morphology of M. Palatoglossus in the 15-week Human Fetus," in *Anatomischer Anzeger* 146, No. 1, 1979, p. 12.)

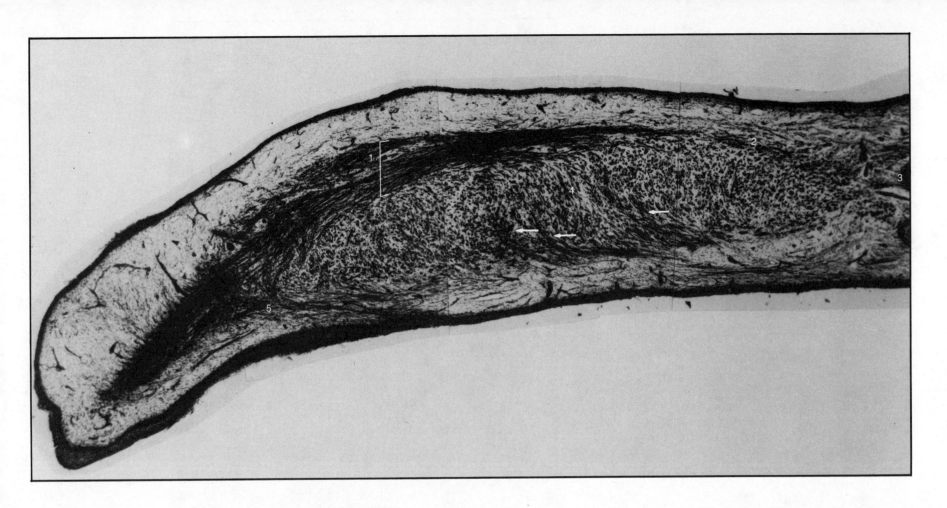

FIGURE 6–5 Sagittal section through velum illustrating course and relationships of uvula muscle. (1) musculus uvulae, (2) palatal aponeurosis, (3) posterior nasal spine, (4) musculature of soft palate, (5) velar raphe, arrows show arches of raphe coursing upward into the musculus uvulae. (Courtesy of H.L. Langdon and K.M. Klueber, "The Longitudinal Fibromuscular Component of the Soft Palate in the 15-week Human Fetus: Musculus Uvulae and Palatine Raphe," in *Cleft Palate Journal* 15, No. 4, 1978, p. 339.)

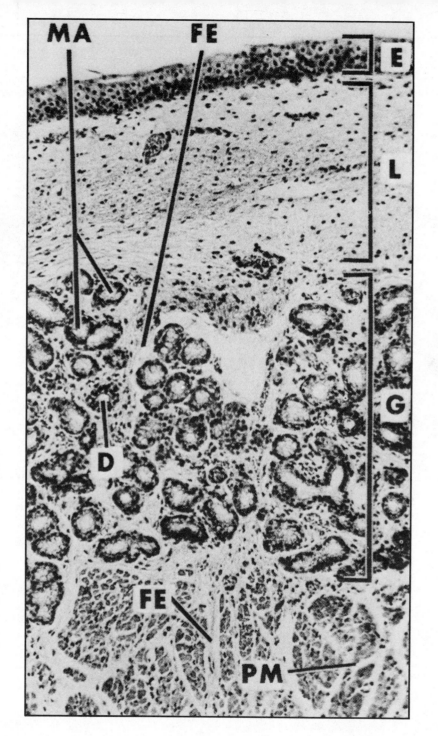

FIGURE 6–6   Coronal section through soft palate
showing layers of tissue which comprise it.
(MA) mucous acini, (FE) fibrous elements, (D) duct of a
mucous gland, (E) epithelium, (L) lamina propria,
(G) glandular submucosa, (PM) palatal muscle fibers.
(Courtesy of D. Vincent Provenza, *Oral Histology*. New
York: Harper & Row, 1964.)

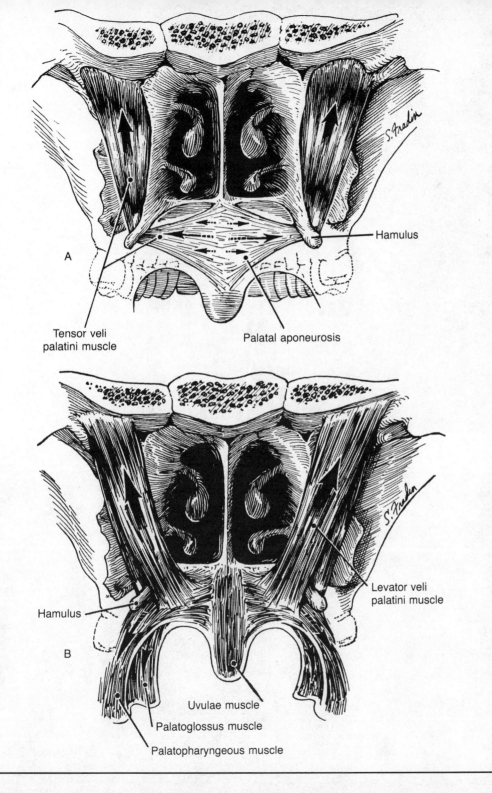

A

Tensor veli
palatini muscle

Hamulus

Palatal aponeurosis

B

Hamulus

Levator veli
palatini muscle

Uvulae muscle

Palatoglossus muscle

Palatopharyngeous muscle

FIGURE 6–7   Line drawings illustrating muscles of soft palate, viewed from behind (pharyngeally). (A) illustrates the tensor veli palatini muscle wrapping around the hamulus and inserting into the palatal aponeurosis. The arrows indicate that when the tensor veli palatini is active, the contracting muscle fibers stretch the palatal aponeurosis. (B) demonstrates levator veli palatini muscle, Musculus uvulae, palatoglossus muscle, and palatopharyngeus muscle. (Courtesy of Raymond J. Nagle and Victor H. Sears, *Dental Prosthetics*. St. Louis: The C.V. Mosby Co., 1958. As reprinted in S. Silverman, *Oral Physiology*. St. Louis: The C.V. Mosby Co., 1961.)

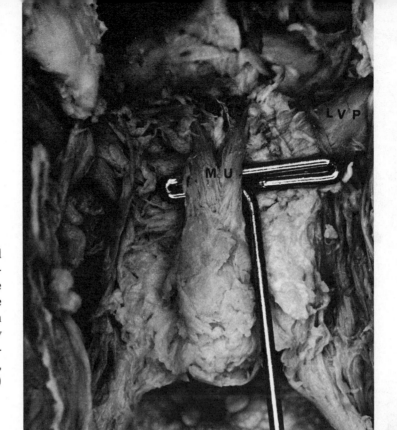

FIGURE 6–8 Nasal surface of soft palate after removal of mucosa from the same specimen as shown in Figure 6–1. The (LVP) levator veli palatini muscle and the paired bundles of the (MU) Musculus uvulae are clearly visible. Note that the blunt probe lies within the fascial plane separating (MU) from (LVP). (Courtesy of Nabil A. Azzam and David P. Keuhn, "The Morphology of Musculus Uvulae," in *Cleft Palate Journal* 14, No. 1, 1977, p. 82.)

FIGURE 6–9 Parasagittal section of older adult human showing undissected (AP) anterior faucial pillar and (PP) posterior faucial pillar, (HP) hard palate, and (T) tongue. Note that the subject was edentulous and the distortion of the lips. The soft palate is in a relatively elevated position. (Courtesy of David P. Keuhn and Nabil A. Azzam, "Anatomical Characteristics of Palatoglossus and the Anterior Faucial Pillar," in *Cleft Palate Journal* 15, No. 4, 1978, p. 351.)

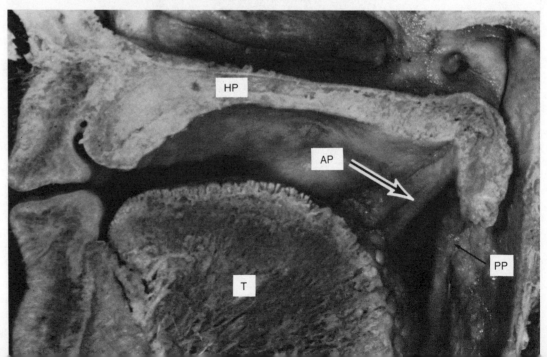

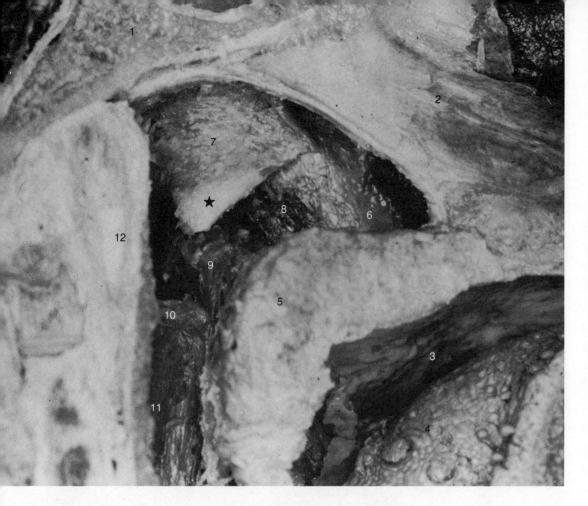

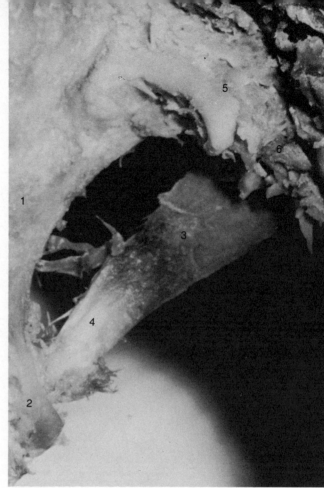

FIGURE 6–10 Dissection of velar and pharyngeal muscles in nasopharynx. (1) body of sphenoid bone, (2) posterior portion of boney nasal septum, (3) oral cavity, (4) dorsum of tongue, (5) soft palate, (6) medial pterygoid plate, (7) auditory tube cartilage (torus tubarius; note its (*) inferior tip), (8) tensor veli palatini muscle, (9) levator veli palatini muscle, (10) superior fibers of superior pharyngeal constrictor muscle which insert into velum, (11) superior pharyngeal constrictor muscle on posterior pharyngeal wall, (12) vertebral column. (Dissection courtesy of Alfred S. Lavorato, Department of Speech Pathology and Audiology, School of Medicine, University of Nevada.)

FIGURE 6–11 Anatomy of tensor veli palatini muscle viewed medially. (1) medial pterygoid plate of sphenoid bone, (2) hamular process, (3) tensor veli palatini muscle and its (4) tendon, which wraps around hamulus and spreads out to form palatal aponeurosis, (5) cartilage of auditory tube, (6) remnants of levator veli palatini muscle. Courtesy of S.R. Rood and W.J. Doyle, Department of Otolaryngology, University of Pittsburgh, School of Medicine.)

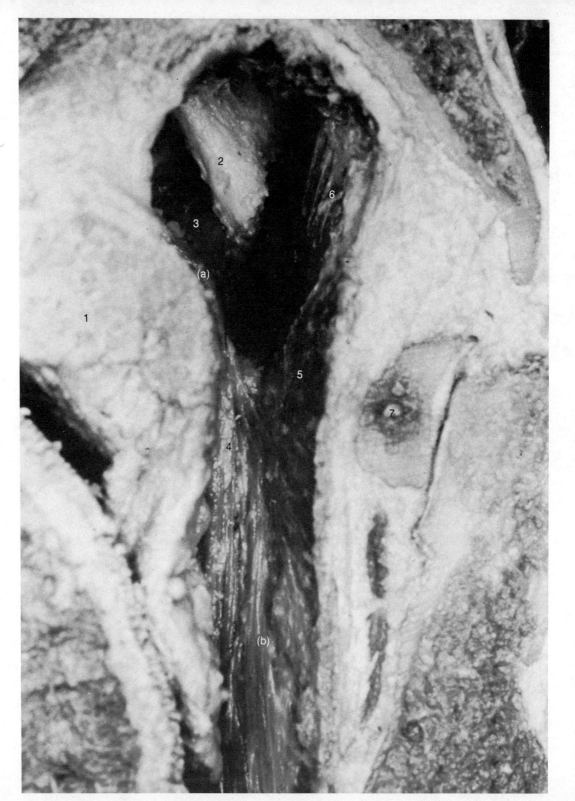

FIGURE 6–12 Dissection showing relationships between velar and pharyngeal wall musculature. (1) soft palate, (2) auditory tube cartilage (torus tubaris), (3) levator veli palatini muscle, (4) palatopharyngeus muscle. Note the anterior extension of fibers (a) and the intermingling of fibers (b) with those of the (5) superior pharyngeal constrictor muscle. (6) longus capitus muscle, (7) portion of atlas (1st cervical vertebra). (Dissection courtesy of Alfred S. Lavorato, Department of Speech Pathology and Audiology, School of Medicine, University of Nevada.)

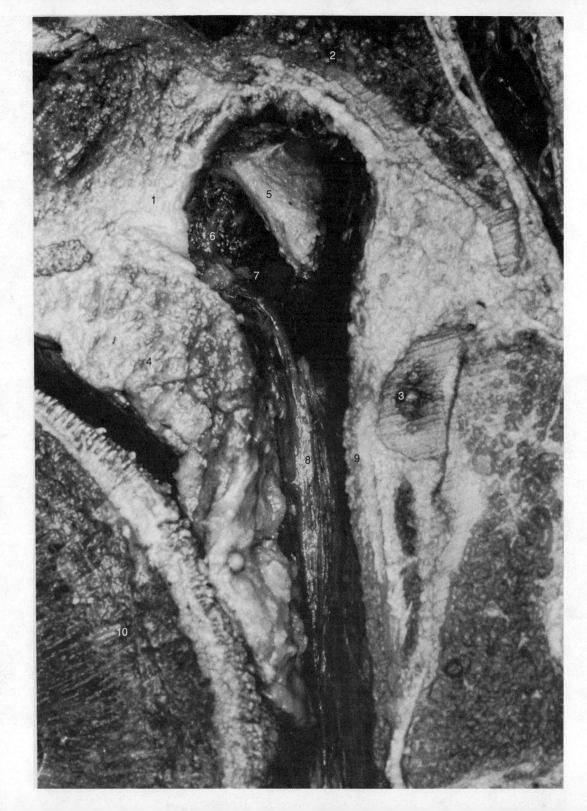

FIGURE 6–13 Dissection of nasopharynx (right side). (1) nasal septum covered with mucosa, (2) body of sphenoid bone, (3) anterior arch of atlas, (4) soft palate, (5) auditory tube cartilage (torus tubarius), (6) tensor veli palatini muscle, (7) levator veli palatini muscle, (8) palatopharyngeus muscle (note slip of muscle coursing over (7) and coursing into the anterior region of the velum), (9) posterior pharyngeal wall, (10) dorsum of tongue. (Dissection courtesy of Alfred S. Lavorato, Department of Speech Pathology and Audiology, School of Medicine, University of Nevada.

THE VELOPHARYNX

111

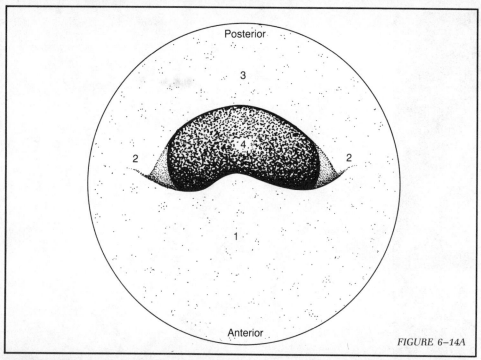

FIGURE 6–14A

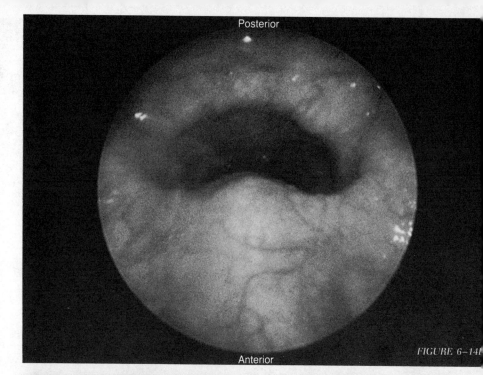

FIGURE 6–14B

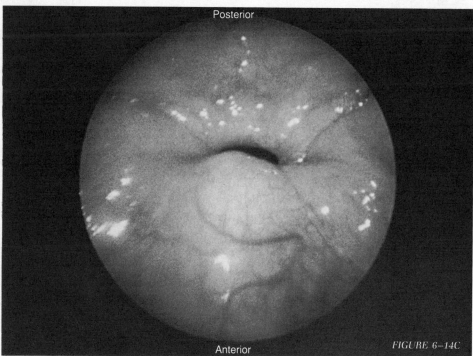

FIGURE 6–14C

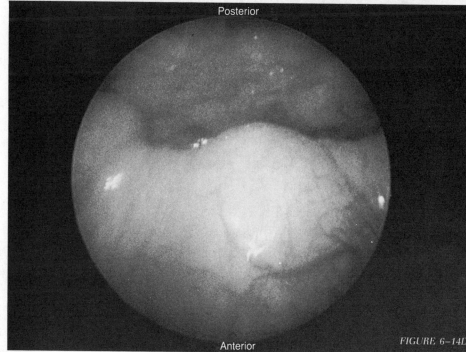

FIGURE 6–14D

THE SPEECH MECHANISM

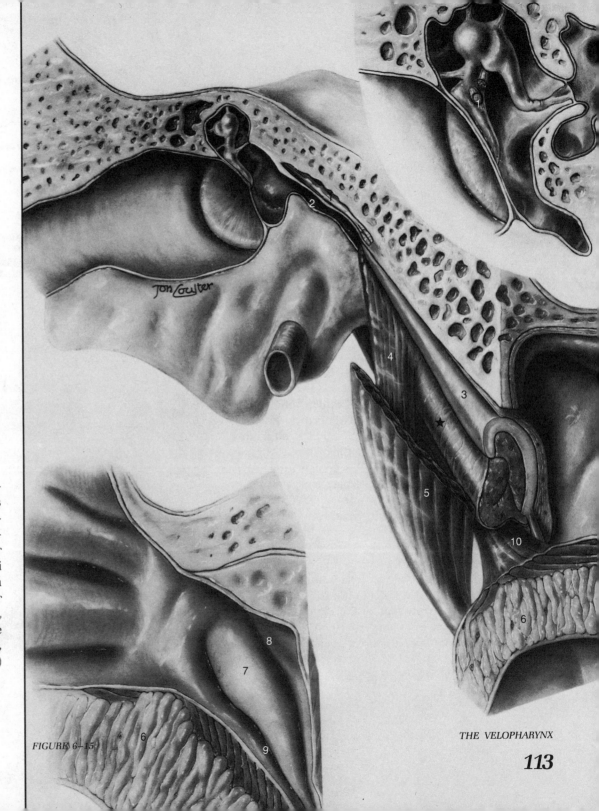

FIGURE 6–14   Nasoendoscopic view of velopharyngeal region. The endoscope was passed through the left nasal cavity and positioned in the nasopharynx superior and anterior to the nasopharyngeal port. (A) is a line drawing illustrating the anatomical features illustrated in the endoscopic photographs. (1) velum, (2) lateral pharyngeal walls, (3) posterior pharyngeal wall, (4) nasopharyngeal port. (B) nasopharyngeal port at rest, (C) partial closure during production of sustained vowel |ʌ|, (D) complete closure during sustained production of |s|. (Photo by K. Clark, R. Linville, and R. Barreras, Department of Otolaryngology and Maxillofacial Surgery, University of Iowa.)

FIGURE 6–15   Schematic of Eustachian tube illustrating cranial base relations and disposition of various muscles. (1) tensor tympani muscle, (2) osseous auditory tube, (3) cartilaginous auditory tube, (*) membranous wall, (4) dilator tubae (medial) portion of tensor veli palatini muscle, (5) tensor (lateral portion) veli palatini muscle, (6) velum, (7) torus tubarius, (8) fossa of Rosenmüller, (9) nasopharyngeal orifice, (10) levator veli palatini muscle. (After W.J. Doyle and S.R. Rood, "Comparison of the Anatomy of the Eustachian Tube in the Rhesus Monkey and Man," *Annals of Otology, Rhinology, and Laryngology* 89, No. 1, 1980, p. 54.)

FIGURE 6–15

FIGURE 6–16   Histologic sections from four regions of
adult human auditory (Eustachian) tube. Insert indicates levels of histological sections represented in the
accompaning photomicrographs. (A) is a cross-sec-
tional view of the human (ET) Eustachian tube, showing the boney part next to the (ART) carotid artery; a
remnant of tubal (CAR) cartilage is still seen in this
area. (B) lies near the tubal isthmus at the (CAR) cartilaginous portion of the (ET) Eustachian tube, (ART)
carotid artery. In (C), the (CAR) cartilaginous portion of
the (ET) Eustachian tube shows tubal (CAR) cartilage,
(AC) accessory cartilage, and tubal (GL) glands; also
shown are (TP) tensor veli palatini muscle, (LP) levator
veli palatini muscle. (D) shows the pharyngeal end of
(ET) Eustachian tube and a thickening of tubal
(CAR) cartilage, as well as (R) Rosenmüller's fossa.
(Magnification × 6; H. & E. stain.) (Courtesy of David J.
Lim, "Functional Morphology of the Lining Membrane
of the Middle Ear and Eustachian Tube," in *Annals of
Otology, Rhinology, and Laryngology* 83, No. 11,
1974, p. 3.)

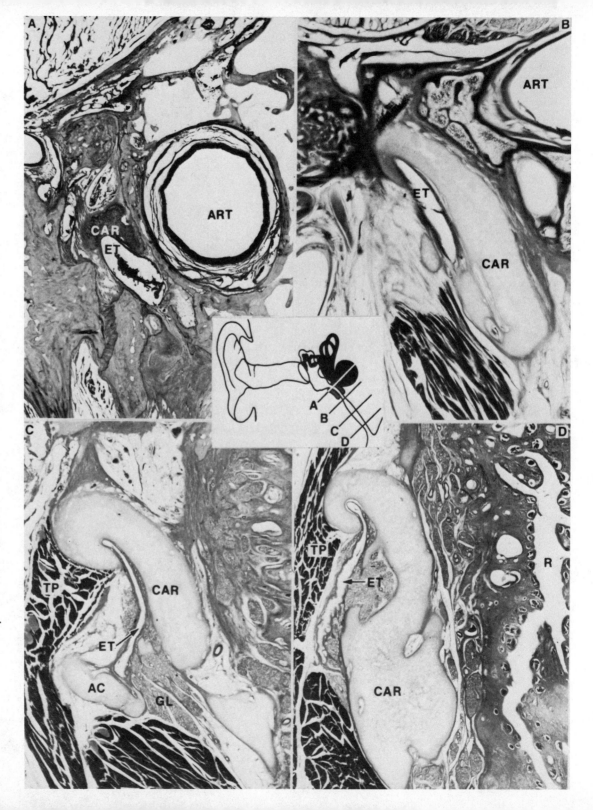

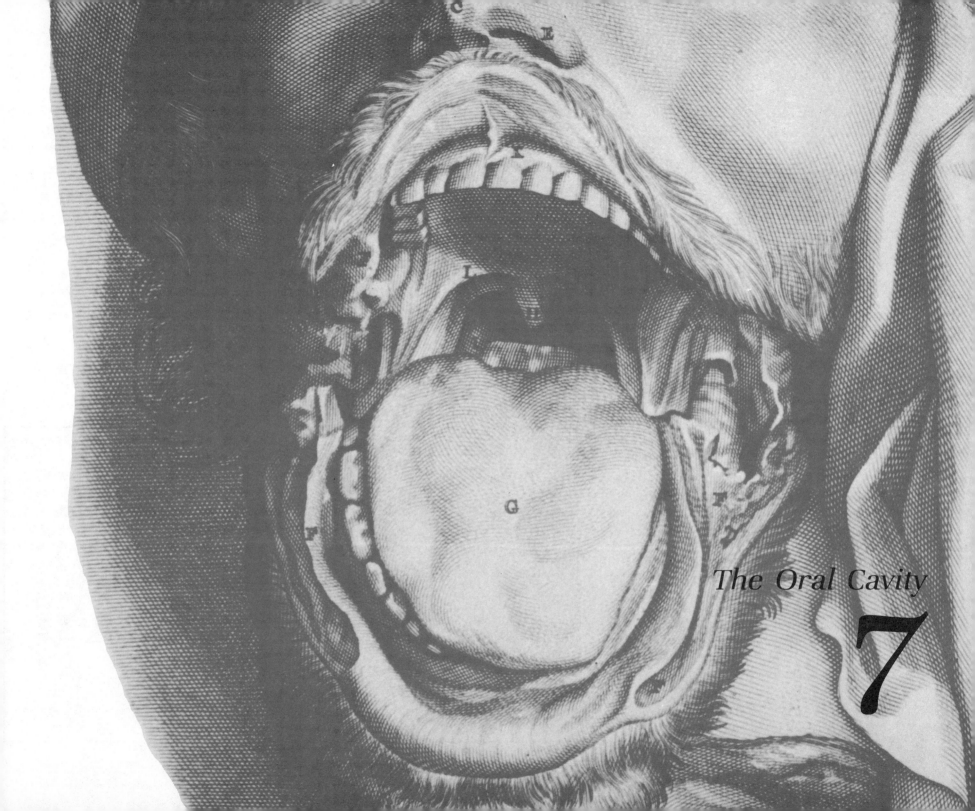

The Oral Cavity

7

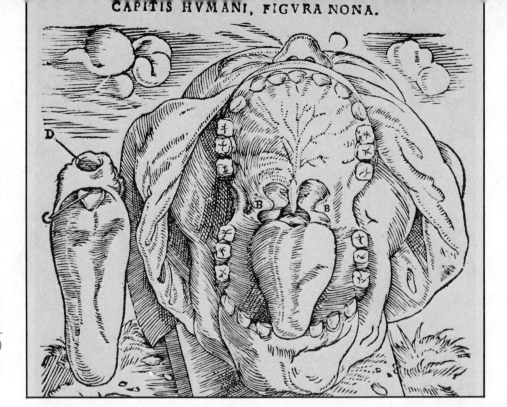

CAPITIS HVMANI, FIGVRA NONA.

FIGURE 7–1   (From Johannes Dryander, *Anatominae*. Marburg: Apud Eucharium Ceruicornum, 1537.)

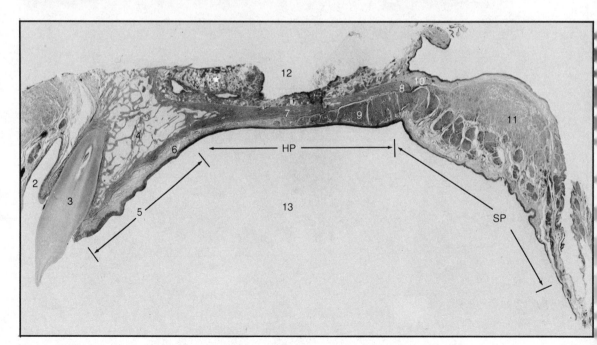

FIGURE 7–2   Photomicrograph of near-midline sagittal section through maxilla and soft palate of 35-year-old male. (1) upper lip, (2) labial vestibule, (3) central incisor tooth, (4) alveolar portion of maxilla, (5) alveolar process with rugae, (6) fatty zone, (7) palatal process of maxilla, (8) posterior nasal spine, (9) glandular zone with mucous secreting cells, (10) palatal aponeurosis, (11) velar muscles, predominately levator veli palatini muscles, (12) nasal cavity with (*) mucosa, (13) oral cavity. (HP) hard palate, (SP) soft palate. (Courtesy of Christopher A. Squier, College of Dentistry, University of Iowa, Iowa City.)

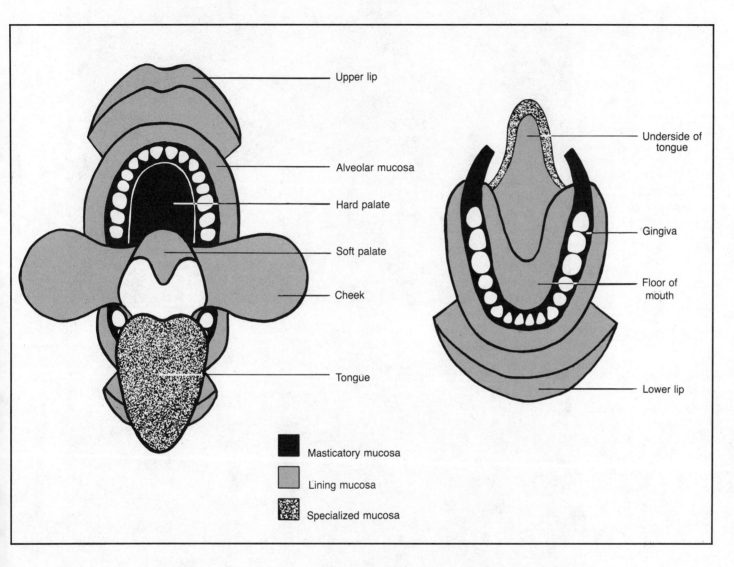

Upper lip

Alveolar mucosa

Hard palate

Soft palate

Cheek

Tongue

Underside of tongue

Gingiva

Floor of mouth

Lower lip

Masticatory mucosa

Lining mucosa

Specialized mucosa

FIGURE 7–3 Diagram to show three main fuctional subdivisions of oral mucosa. (Modified from C.A. Squier, N.W. Johnson, and R.M. Hoops, *Human Oral Mucosa: Development, Structure, and Function.* Oxford: Blackwell Scientific Publications, Ltd., 1976. Original version in B. Roed-Petersen and G. Renstrup, "The Topographical Classification of the Oral Mucosa Suitable for Electronic Data Processing: Its Application to 560 Leudoplakias," in *Acta Odontologica Scandinavia* 27, No. 6, December 1969, p. 683.)

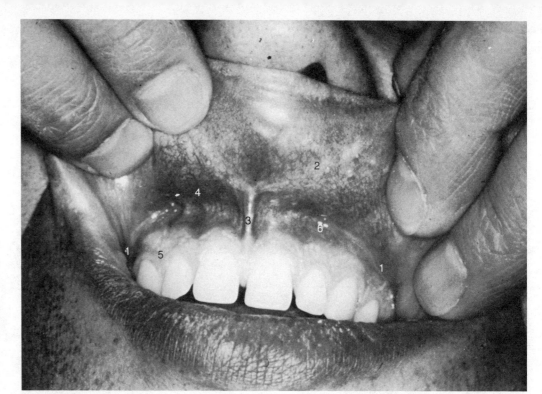

FIGURE 7–4 Upper lip elevated and retracted to expose underlying vestibule and gingiva of maxilla. (1) vestibule, (2) mucosa of upper lip, (3) labial frenulum, (4) mucolabial (vestibular) fold, (5) attached (or true) gingiva, (6) alveolar mucosa. (Courtesy of Robert B. Purdy, Department of Oral Diagnosis, University of Tennessee Center for the Health Sciences, Memphis.)

FIGURE 7–5 Lower lip depressed to illustrate vestibule and gingiva of mandible. (1) lower lip mucosa with labial gland openings, (2) labial frenulum, (3) alveolar mucosa with mucolabial (vestibular) folds, (4) vestibule of mandible, (5) attached (true) gingiva. (Courtesy of Robert B. Purdy, Department of Oral Diagnosis, University of Tennessee Center for the Health Sciences, Memphis.)

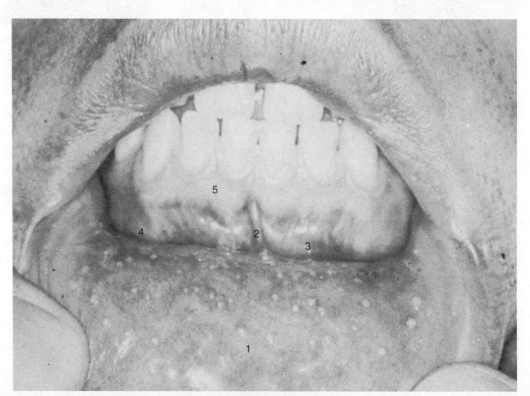

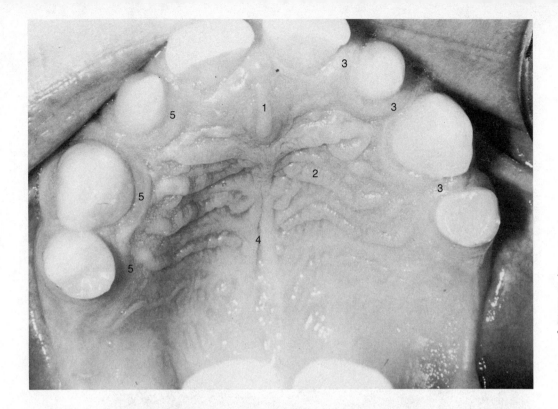

FIGURE 7–6   Hard palate of child. (1) incisive papilla, (2) rugae, (3) alveolar process, (4) palatine raphe, (5) palatal (lingual) gingiva. (Courtesy of Robert B. Purdy, Department of Oral Diagnosis, University of Tennessee Center for the Health Sciences, Memphis.)

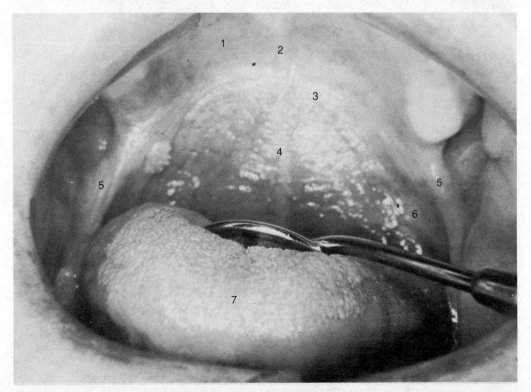

FIGURE 7–7   Juncture of hard and soft palates and their relationships to faucial pillars. (1) hard palate, (2) median palatal raphe, (3) posterior border of hard palate, (4) soft palate, (5) anterior and (6) posterior faucial pillars (note benign lesion on subject's right side), (7) tongue (dorsum). (Courtesy of Robert B. Purdy, Department of Oral Diagnosis, University of Tennessee Center for the Health Sciences, Memphis.)

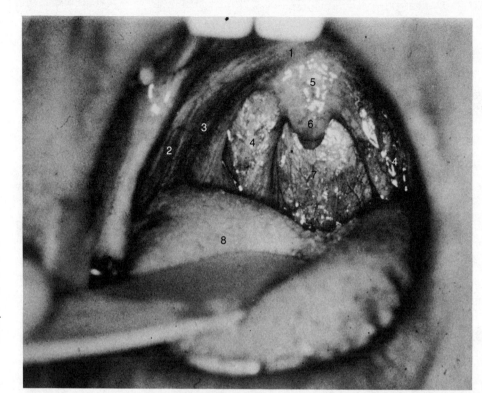

FIGURE 7–8 Peroral view of oral cavity. (1) hard palate, (2) buccal (cheek) mucosa, (3) anterior (palatoglossal) faucial pillar, (4) posterior (palatopharyngeal) faucial pillar, (5) soft palate, (6) uvula, (7) posterior pharyngeal wall, (8) tongue. (Courtesy of Robert B. Purdy, Department of Oral Diagnosis, University of Tennessee Center for the Health Sciences, Memphis.)

FIGURE 7–9 Close-up of posterior region of oral cavity. (1) anterior (palatoglossal) faucial pillar, (2) posterior (palatopharyngeal) faucial pillar, (3) tonsilar fossa, (4) uvula, (5) soft palate, (6) posterior pharyngeal wall. (Courtesy of Robert B. Purdy, Department of Oral Diagnosis, University of Tennessee Center for the Health Sciences, Memphis.)

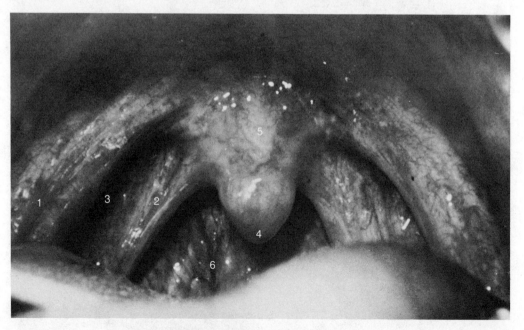

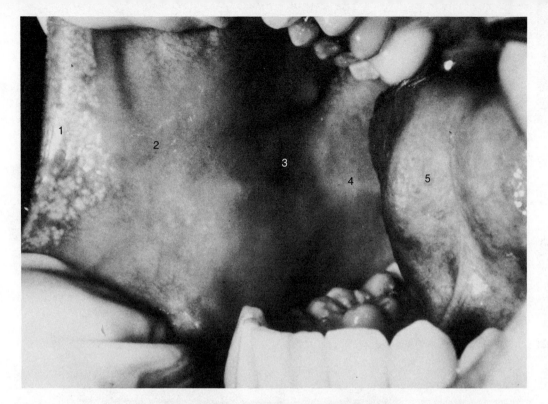

FIGURE 7–10 Right lateral (buccal) wall of oral cavity. (1) glands in labial mucosa, (2) buccal mucosa, (3) region of pterygomandibular raphe, (4) region of lateral wall formed by fibers of superior pharyngeal constrictor muscle, (5) elevated tongue showing lingual frenulum. (Courtesy of Robert B. Purdy, Department of Oral Diagnosis, University of Tennessee Center for the Health Sciences, Memphis.)

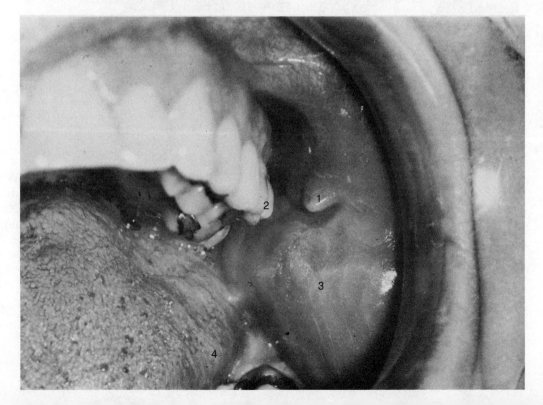

FIGURE 7–11 Buccal mucosa (left side). (1) papilla and orifice of parotid (Stensen's) duct, (2) second molar, (3) buccal mucosa, (4) lateral margin of tongue. (Courtesy of Robert B. Purdy, Department of Oral Diagnosis, University of Tennessee Center for the Health Sciences, Memphis.)

THE ORAL CAVITY

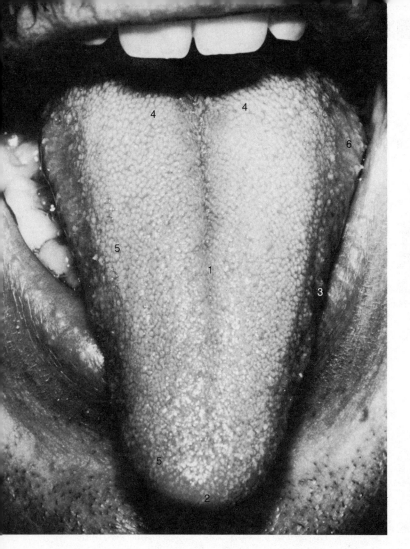

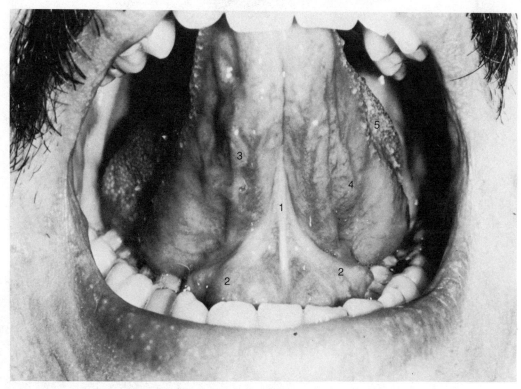

FIGURE 7–12 Anatomical characteristics of dorsum of body of tongue. Note that the dorsum contains numerous projections or papillae. (1) median sulcus, (2) apex, (3) lateral margin, (4) filiform papillae, (5) fungiform papillae, (6) foliate papillae. (Photo by Joel C. Kahane.)

FIGURE 7–13 Undersurface of tongue shown with apex of tongue elevated to alveolar ridge. (1) lingual frenulum, (2) sublingual folds, (3) fimbriated folds, (4) lingual mucosa, (5) lingual mucosa with tastebuds on lateral surface of tongue dorsum. (Photo by Joel C. Kahane.)

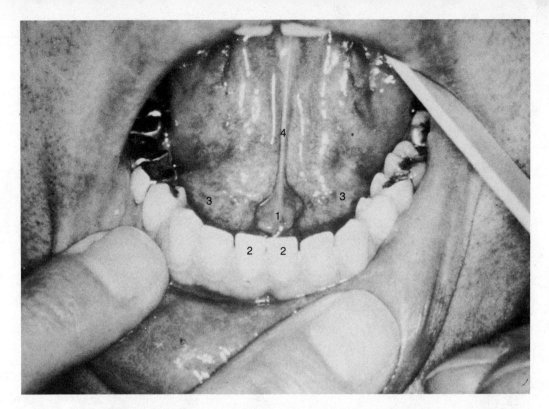

FIGURE 7–14 Floor of mouth. (1) sublingual papilla (coruncle) containing openings of submandibular ducts, (2) central incisors, (3) sublingual folds, (4) lingual frenulum. (Courtesy of Robert B. Purdy, Department of Oral Diagnosis, University of Tennessee Center for the Health Sciences, Memphis.)

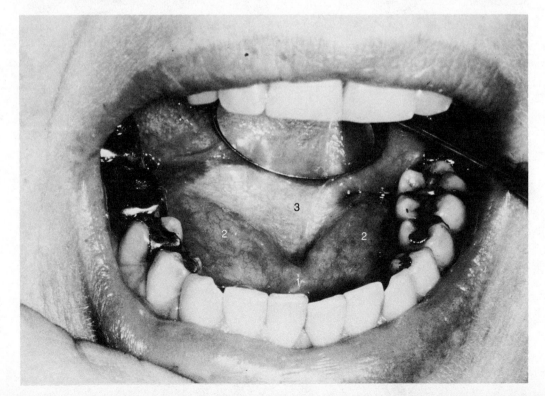

FIGURE 7–15 Floor of mouth with tongue retracted. (1) sublingual papilla, (2) sublingual folds, (3) sublingual mucosa. (Courtesy of Robert B. Purdy, Department of Oral Diagnosis, University of Tennessee Center for the Health Sciences, Memphis.)

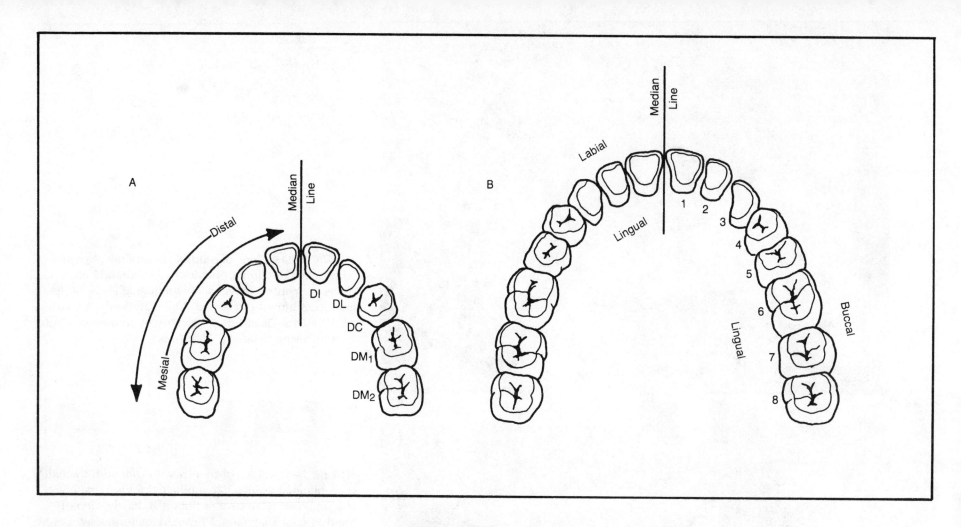

FIGURE 7–16 (A) arrangement of deciduous teeth in dental arch. (DI) deciduous central incisor, (DL) deciduous lateral incisor, (DC) deciduous cuspid, (DM₁) 1st deciduous molar, (DM₂) 2nd deciduous molar. (B) identification of permanent teeth and their relationship within dental arch. (1) central incisor, (2) lateral incisor, (3) cuspid (canine), (4) 1st bicuspid (premolar), (5) 2nd bicuspid (premolar), (6) 1st molar, (7) 2nd molar, (8) 3rd molar (wisdom tooth). (Courtesy of Richard H. Barrett and Marvin L. Hanson, *Oral Myofunctional Disorders*, 2nd Ed. St. Louis: The C.V. Mosby Co., 1978.)

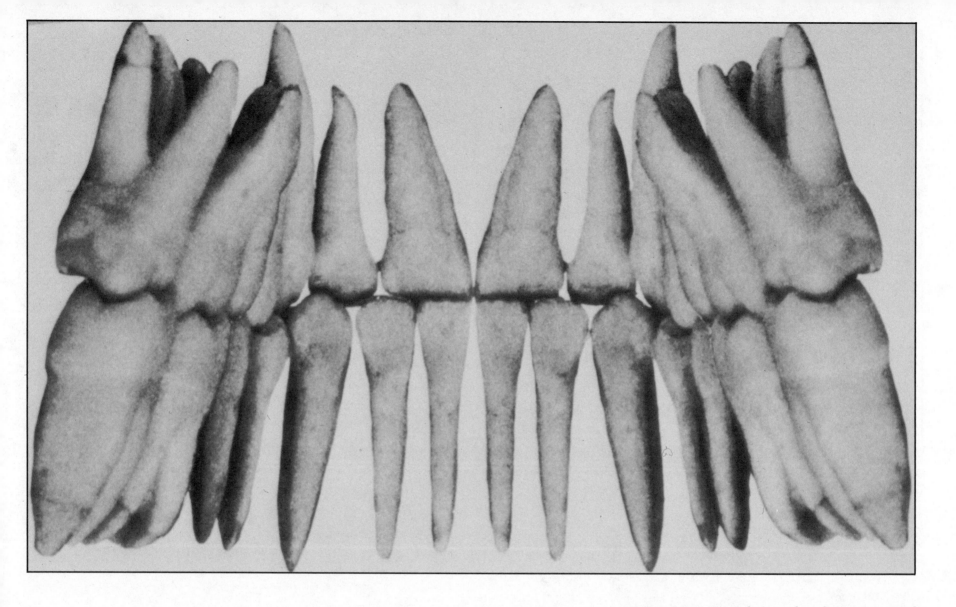

FIGURE 7–17 Lingual view of teeth in intercuspal position. (Courtesy of Bertram Kraus, Ronald Jordan, and Leonard Abrams, *Dental Anatomy and Occlusion*. Baltimore: The Williams and Wilkins Co., 1969.)

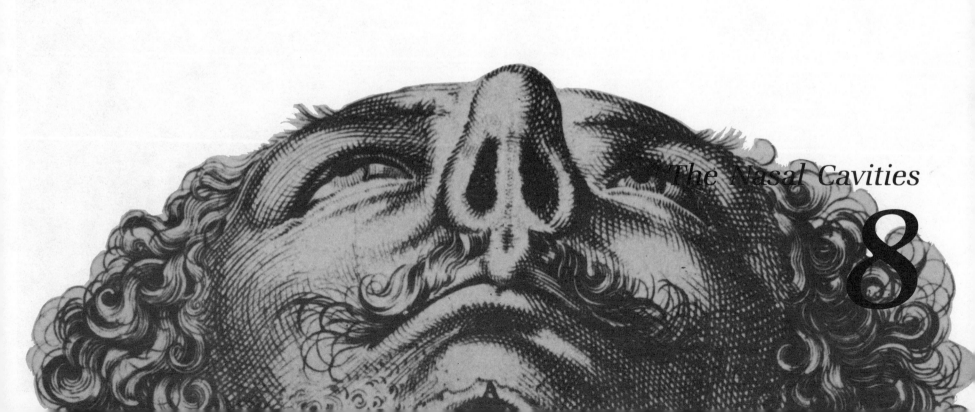

The Nasal Cavities

8

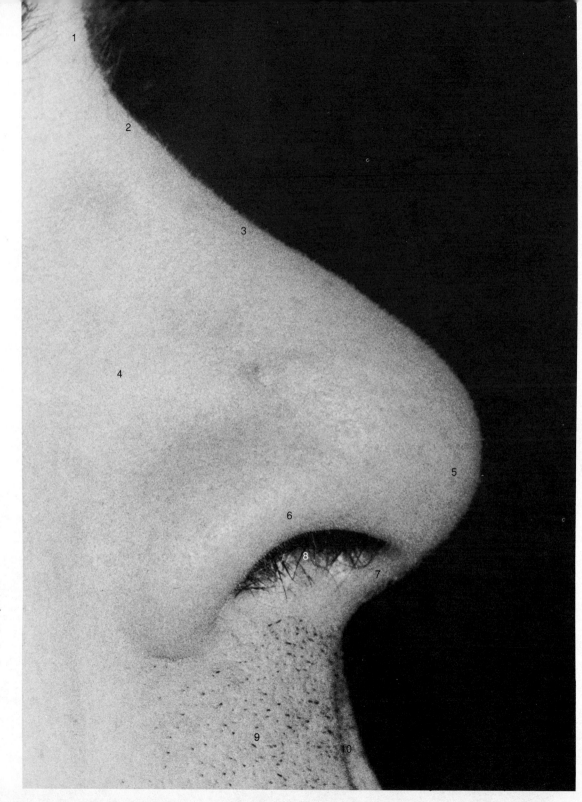

FIGURE 8–1   Lateral view of external nose and upper
lip. (1) root, (2) bridge, (3) dorsum, (4) side, (5) tip,
(6) ala, (7) columella (mobile septum), (8) right naris,
(9) upper lip, (10) philtrum.

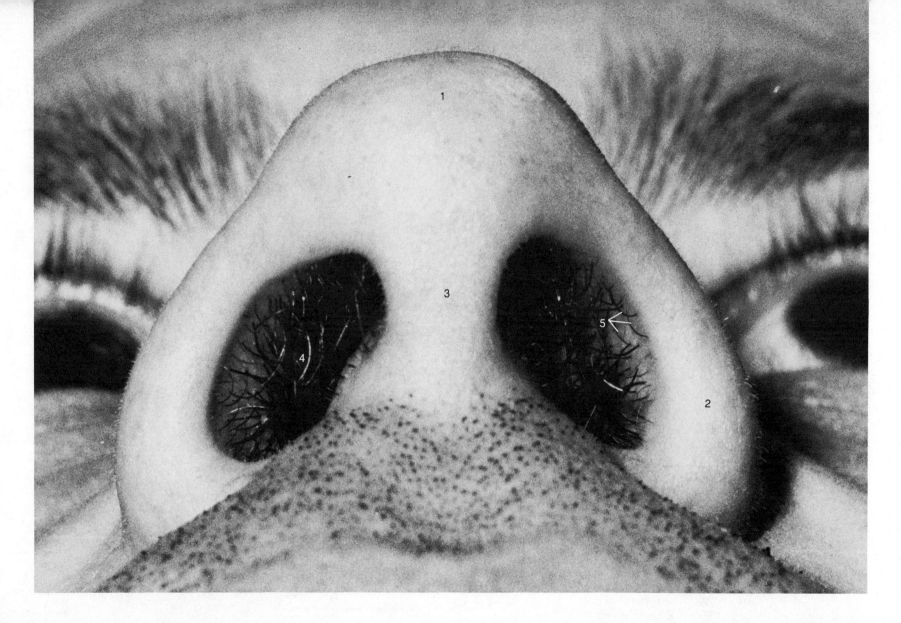

FIGURE 8–2 Inferior view of nose. (1) tip, (2) ala, (3) columella (mobile septum), (4) naris, (5) vestibule containing vibrissae or hairs.

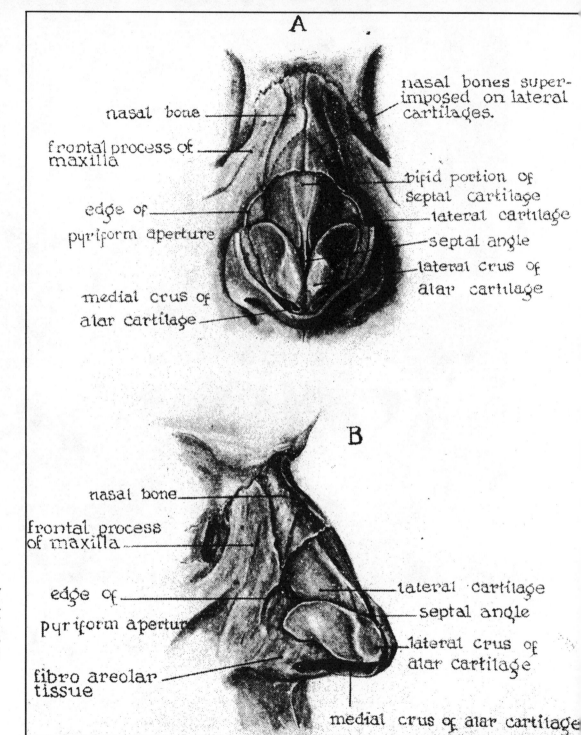

FIGURE 8–3 Anatomy of cartilagenous and boney framework of external aspect of nose. (Courtesy of J.M. Converse, "The Cartilagenous Structures of the Nose," in *Annals of Otology, Rhinology, and Laryngology* 64, No. 1, 1955, p. 222.)

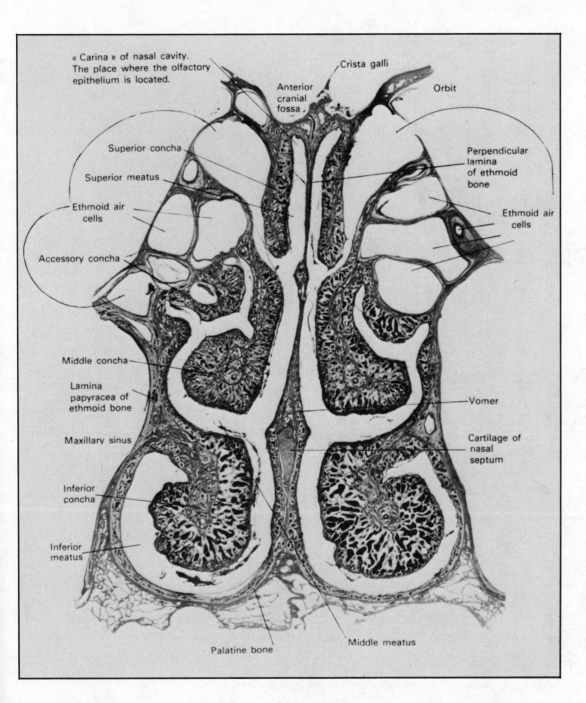

« Carina » of nasal cavity. The place where the olfactory epithelium is located.

Crista galli

Anterior cranial fossa

Orbit

Superior concha

Superior meatus

Ethmoid air cells

Accessory concha

Perpendicular lamina of ethmoid bone

Ethmoid air cells

Middle concha

Lamina papyracea of ethmoid bone

Maxillary sinus

Vomer

Cartilage of nasal septum

Inferior concha

Inferior meatus

Palatine bone

Middle meatus

FIGURE 8–4 Frontal section of nose from a location deep in nasal cavity. (Courtesy of Hans Elias, Joun Pauly, and E. Robert Burns, *Histology and Human Microanatomy*, 4th ed. Padova, Italy: Piccin Medical Books, 1978.)

THE NASAL CAVITIES

131

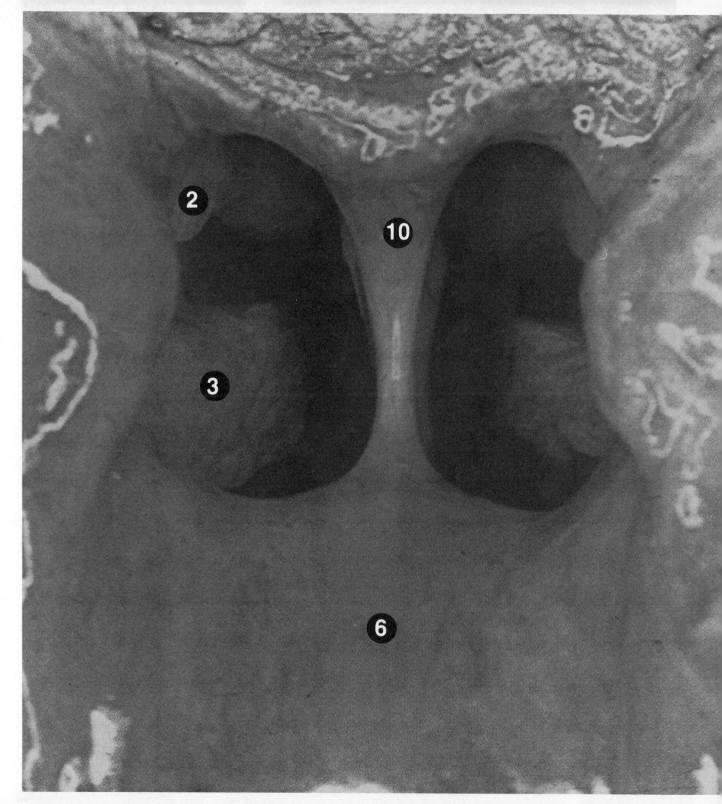

FIGURE 8–5   Posterior view of nasal choanae. (2) middle concha, (3) inferior concha, (6) soft palate, (10) nasal septum. (Courtesy of Chihiro Yokochi and Johannes W. Rohen, *Photographic Anatomy of the Human Body*, 2nd Ed. Tokyo: Igakua-Shoin, Ltd., 1978.)

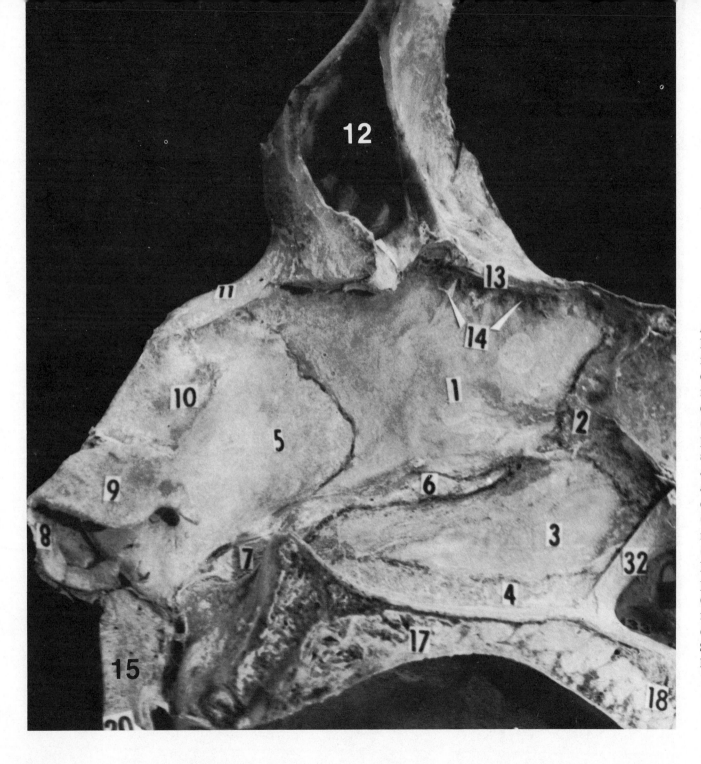

FIGURE 8–6 Anatomy of cartilages and bones of nasal cavity. (1) perpendicular plate of ethmoid, (2) rostrum of sphenoid, (3) vomer, (4) nasal crest of palatine bone and maxilla, (5) septal cartilage and (6) its posterior recess, (7) vomeronasal cartilage, (8) medial crus and (9) lateral crus of greater alar cartilage, (10) lateral nasal cartilage, (11) nasal bone, (12) frontal air sinus, (13) cribriform plate of ethmoid, (14) olfactory nerves, (15) upper lip, (16) soft palate, (17) hard palate. (Courtesy of the Anatomy Museum of the Department of Anatomy and Cell Biology, University of Pittsburgh, School of Medicine, Pittsburgh.)

THE NASAL CAVITIES

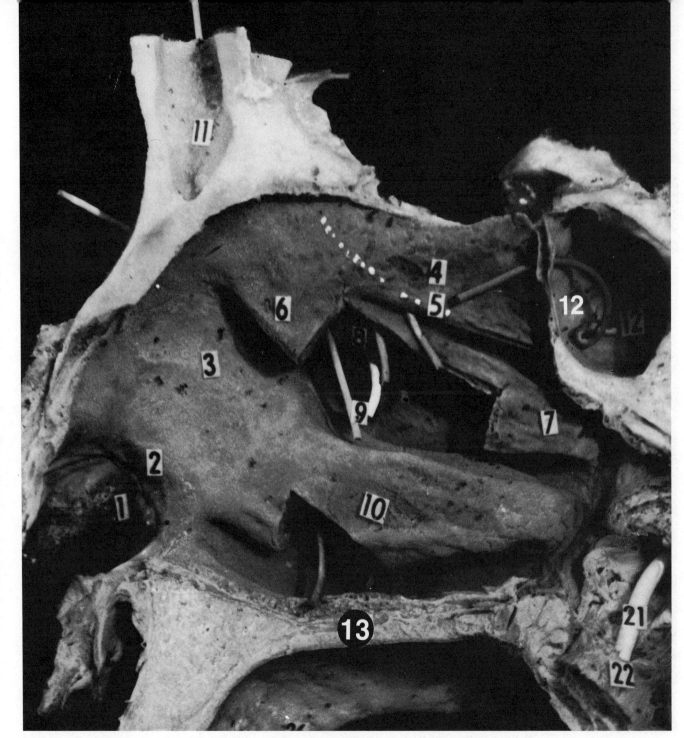

FIGURE 8–7 Lateral wall of nasal cavity. (1) vestibule of nose lined with protective hairs (vibrissae), (2) limen nasi, (3) olfactory sulcus (passageway of inhaled air), (4) olfactory area, (5) superior nasal concha, (6)–(7) middle nasal concha, (8) ethmoidal bulla, (9) probes passing through hiatus semilunaris into maxillary air sinus and along frontonasal duct into (11) frontal air sinus, (10) inferior nasal concha (note probe from nasolacrimal duct opening into the inferior meatus), (12) sphenoidal air sinus with probe in its sphenoethmoidal recess, and (13) hard palate. (Courtesy of the Anatomy Museum of the Department of Anatomy and Cell Biology, University of Pittsburgh, School of Medicine, Pittsburgh.)

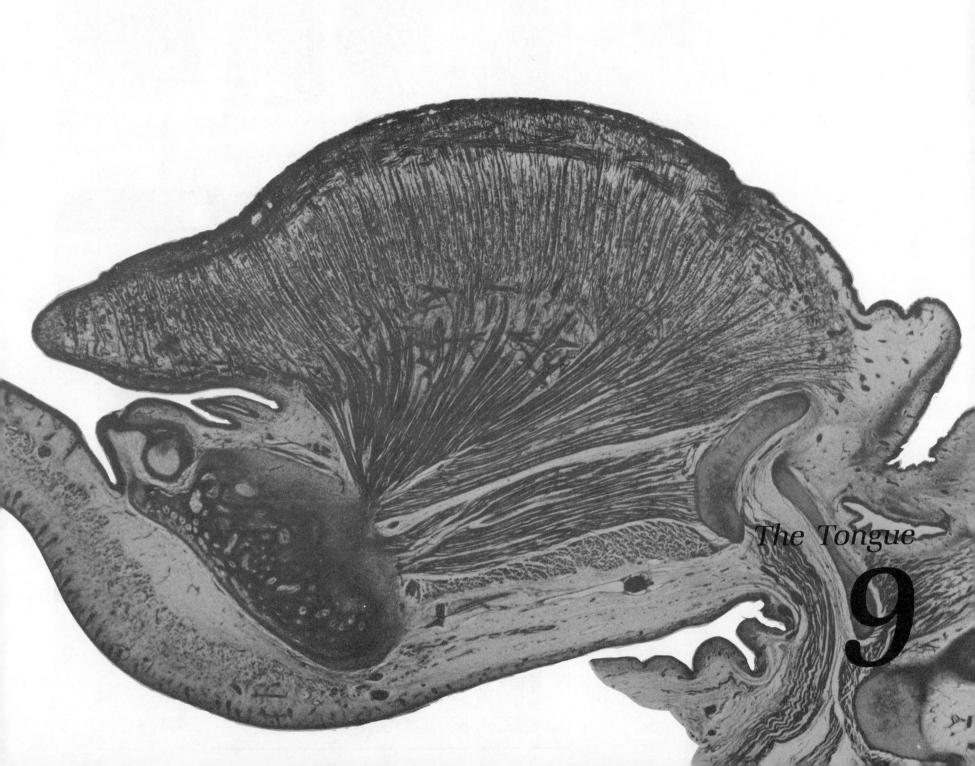

The Tongue

9

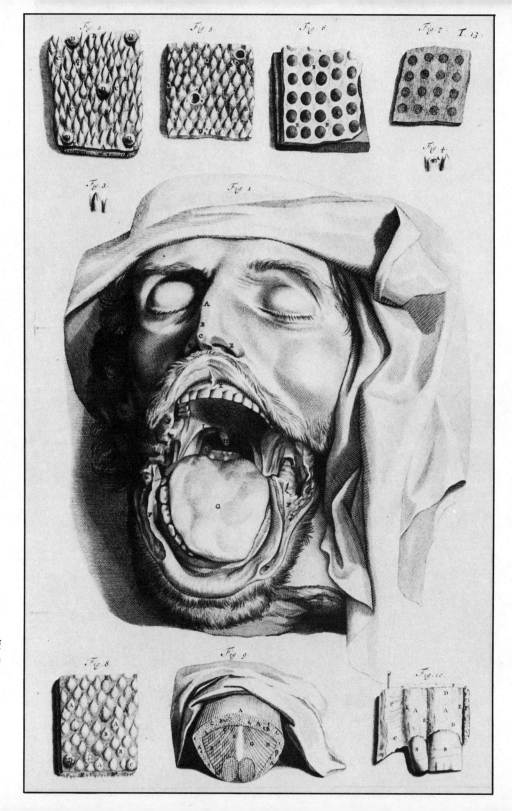

FIGURE 9–1   (From Govard Bidlvo, *Anatoma Humani Corporis*. Amsterdam: Johannis A. Someren, 1685.)

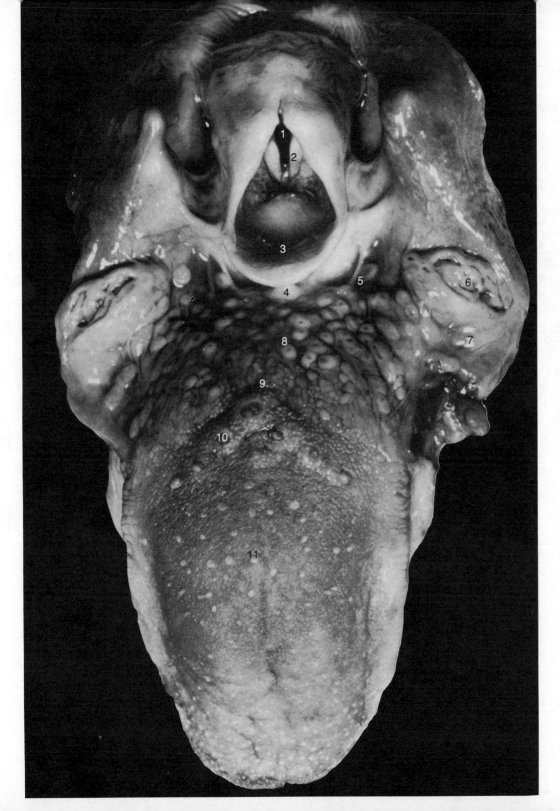

FIGURE 9–2   Human tongue and pharynx viewed from above. (1) rima glottidis, (2) vocal folds, (3) epiglottis, (4) median and (5) lateral glossoepiglottic folds, (6) palatine tonsils, (7) palatoglossus muscle, (8) root of tongue with lingual tonsils, (9) foramen cecum, (10) circumvallate papillae, (11) body of tongue covered with papillae. The valleculae are found between (4) and (5) but are not shown in this preparation because of the overhang of the epiglottis. (Courtesy of Chihiro Yokochi, *Photographic Anatomy of the Human Body*, 1st Ed. Tokyo: Igaku-Shoin, Ltd., 1971.)

THE TONGUE

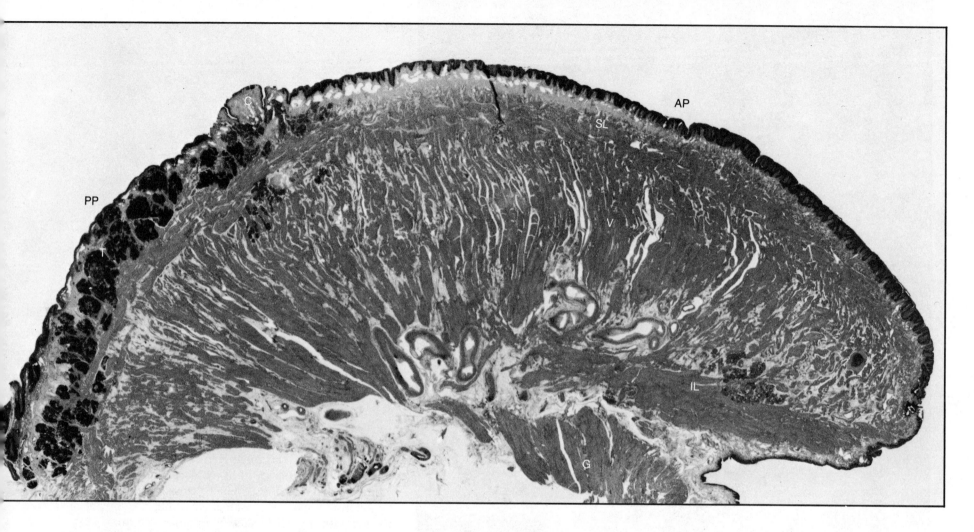

FIGURE 9–3 Photomicrograph of a near-midline sagittal section through tongue of 55-year-old human. The (AP) anterior part or body of the tongue is separated from the (PP) posterior part or base by a (C) circumvallate papilla. There is a large mass of lymphoid tonsillar tissue in the base. Fibers of the (V) vertical, (SL) superior longitudinal, and (IL) inferior longitudinal intrinsic tongue muscles are evident. Some (G) genioglossus fibers is also present. (Courtesy of Christopher A. Squier, College of Dentistry, University of Iowa, Iowa City.)

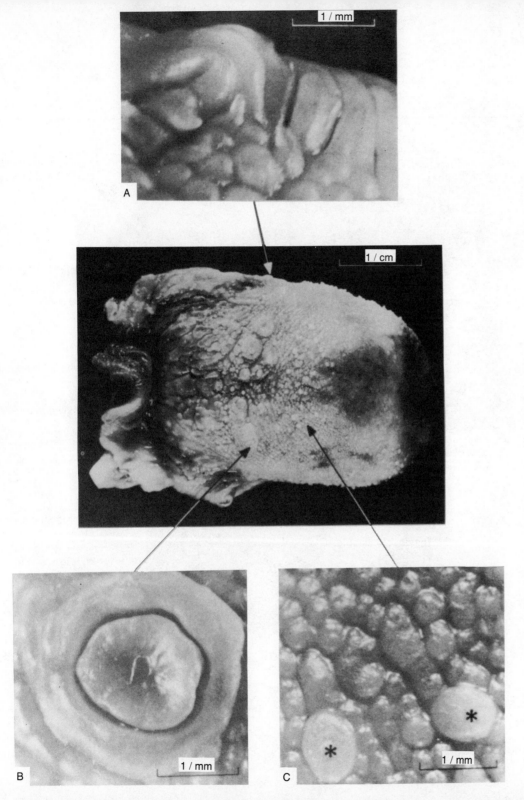

FIGURE 9–4   Dorsal surface of a child's tongue (center), showing distribution and types of lingual papillae. The (a) ridge-shaped foliate papillae are located laterally while (b) circumvallate papillae are situated in a row in front of the sulcus terminalis. Fungiform papillae are interspersed among the numerous filiform papillae on the anterior of the tongue, two of which are shown (*) in (c). (Courtesy of C.A. Squier, N.W. Johnson, and R.M. Hoops, *Human Oral Mucosa: Development, Structure, and Function*. Oxford: Blackwell Scientific Publications, Ltd., 1976.)

THE TONGUE

139

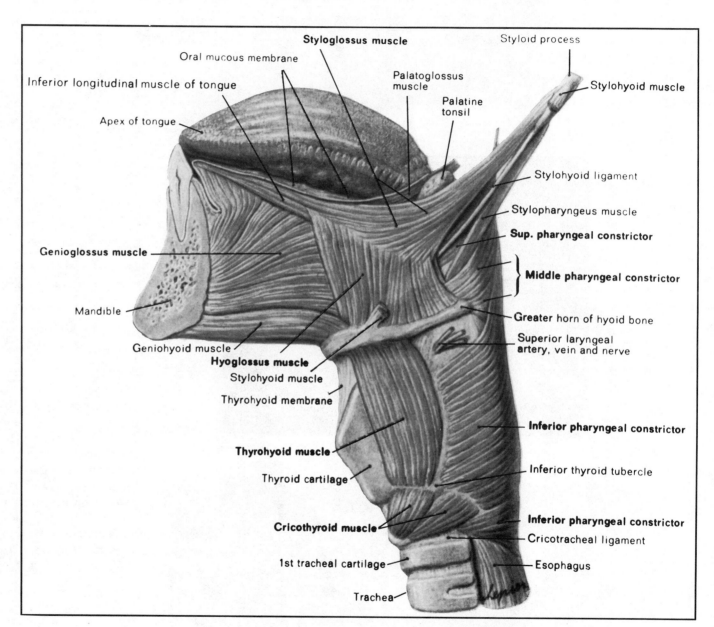

FIGURE 9–5 Lateral view of extrinsic muscles of tongue. (From Carmine D. Clemente, *Anatomy: A Regional Atlas of the Human Body*, 2nd Ed. Baltimore: Urban & Swarzenberg, 1981.)

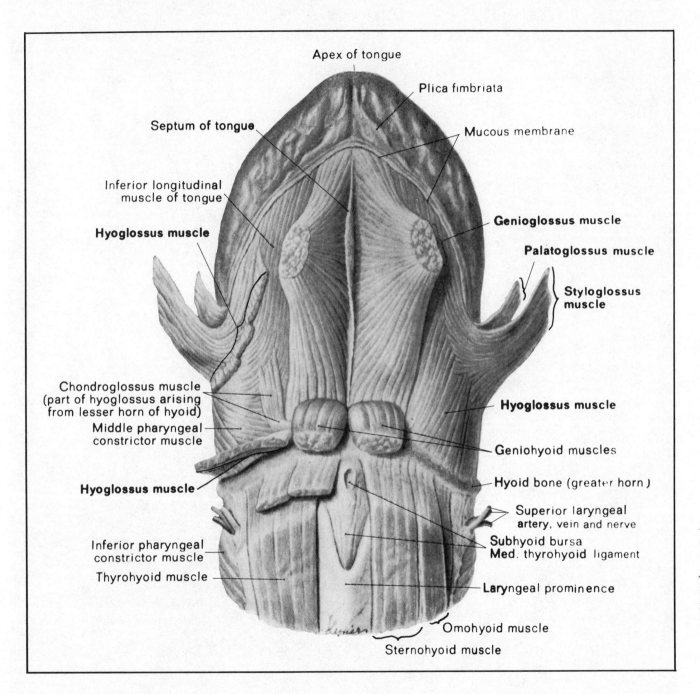

Apex of tongue

Plica fimbriata

Septum of tongue

Mucous membrane

Inferior longitudinal muscle of tongue

Genioglossus muscle

Hyoglossus muscle

Palatoglossus muscle

Styloglossus muscle

Chondroglossus muscle (part of hyoglossus arising from lesser horn of hyoid)

Hyoglossus muscle

Middle pharyngeal constrictor muscle

Geniohyoid muscles

Hyoglossus muscle

Hyoid bone (greater horn)

Superior laryngeal **artery,** vein and nerve

Subhyoid bursa
Med. thyrohyoid ligament

Inferior pharyngeal constrictor muscle

Thyrohyoid muscle

Laryngeal prominence

Omohyoid muscle

Sternohyoid muscle

FIGURE 9–6 Extrinsic muscles of tongue, viewed from below. (From Carmine D. Clemente, *Anatomy: A Regional Atlas of the Human Body,* 2nd Ed. Baltimore: Urban & Schwarzenberg, 1981.)

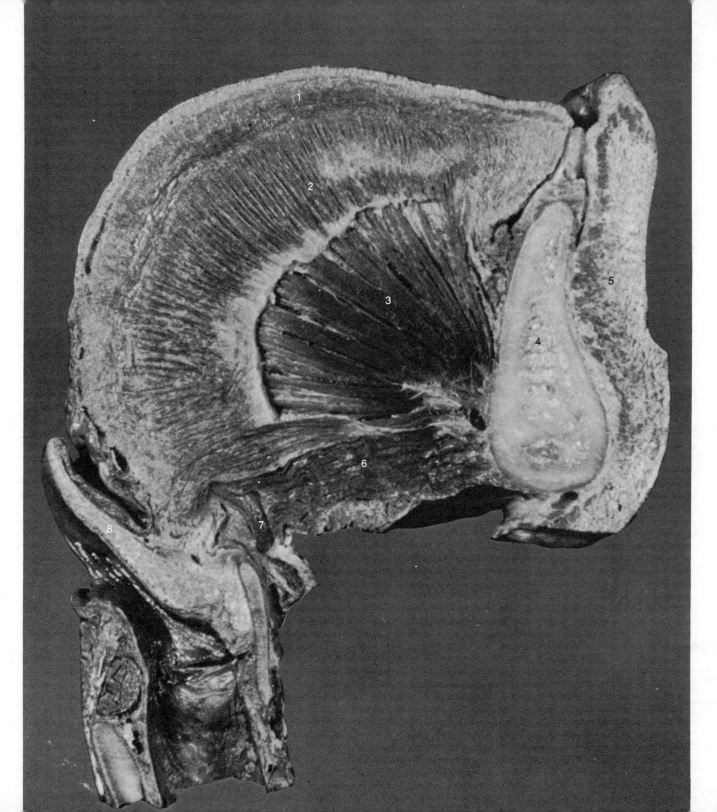

FIGURE 9–7 Medial view of a sagittally sectioned human tongue. (1) superior longitudinal muscle, (2) transverse lingual and vertical lingual muscles, (3) genioglossus muscle, (4) mandible, (5) lower lip, (6) geniohyoid muscle, (7) hyoid bone, (8) epiglottis. (Courtesy of Chihiro Yokochi and Johannes W. Rohen, *Photographic Anatomy of the Human Body*, 2nd Ed. Tokyo: Igaku-Shoin, Ltd., 1978.)

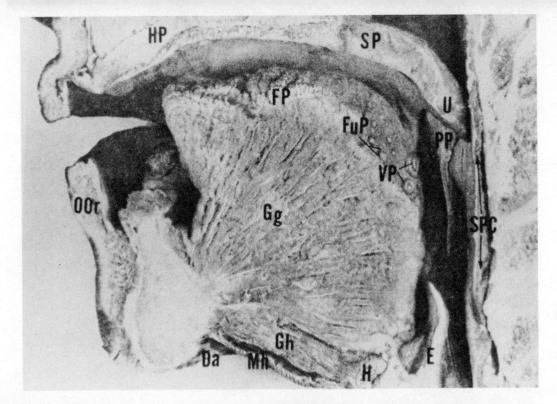

FIGURE 9–8 Sagittal section of mouth from an aged, edentulous specimen. (HP) hard palate, (SP) soft palate, (U) uvula, (OOr) lower lip, (FP) foliate papillae, (FuP) fungiform papillae, (VP) circum vallate papillae, (PP) palatopharyngeus muscle, (SPC) superior pharyngeal constrictor muscle, (Gg) genioglossus muscle, (Da) anterior belly of digastric muscle, (Mh) mylohyoid muscle, (Gh) geniohyoid muscle, (H) hyoid bone, (E) epiglottis. (Courtesy of A.L. Martone and L.F. Edwards, "Anatomy of the Mouth and Related Structures: Part III, Functional Anatomical Considerations," in *Journal of Prosthetic Dentistry* 12, No. 2, 1962, p. 208.)

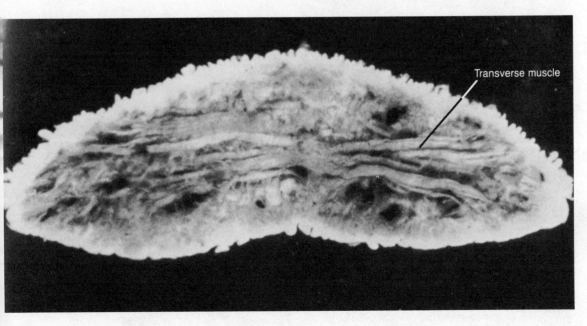

Transverse muscle

FIGURE 9–9 Coronal dissection of fetal human tongue just posterior to the lip. (Courtesy of Leon H. Strong, "Muscle Fibers of the Tongue Functional in Consonant Production," in *Anatomical Record* 126, No. 1, September 1956, p. 75.)

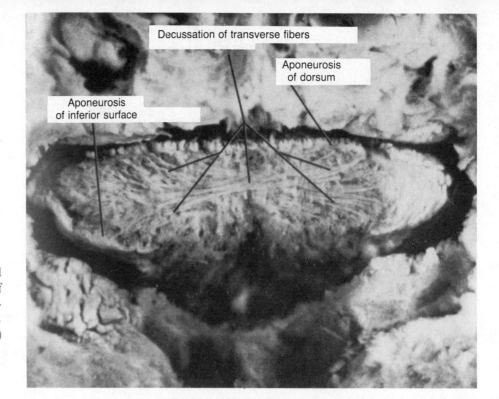

FIGURE 9–10 Frontal section from human fetal tongue just posterior to the frenulum. (Courtesy of Leon H. Strong, "Muscle Fibers of the Tongue Functional in Consonant Production," in *Anatomical Record* 126, No. 1, September 1956, p. 75.)

FIGURE 9–11 Coronal dissection of human tongue just posterior to the lip, from a 38-day-old human specimen. The transverse muscle fibers are shown to decussate through the midline. (Courtesy of Leon H. Strong, "Muscle Fibers of the Tongue Functional in Consonant Production," in *Anatomical Record* 126, No. 1, September 1956, p. 77.)

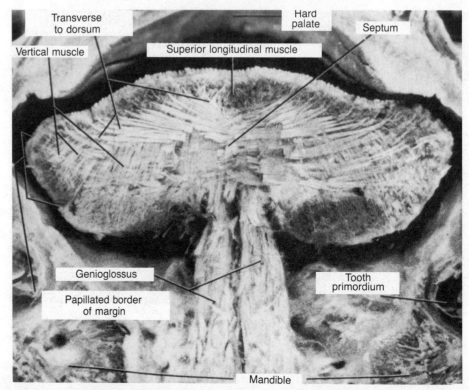

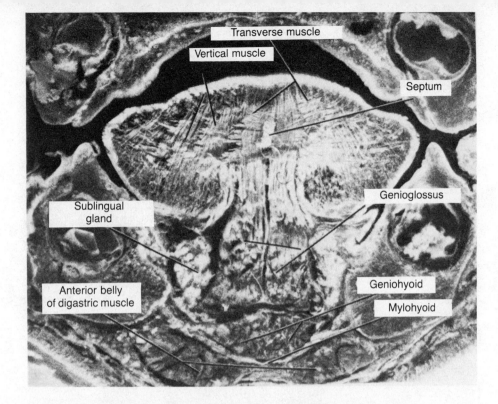

FIGURE 9–12 Coronal dissection of human fetal tongue through the midline of the dorsum. (Courtesy of Leon H. Strong, "Muscle Fibers of the Tongue Functional in Consonant Production," in *Anatomical Record* 126, No. 1, September 1956, p. 79.)

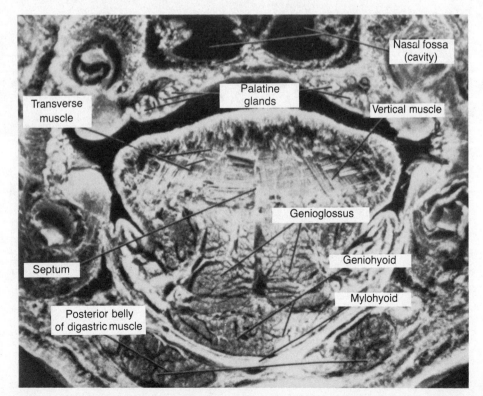

FIGURE 9–13 Coronal section of fetal human tongue through the 1st molar. (Courtesy of Leon H. Strong, "Muscle Fibers of the Tongue Functional in Consonant Production," in *Anatomical Record* 126, No. 1, September 1956, p. 79.)

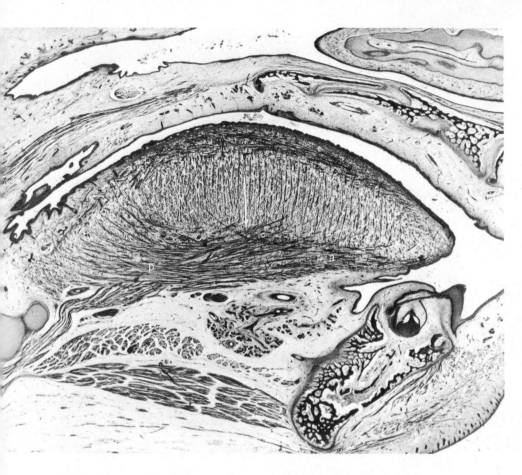

FIGURE 9–14 Parasagittal section through tongue illustrating the two segments (a, p) of the inferior longitudinal muscle. (The tip of the tongue is situated at right of the photograph). Note the area of junction (arrow) of the two segments; also the insertions of the fibers of the posterior segment into the lamina propria of the posterior third of the tongue. (Courtesy of Y.M. Barnwell, H.L. Langdon, and K.M. Klueber, "The Anatomy of the Intrinsic Musculature of the Tongue in the Early Human Fetus: Part 2," in *International Journal of Oral Myology* 4, No. 4, 1978, p. 6.)

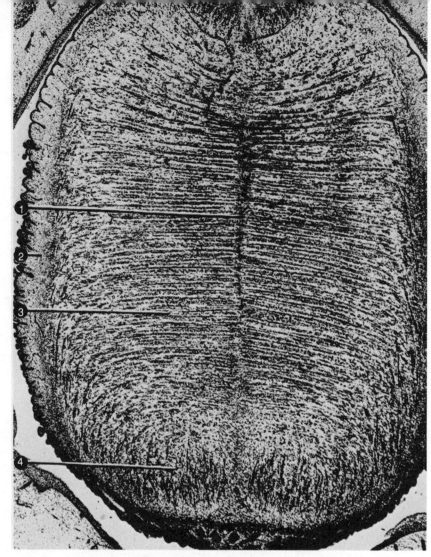

FIGURE 9–15 Photomicrograph of transverse section of the tongue from a $3\frac{1}{2}$-month human fetus. (1) median fibrous septum, (2) longitudinal muscle fibers, (3) transverse muscle fibers, (4) vertical muscle fibers. (Courtesy of Moses Diamond, *Dental Anatomy Including Anatomy of the Head and Neck*, 3rd Ed. New York: Macmillan Publishing Co., Inc., 1952.)

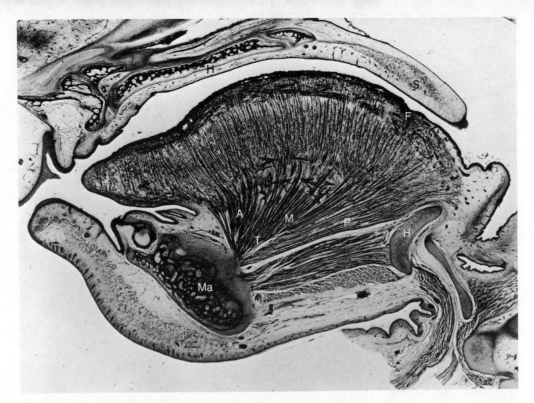

FIGURE 9–16 Parasagittal section through tongue of a 15-week human fetus illustrating the deposition of genioglossal fibers into (A) anterior, (M) middle, and (P) posterior components. (Ma) mandible, (H) hyoid complex, (F) foramen cecum, (T) tendon, (H) hard palate, (S) soft palate. (Courtesy of H.L. Langdon, K.M. Klueber, and Y.M. Barnwell, "The Anatomy of M. Genioglossus in the 15-week Human Fetus," in *Anatomy and Embryology* 155, No. 1, December 1978, p. 109.)

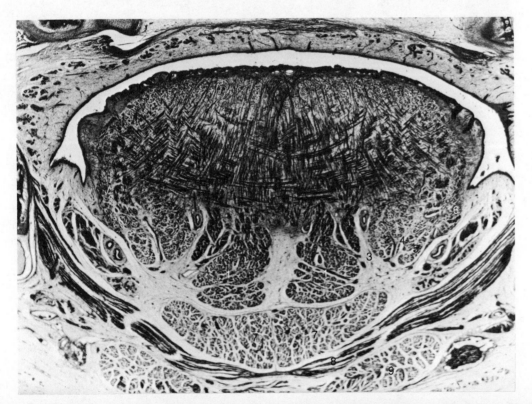

FIGURE 9–17 Coronal section through midpart of tongue. (1) genioglossus, (2) inferior longitudinal muscle, (3) paramedian and (4) lateral septa, (5) hyoglossus muscle, (6) styloglossus muscle, (7) geniohyoid muscle, (8) mylohyoid muscle, (9) anterior digastric muscle. (Courtesy of Y.M. Barnwell, H.L. Langdon, and K.M. Klueber, "The Anatomy of the Intrinsic Musculature of the Tongue in the Early Human Fetus: Part 2," in *International Journal of Oral Myology* 4, No. 4, 1978, p. 7.)

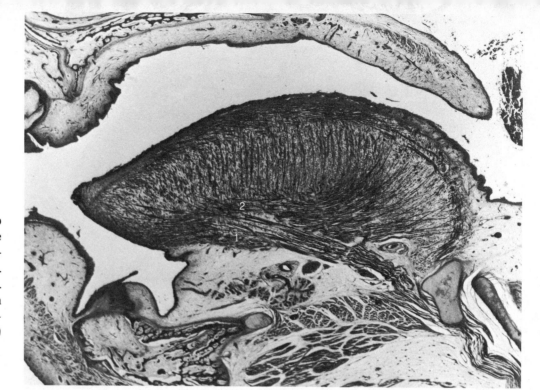

FIGURE 9–18   Parasagittal section, located lateral to Figure 9–19 showing course of (1) hyoglossus muscle as it runs distally in the tongue to parallel the (2) anterior segment of the inferior longitudinal muscle. (Courtesy of Y.M. Barnwell, H.L. Langdon, and K.M. Klueber, "The Intrinsic Musculature of the Tongue in the Early Human Fetus: Part 2," in *International Journal of Oral Myology* 4, No. 4, 1978, p. 7.)

FIGURE 9–19   Parasagittal section through tongue showing interrelationship between fibers of the (1) superior longitudinal muscle and (2) hyoglossus muscle. (Courtesy of Y.M. Barnwell, K.M. Klueber, and H.L. Langdon, "The Anatomy of the Intrinsic Musculature of the Tongue in the Early Human Fetus: Part 1," in *International Journal of Oral Myology* 4, No. 3, 1978, p. 7.)

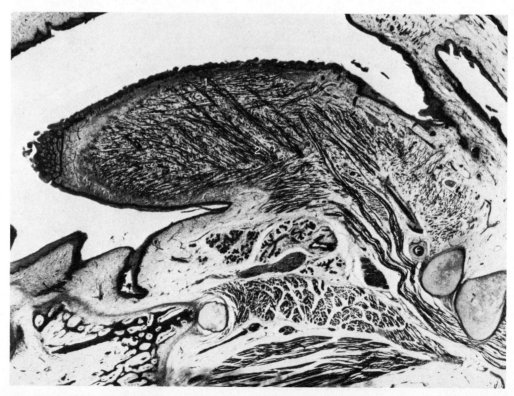

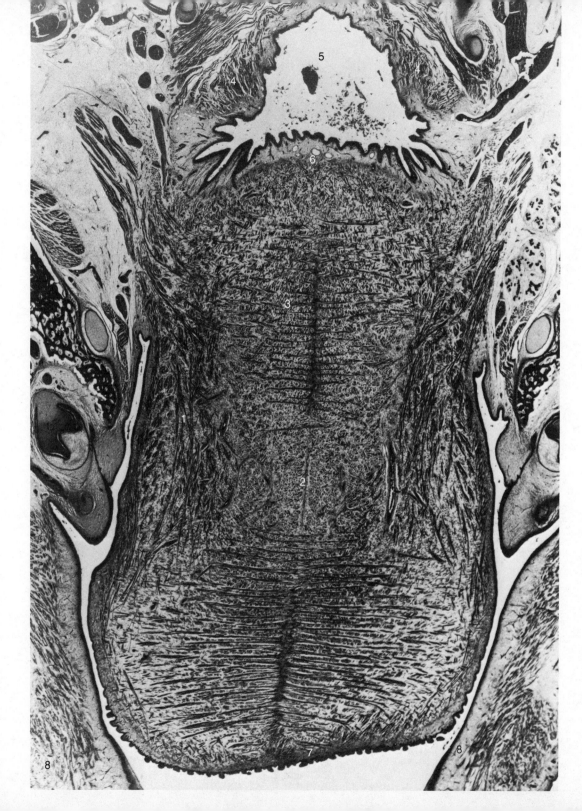

FIGURE 9–20 Horizontal section through the tongue of a 15-week human fetus illustrating the course of styloglossus muscle in the tongue and its relationship to the transverse lingual muscle. (1) styloglossus muscle, (2) lingual septum, (3) transverse lingual muscle, (4) middle pharyngeal constrictor muscle, (5) oropharynx, (6) root of tongue, (7) tip of tongue, (8) mandible. (Courtesy of H.L. Langdon and Y.M. Barnwell, Department of Anatomy and Histology, University of Pittsburgh, School of Dental Medicine, Pittsburgh.)

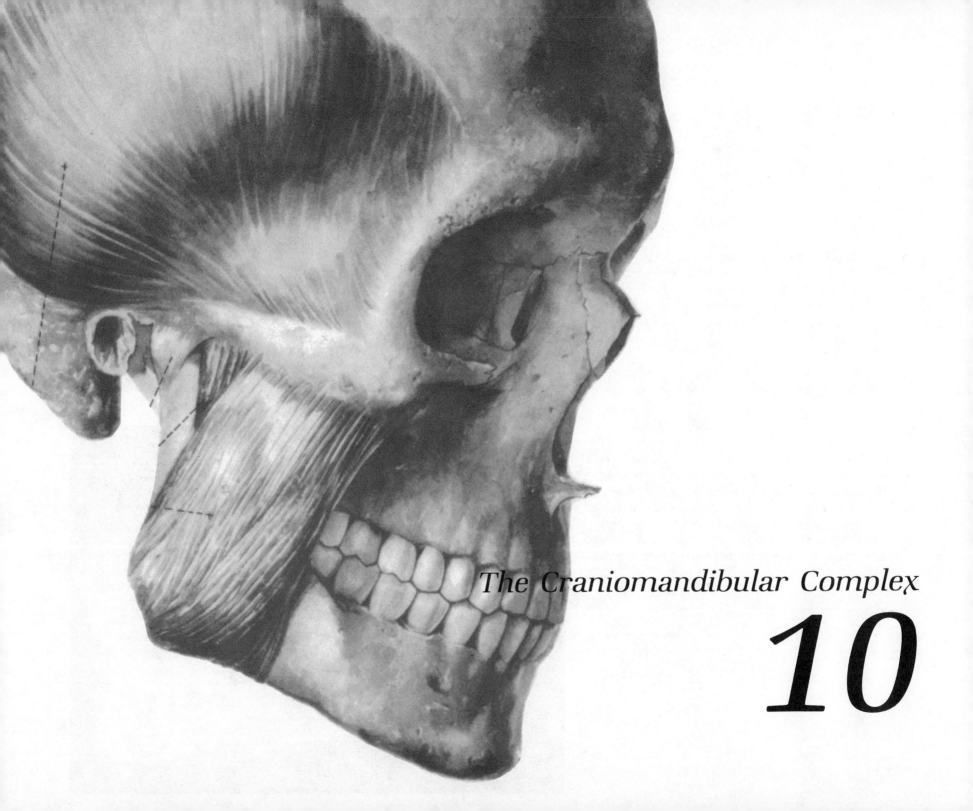

The Craniomandibular Complex

10

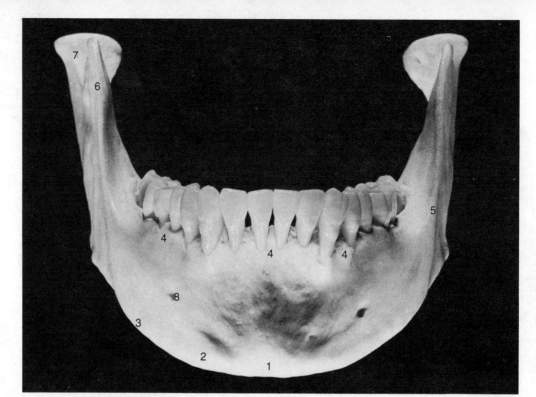

FIGURE 10–1   Anterior aspect of mandible. (1) symphysis menti, (2) mental tubercle, (3) inferior border, (4) alveolar process, (5) oblique line, (6) coronoid process, (7) condyloid process, (8) mental foramen. (Photo by Paul Reimann, Department of Anatomy, University of Iowa.)

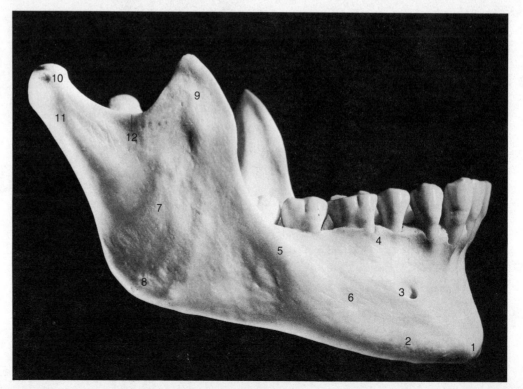

FIGURE 10–2   Lateral aspect of mandible. (1) mental protuberance, (2) mental tubercle, (3) mental foramen, (4) alveolar process, (5) oblique lines, (6) body, (7) ramus, (8) angle, (9) coronoid process, (10) condyloid process, (11) neck, (12) semilunar (mandibular) notch. (Photo by Paul Reimann, Department of Anatomy, University of Iowa.)

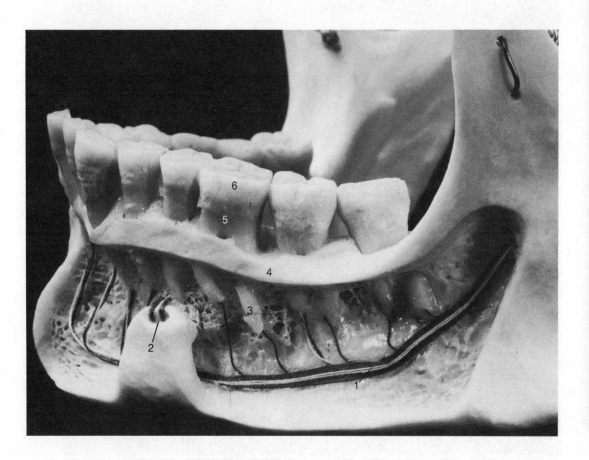

FIGURE 10–3 Lateral view of body of mandible with outer layer of bone removed to show blood and nerve supply to the teeth. (1) inferior alveolar nerve (white line) and artery and vein (dark lines), (2) mental foramen with nerve and vessels passing through it, (3) root of tooth, (4) alveolar process, (5) neck of tooth, (6) crown of tooth. (Photo by Paul Reimann, Department of Anatomy, University of Iowa.)

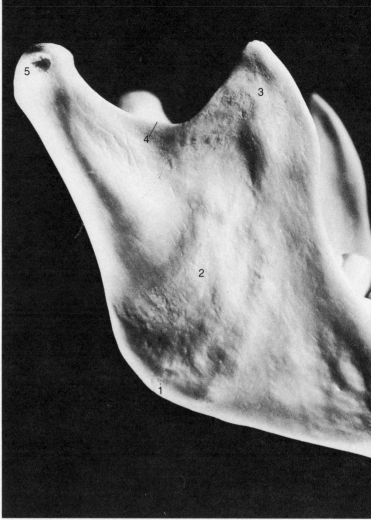

FIGURE 10–4 Ramus (right) of mandible. (1) angle, (2) ramus, (3) coronoid process, (4) mandibular (semilunar) notch, (5) condyloid process (condyle). (Photo by Paul Reimann, Department of Anatomy, University of Iowa.)

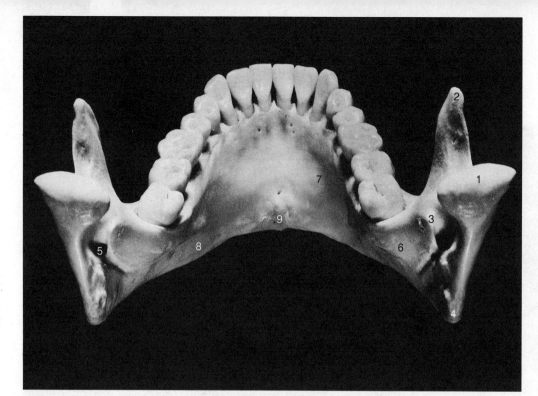

FIGURE 10–5   Posterior view of mandible. (1) condyloid process, (2) coronoid process, (3) ramus, (4) angle, (5) left mandibular foramen, (6) part of mylohyoid line, (7) body of mandible, (8) sublingual fossa, (9) genial tubercles. (Photo by Paul Reimann, Department of Anatomy, University of Iowa.)

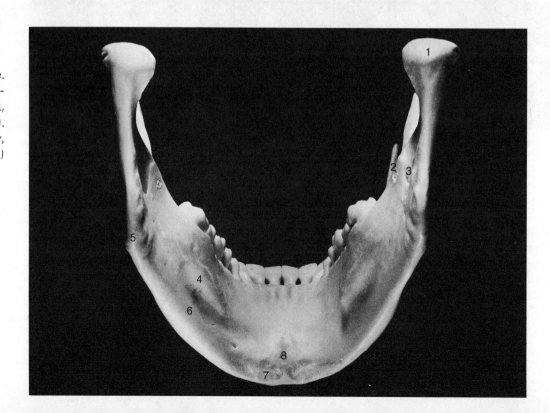

FIGURE 10–6   Posteroinferior view of mandible. (1) condyloid process, (2) lingula, (3) mandibular foramen, (4) mylohyoid line, (5) angle, (6) sublingual fossa, (7) digastric fossa, (8) genial tubercle (mental spine). (Photo by Paul Reimann, Department of Anatomy, University of Iowa.)

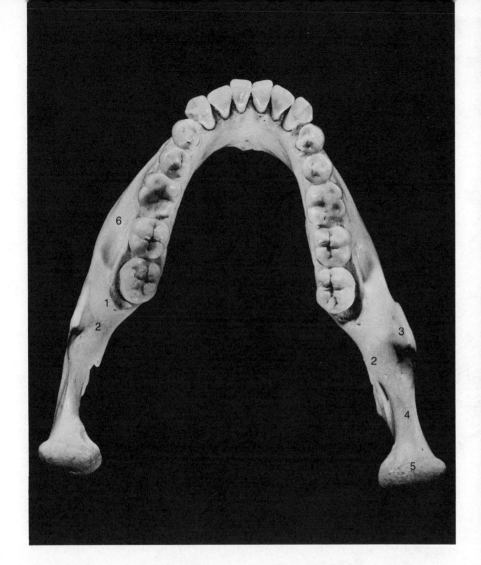

FIGURE 10–7 Superior aspect of mandible; note teeth in sockets of alveolar process. (1) retromolar triangle, (2) temporal crest, (3) coronoid process, (4) neck of mandible, (5) condyloid process, (6) body of mandible. (Photo by Paul Reimann, Department of Anatomy, University of Iowa.)

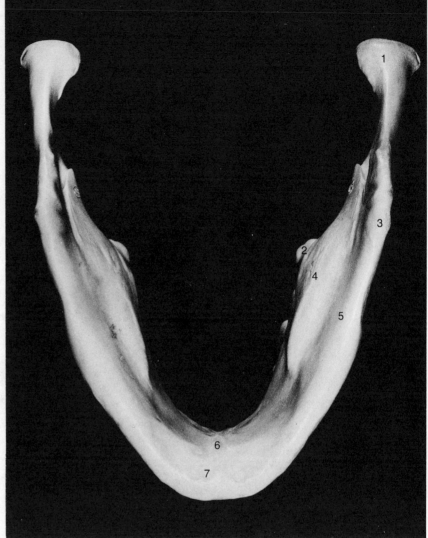

FIGURE 10–8 Inferior aspect of mandible. (1) condyloid process, (2) coronoid process, (3) angle, (4) mylohyoid line, (5) submandibular fossa, (6) genial tubercles (mental spines), (7) digastric fossa. (Photo by Paul Reimann, Department of Anatomy, University of Iowa.)

THE CRANIOMANDIBULAR COMPLEX

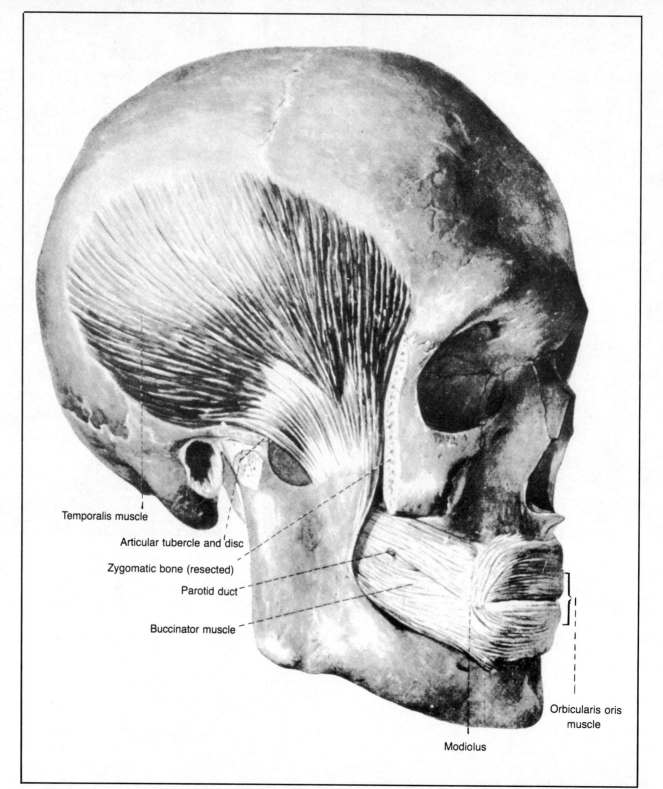

FIGURE 10–9 Temporalis muscle viewed from right side. The zygomatic arch has been removed. The temporomandibular joint has been sectioned longitudinally, and the most superficial fibers of the temporalis muscle have been removed. (Courtesy of W. Spalteholz and R. Spanner, *Atlas of Human Anatomy*, 16th Ed. Philadelphia: F.A. Davis Company, 1967 (English). Amsterdam: Scheltema, Holkema, and Vermeulen 1967, (Dutch).)

Temporalis muscle

Articular tubercle and disc

Zygomatic bone (resected)

Parotid duct

Buccinator muscle

Orbicularis oris muscle

Modiolus

THE SPEECH MECHANISM

156

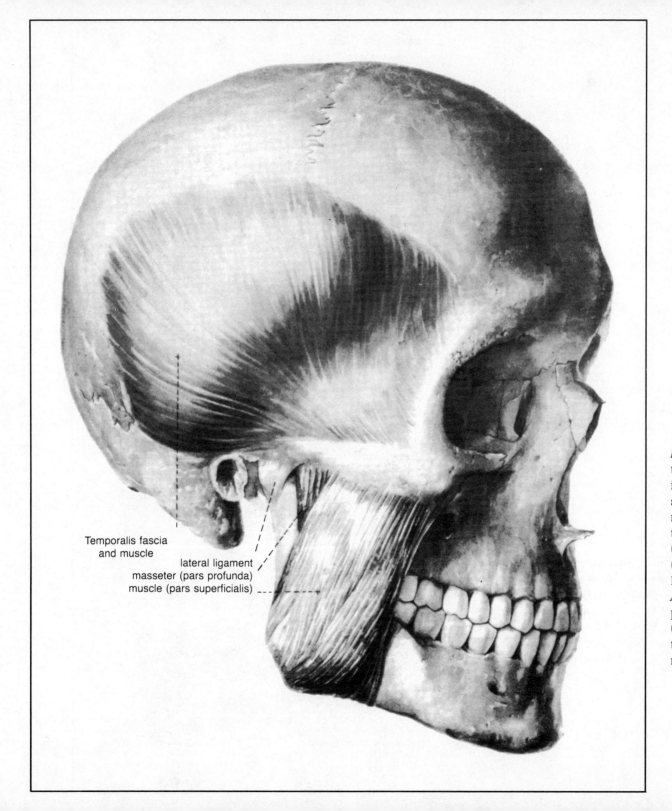

Temporalis fascia
and muscle

lateral ligament
masseter (pars profunda)
muscle (pars superficialis)

FIGURE 10–10 Masseter and temporalis muscles. Temporalis is shown covered by its fascial sheath. Both the deep part of masseter (pars profunda) and the main body of masseter (pars superficialis) are shown. (Courtesy of W. Spalteholz and R. Spanner, *Atlas of Human Anatomy*, 16th Ed. Philadelphia: F.A. Davis Company, 1967 (English). Amsterdam: Scheltema, Holkema, and Vermeulen, 1967 (Dutch).)

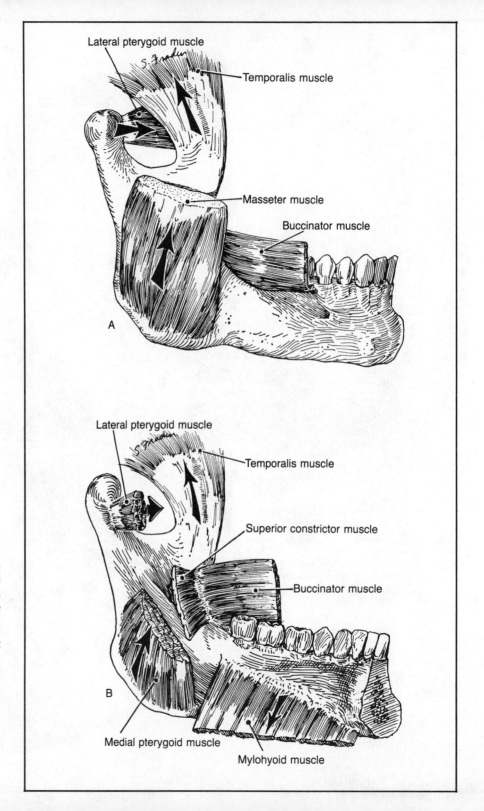

FIGURE 10–11 Muscles inserting into mandible, viewed (A) laterally and (B) medially. Arrows indicate the direction of muscle fibers for most muscles. (Courtesy of Raymond J. Nagle and Victor H. Sears, *Dental Prosthetics*; St. Louis: The C.V. Mosby Co., 1958. As reprinted in S. Silverman, *Oral Physiology*; St. Louis: The C.V. Mosby Co., 1961.)

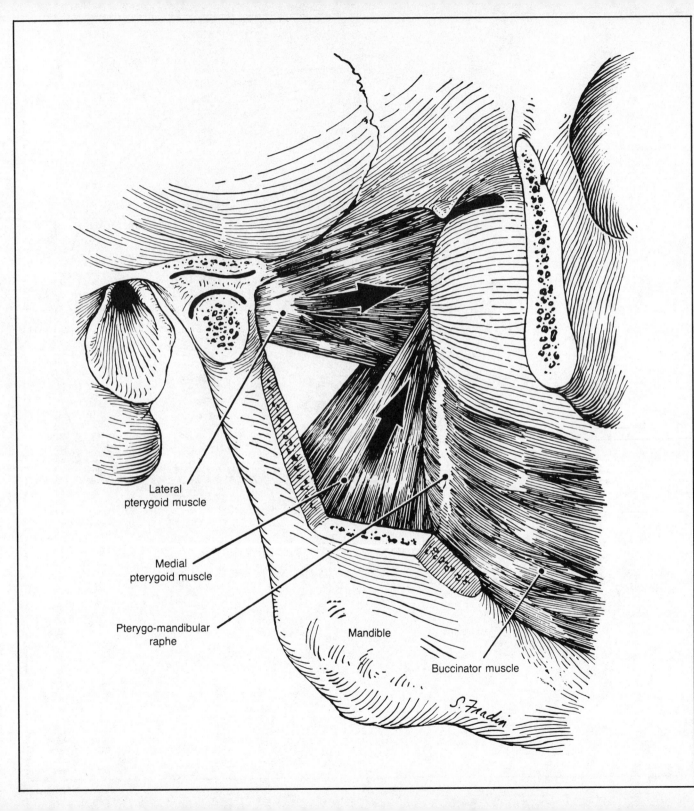

Lateral pterygoid muscle

Medial pterygoid muscle

Pterygo-mandibular raphe

Mandible

Buccinator muscle

FIGURE 10–12 Lateral and medial pterygoid muscles, viewed laterally. The coronoid process of the mandible and the zygomatic process have been removed. The two parts of the lateral pterygoid muscle are not very distinct in this figure; however, it can be seen that some fibers insert into the capsular ligament of the temporomandibular joint, and others insert into the condyloid process. (Courtesy of Raymond J. Nagle and Victor H. Sears, *Dental Prosthetics*; St. Louis: The C.V. Mosby Co., 1958. As reprinted in S. Silverman, *Oral Physiology*; St. Louis: The C.V. Mosby Co., 1961.)

THE CRANIOMANDIBULAR COMPLEX

159

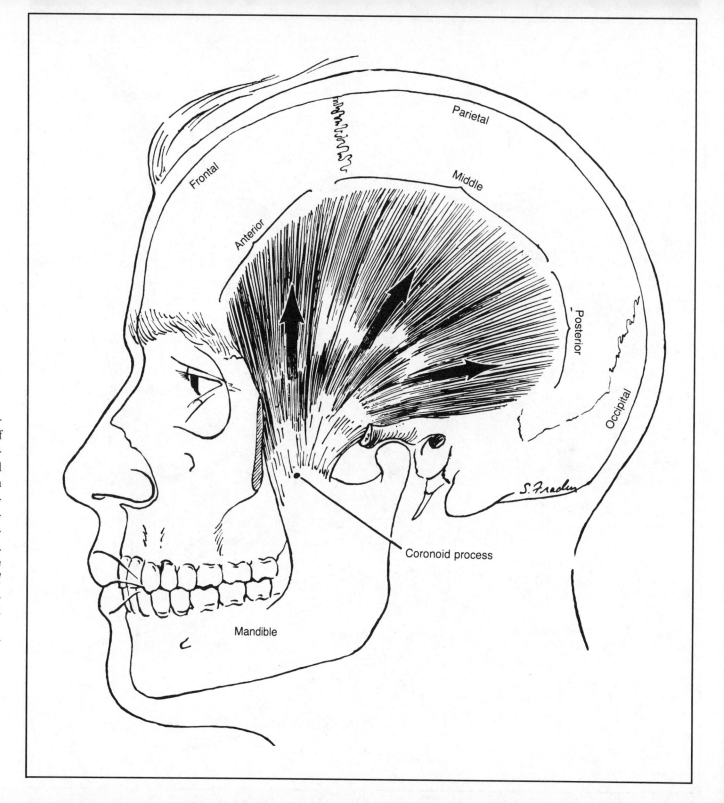

FIGURE 10–13 Anterior, middle, and posterior divisions of temporalis muscle. Arrows reflect the differences in general orientation of muscle fibers. In contrast to this tripartite division, a bipartite division (anterior and posterior) of temporalis is sometimes seen. (Courtesy of Raymond J. Nagle and Victor H. Sears, *Dental Prosthetics*; St. Louis: The C.V. Mosby Co., 1958. As reprinted in S. Silverman, *Oral Physiology*; St. Louis: The C.V. Mosby Co., 1961.)

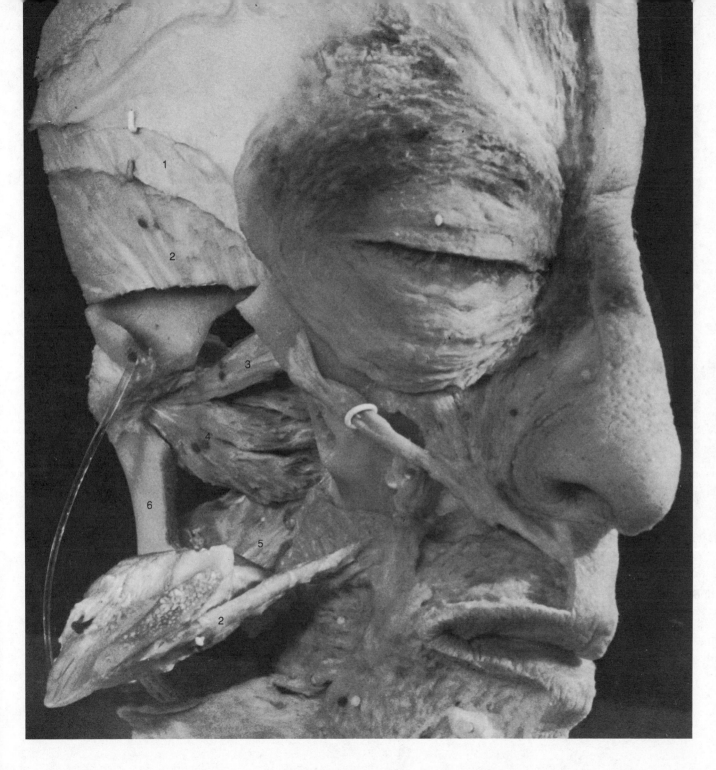

FIGURE 10–14 Muscles of mastication. The right ramus of the mandible and the temporalis muscle have been cut and parts of them are reflected downward. (1) temporalis fascia, (2) temporalis muscle, (3) superior and (4) inferior portions of the lateral pterygoid muscle, (5) medial pterygoid muscle, (6) posterior border of ramus of mandible. (Courtesy of P.A. Knudsen, Royal Dental College, Aarhaus, Denmark; as reprinted in Bertram Kraus, Ronald Jordan, and Leonard Abrams, *Dental Anatomy and Occlusion.* Baltimore: The Williams and Wilkins Co., 1969.)

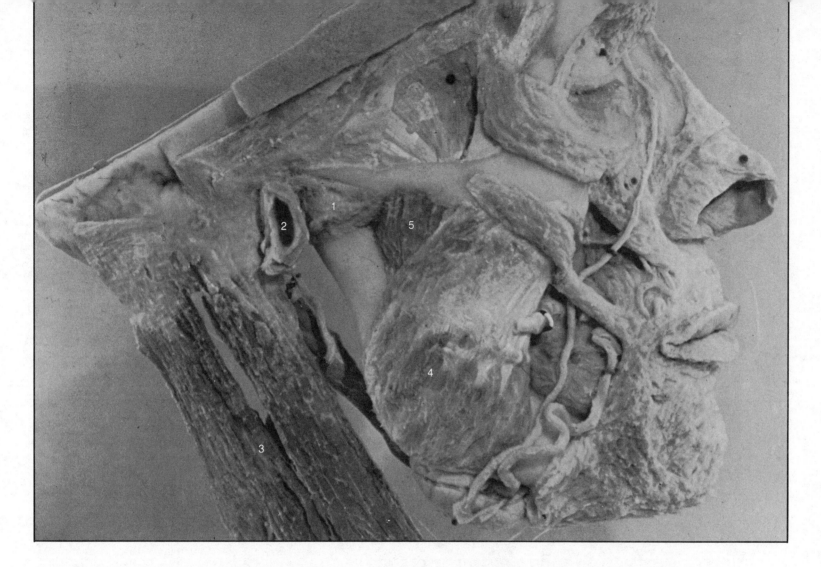

FIGURE 10–15   Dissection of skull, side view, showing (1) capsule of the temporomandibular joint just anterior to the (2) external auditory meatus. The (3) insertion of the sternocleidomastoid muscle is posterior to the external auditory meatus. The (4) main body of the masseter muscle is anterior to the much smaller (5) deep part of masseter. (Courtesy of P.A. Knudsen, Royal Dental College, Aarhus, Denmark; as reprinted in Bertram Kraus, Ronald Jordan, and Leonard Abrams, *Dental Anatomy and Occlusion*. Baltimore: The Williams and Wilkins Co., 1969.)

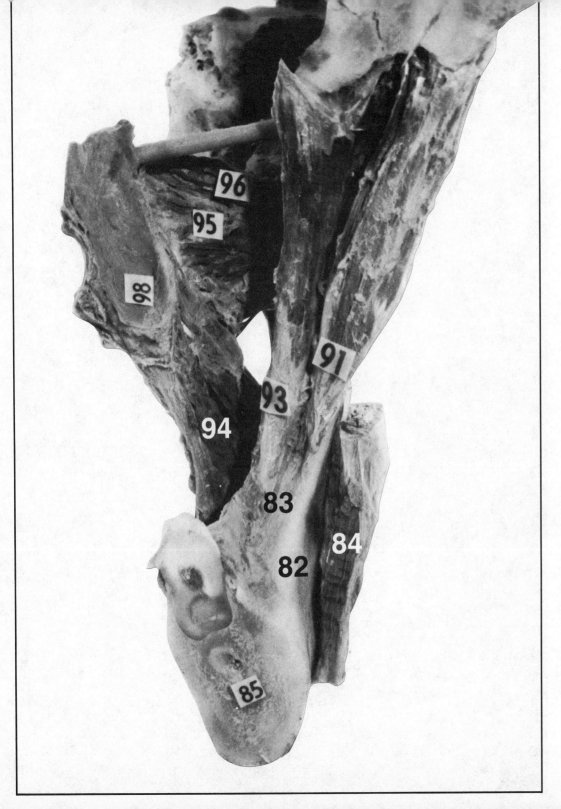

FIGURE 10–16 Anterior view of muscles of mastication and their attachment to mandible and sphenoid bones on left side. (91) superficial and (93) deep tendons of temporalis muscle attaching to anterior border of coronoid process, (82) mandibular ramus and (83) temporal crest of mandible, (84) portion of masseter muscle, (85) body of mandible cut through molar tooth, (95) inferior and (96) superior heads of lateral pterygoid muscle, (94) medial pterygoid muscle, (98) portion of sphenoid bone. (Courtesy of the Anatomy Museum of the Department of Anatomy and Cell Biology, University of Pittsburgh, School of Medicine, Pittsburgh.)

THE CRANIOMANDIBULAR COMPLEX

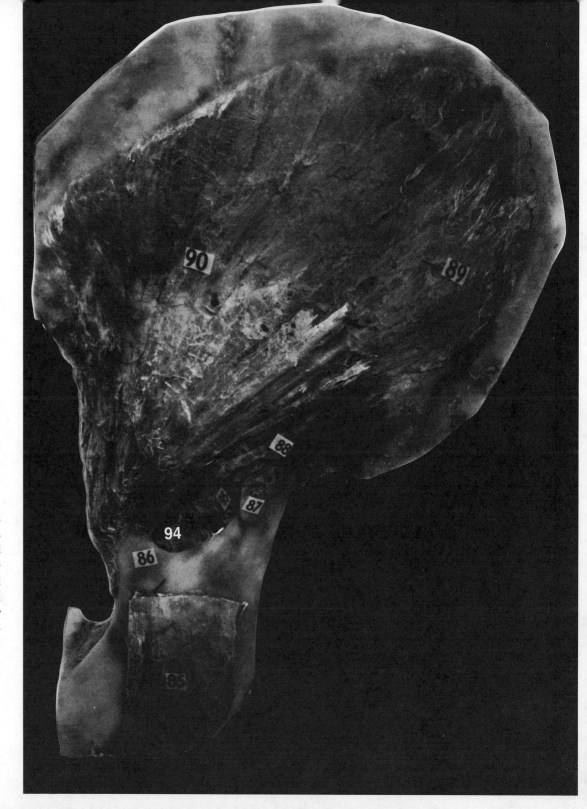

FIGURE 10–17   Lateral view of muscles of mastication and their attachment to mandible on left side. (85) portion of masseter muscle, (86) coronoid and (87) condyloid processes of mandible, (88) part of zygomatic process of temporal bone, (89) posterior and (90) anterior fibers of temporalis muscle, (94) medial pterygoid muscle, (95) lateral pterygoid muscle (lower head). (Courtesy of the Anatomy Museum of the Department of Anatomy and Cell Biology, University of Pittsburgh, School of Medicine, Pittsburgh.)

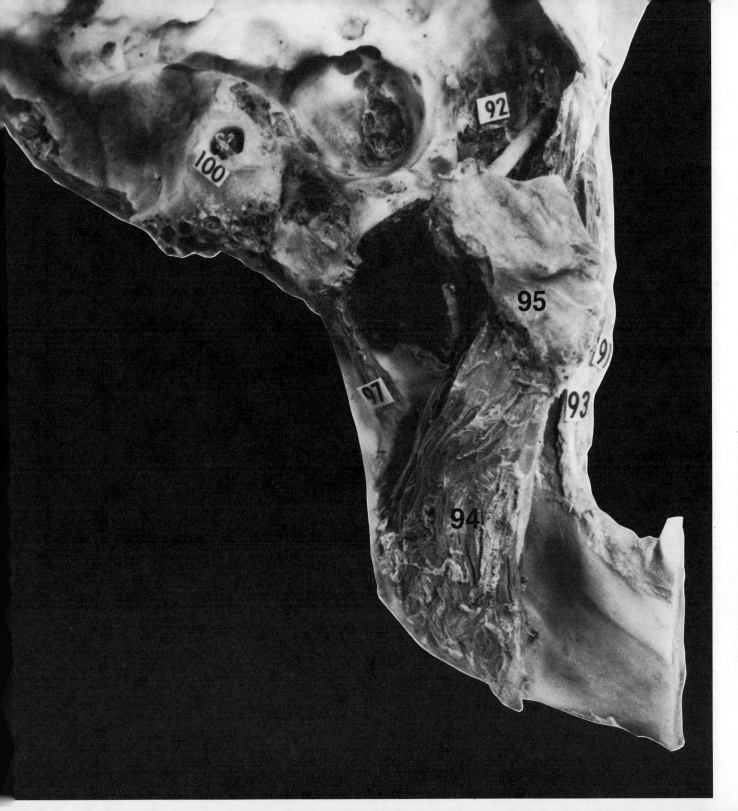

FIGURE 10–18 Medial view of mandible and base of skull. (91) superficial tendon, (92) sphenoidal origin, and (93) deep tendon of temporalis muscle; (94) medial pterygoid muscle; (95) lateral pterygoid plate of sphenoid bone; (97) sphenomandibular ligament, (100) internal auditory meatus. (Courtesy of the Anatomy Museum of the Department of Anatomy and Cell Biology, University of Pittsburgh, School of Medicine, Pittsburgh.)

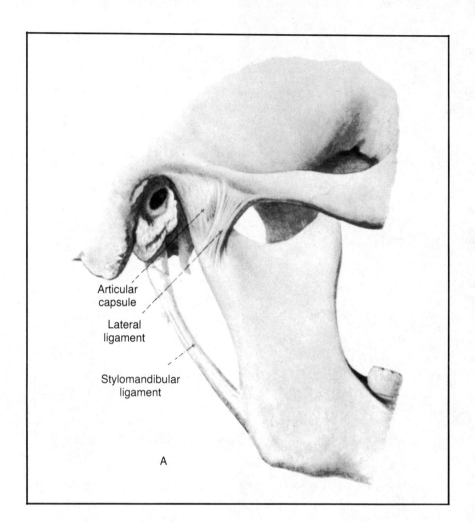

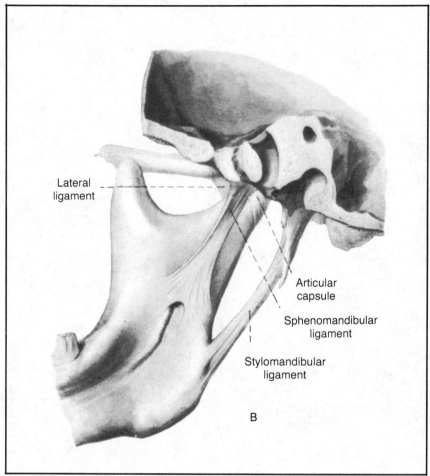

FIGURE 10–19   Right temporomandibular joint showing fibrous articular capsule and ligaments, (a) lateral aspect and (b) medial aspect. (Courtesy of W. Spalteholz and R. Spanner, *Atlas of Human Anatomy*, 16th Ed. Philadelphia: F.A. Davis Company, 1967 (English). Amsterdam: Scheltema, Holkema, and Vermeulen, 1967 (Dutch).)

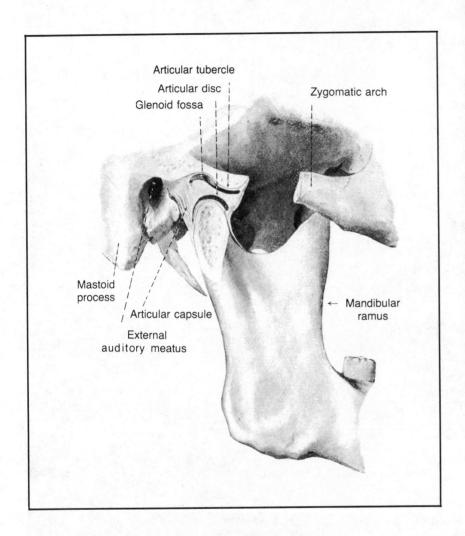

FIGURE 10–20 Longitudinal section of temporomandibular joint showing articular disc with articular surfaces slightly pulled apart. (Courtesy of W. Spalteholz and R. Spanner, *Atlas of Human Anatomy*, 16th Ed. Philadelphia: F.A. Davis Company, 1967 (English). Amsterdam: Scheltema, Holkema, and Vermeulen, 1967 (Dutch).)

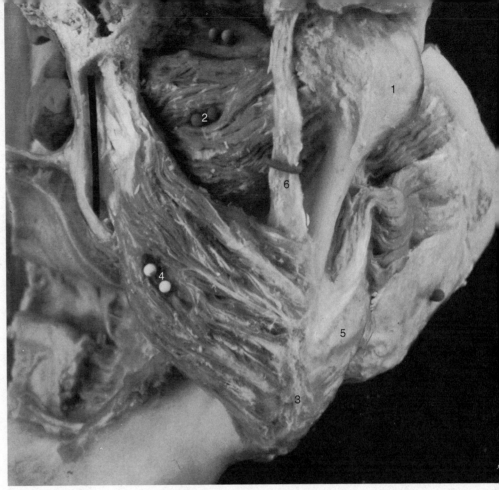

FIGURE 10–21 Capsule of (1) temporomandibular joint, viewed from behind. Note the (2) lateral pterygoid muscle and the muscular sling around the angle of the (3) mandible formed by the (4) medial pterygoid muscle and the (5) masseter. The (6) stylomandibular ligament is also shown. Courtesy of P.A. Knudsen, Royal Dental College, Aarhus, Denmark; reprinted in Bertram Kraus, Ronald Jordan, and Leonard Abrams, *Dental Anatomy and Occlusion*. Baltimore: The Williams and Wilkins Co., 1969.)

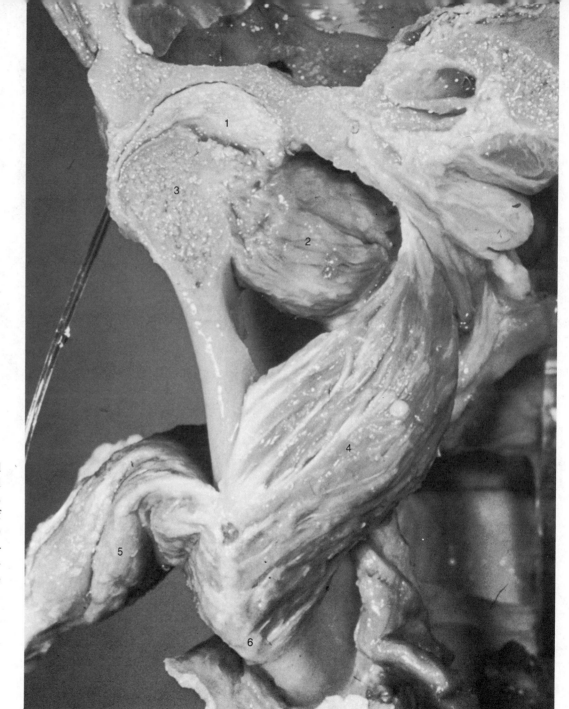

FIGURE 10–22 Right temporomandibular joint, viewed from behind. The joint has been opened by a vertical pole-to-pole section of the condyle. The (1) disc is thicker medially than laterally. The inferior portion of the (2) lateral pterygoid muscle is shown inserting into the (3) condyloid process. The (4) medial pterygoid muscle and the (5) masseter muscle (shown reflected downward) form a muscular sling around the angle of the (6) mandible. (Courtesy of P.A. Knudsen, Royal Dental College, Aarhus, Denmark; as reprinted in Bertram Kraus, Ronald Jordan, and Leonard Abrams, *Dental Anatomy and Occlusion.* Baltimore: The Williams and Wilkins Co., 1969.)

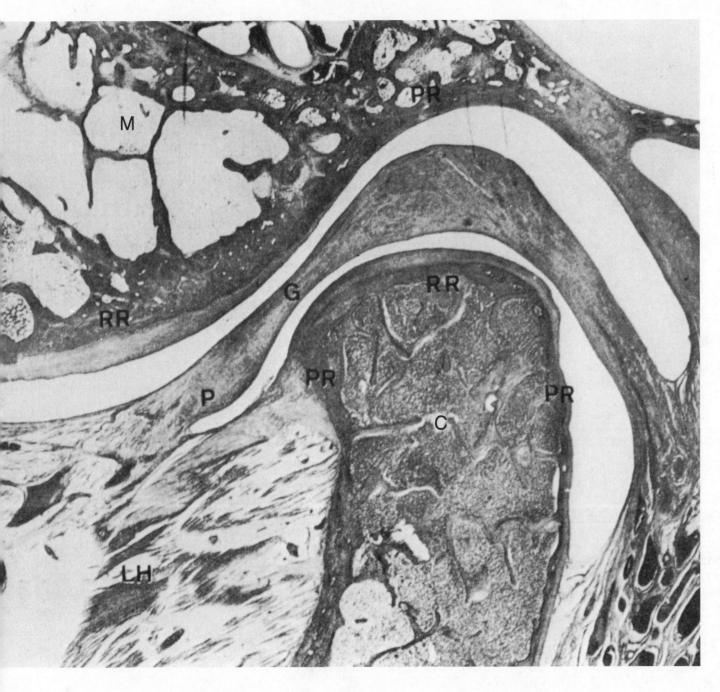

FIGURE 10–23 Sagittal section of temporomandibular joint approximately at midline. The (M) mastoid portion of the temporal bone and the (C) condyloid process are marked for areas of (PR) progressive remodelling and (RR) regressive remodelling. The disc (meniscus) is labelled on the (P) pemenisci and (G) pars gracilis menisci. (LH) fibers from the inferior head of the lateral pterygoid muscle. (Luxol fast blue and H. & E. stains.) (Courtesy of C.J. Griffin, R. Hawthorne, and R. Harris, "Anatomy and Histology of the Human Temporomandibular Joint," in Vol. 4, C.J. Griffin and R. Harris (Eds.), *The Temporomandibular Joint Syndrome: The Masticatory Apparatus of Man in Normal and Abnormal Function*, of Howard M. Myers (Series Ed.), *Monographs in Oral Science*. Basel, Switzerland: S. Karger AG, 1975, p. 16.)

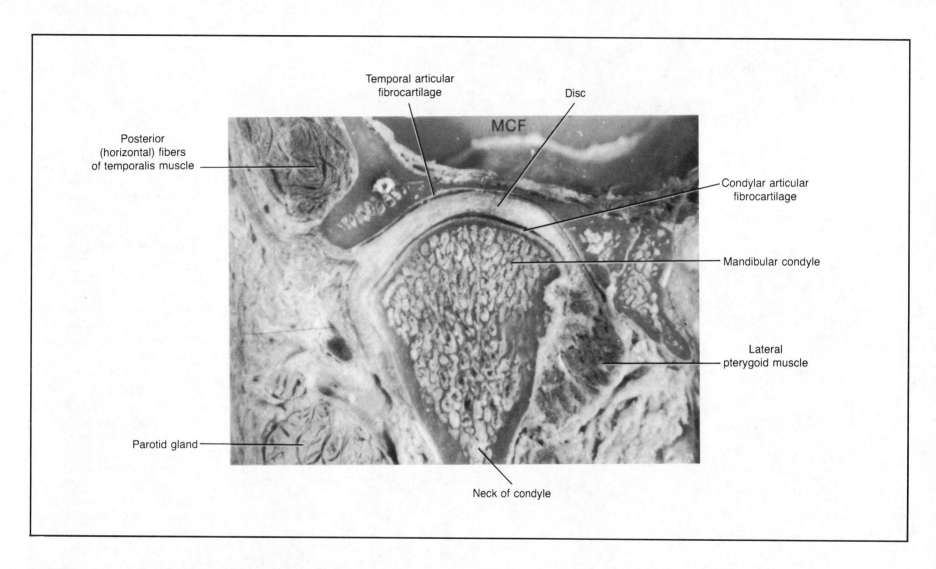

FIGURE 10–24   Coronal section of temporomandibular
joint. (Courtesy of B. Liebgott, *Anatomical Basis of Dentistry*. Philadelphia: W.B. Saunders Company, 1982.)

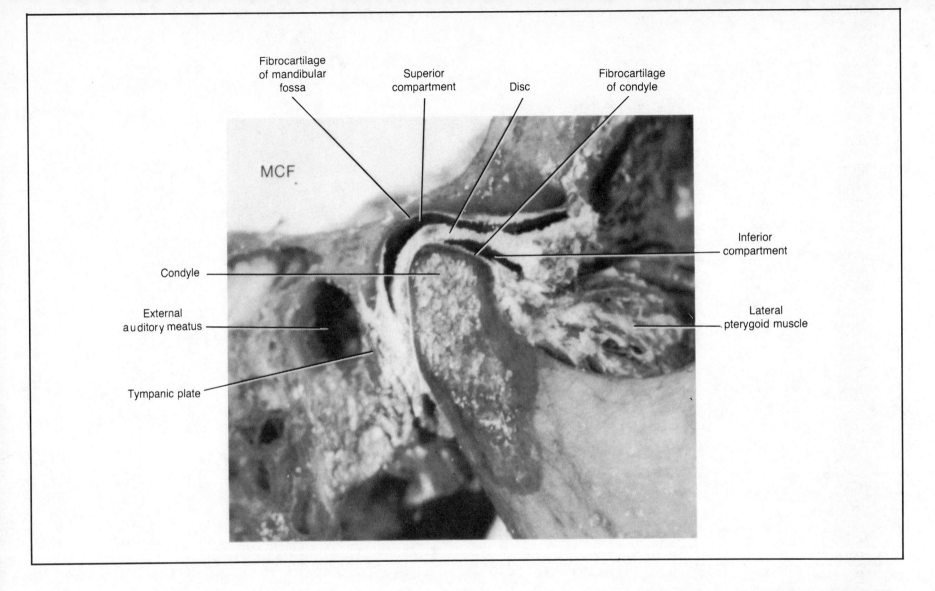

Fibrocartilage of mandibular fossa

Superior compartment

Disc

Fibrocartilage of condyle

MCF

Inferior compartment

Condyle

External auditory meatus

Lateral pterygoid muscle

Tympanic plate

FIGURE 10–25 Sagittal section of temporomandibular joint. (Courtesy of B. Liebgott, *Anatomical Basis of Dentistry.* Philadelphia: W.B. Saunders Company, 1982.)

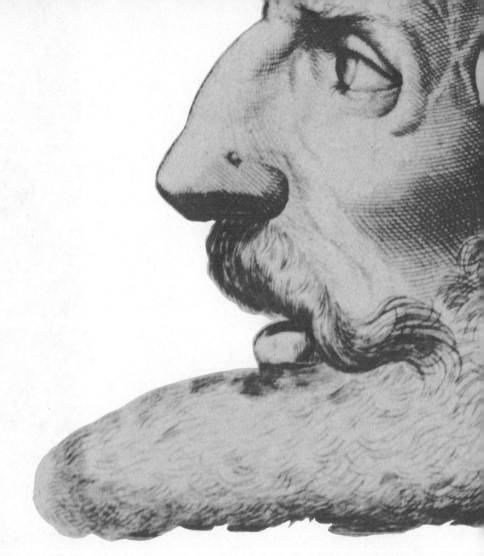

The Face

11

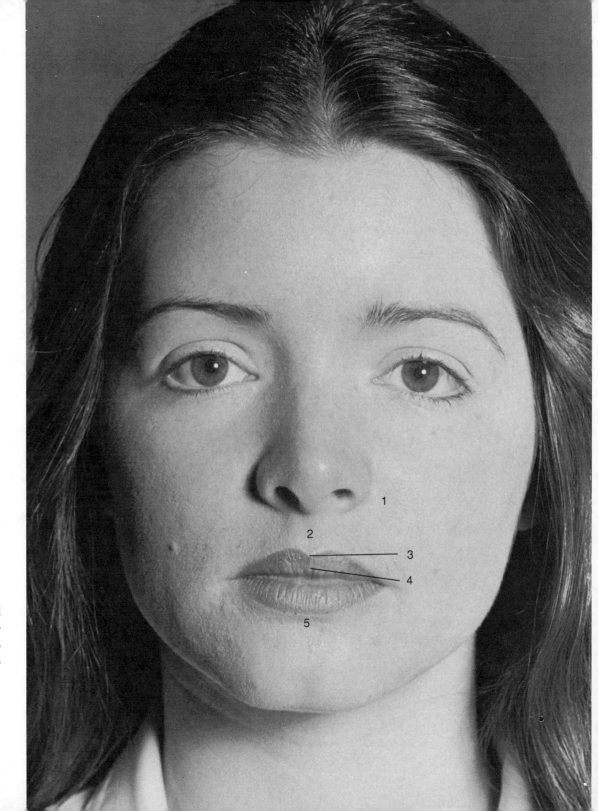

FIGURE 11–1 Adult female face illustrating external
morphologic features. (1) nasolabial groove, (2) philtrum, (3) cupids bow, (4) tubercle of upper lip,
(5) labiomental groove.

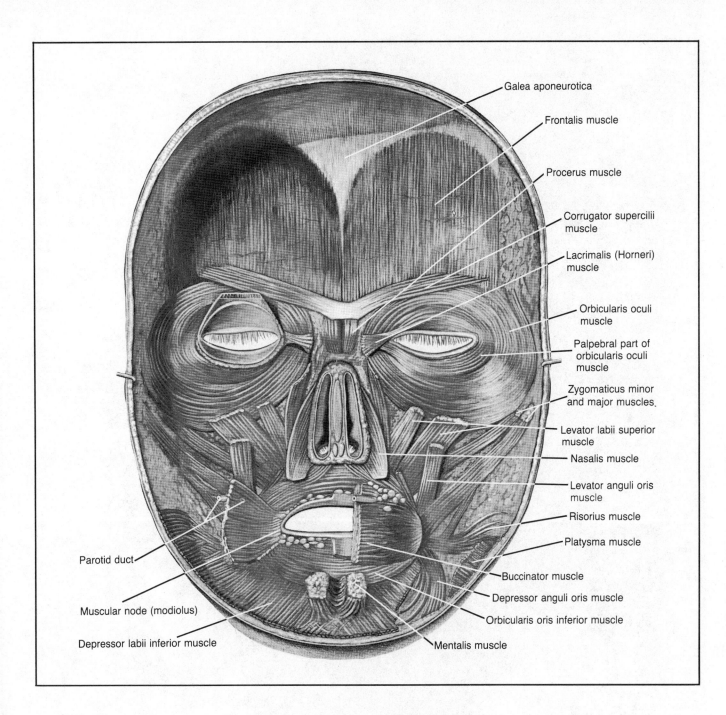

Galea aponeurotica

Frontalis muscle

Procerus muscle

Corrugator supercilii muscle

Lacrimalis (Horneri) muscle

Orbicularis oculi muscle

Palpebral part of orbicularis oculi muscle

Zygomaticus minor and major muscles.

Levator labii superior muscle

Nasalis muscle

Levator anguli oris muscle

Risorius muscle

Platysma muscle

Buccinator muscle

Depressor anguli oris muscle

Orbicularis oris inferior muscle

Parotid duct

Muscular node (modiolus)

Depressor labii inferior muscle

Mentalis muscle

FIGURE 11–2 Illustration of facial muscles removed as a mask, viewed from skeletal side. The right buccinator muscle has been reflected medially so that its superficial surface may be seen. (From Eduard Pernkopf, *Atlas of Topographical and Applied Anatomy*, 2nd Rev. Ed., Vol. 1. Munich and Baltimore: Urban and Schwarzenberg, 1980.)

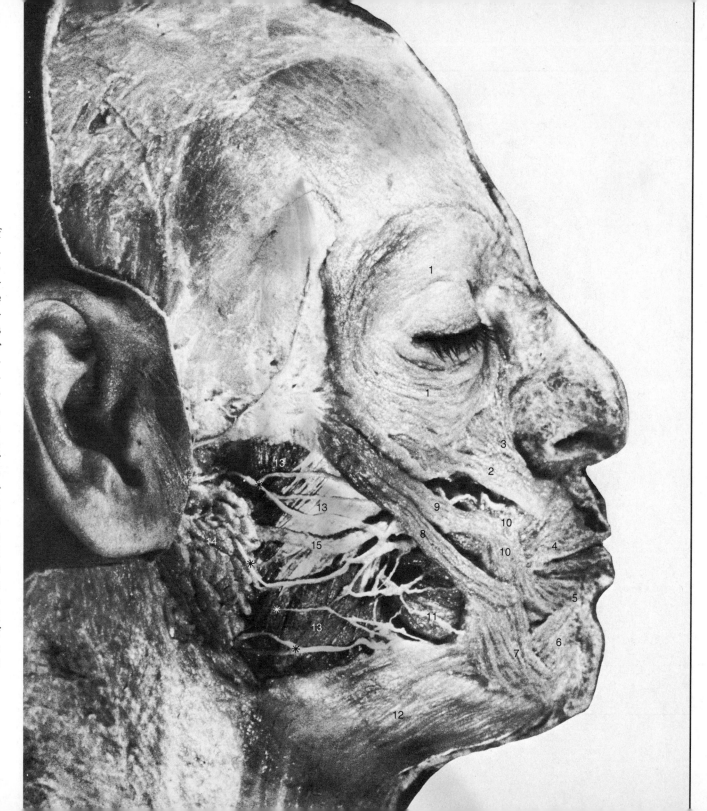

FIGURE 11–3 Dissection of face, viewed from right side. (1) orbicularis oculi muscle, (2) levator labii superior muscle, (3) levator labii alaeque nasi, (4) orbicularis oris superior muscle, (5) orbicularis oris inferior muscle, (6) depressor labii inferioris muscle, (7) depressor anguli oris, (8) zygomaticus major muscle, (9) zygomaticus minor muscle, (10) levator anguli oris muscle, (11) buccinator muscle, (12) platysma muscle (posterior fibers removed to reveal underlying structures), (13) masseter muscle, (14) parotid gland, (15) parotid duct, (*) branches of facial nerve which have pierced the parotid gland and are spreading out to innervate facial musculature. (Dissection by Nedzad Gluhbegovic, Department of Anatomy and Embryology, University of Utrecht, Utrecht, The Netherlands.)

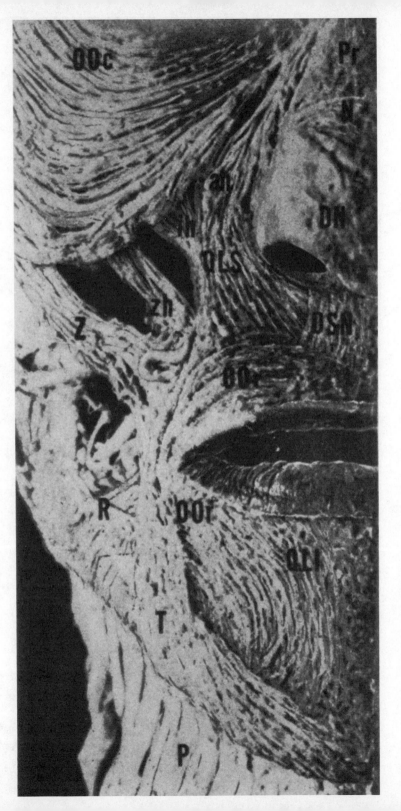

FIGURE 11-4 Dissection of right-side facial musculature, viewed from front. (OOc) orbicularis oculi muscle; (Pr) procerus muscle; (N) nasalis muscle; (DN) dilatoris naris muscle; (DSN) depressor septi nasi muscle; three parts of the (QLS) levator labii superior muscle: (ah) levator labii superior alaeque nasi, (ih) infraorbital head, (zh) zygomaticus minor muscle; (Z) zygomaticus major muscle; (OOr) orbicularis oris superior muscle; (R) risorius muscle; (OOi) orbicularis oris inferior muscle; (QLI) depressor labii inferior muscle; (T) depressor anguli oris muscle; (P) platysma muscle. (Courtesy of Alexander L. Martone, "Anatomy of Facial Expression and its Prosthetic Significance," in *Journal of Prosthetic Dentistry* 12, No. 6, 1962, p. 1027.)

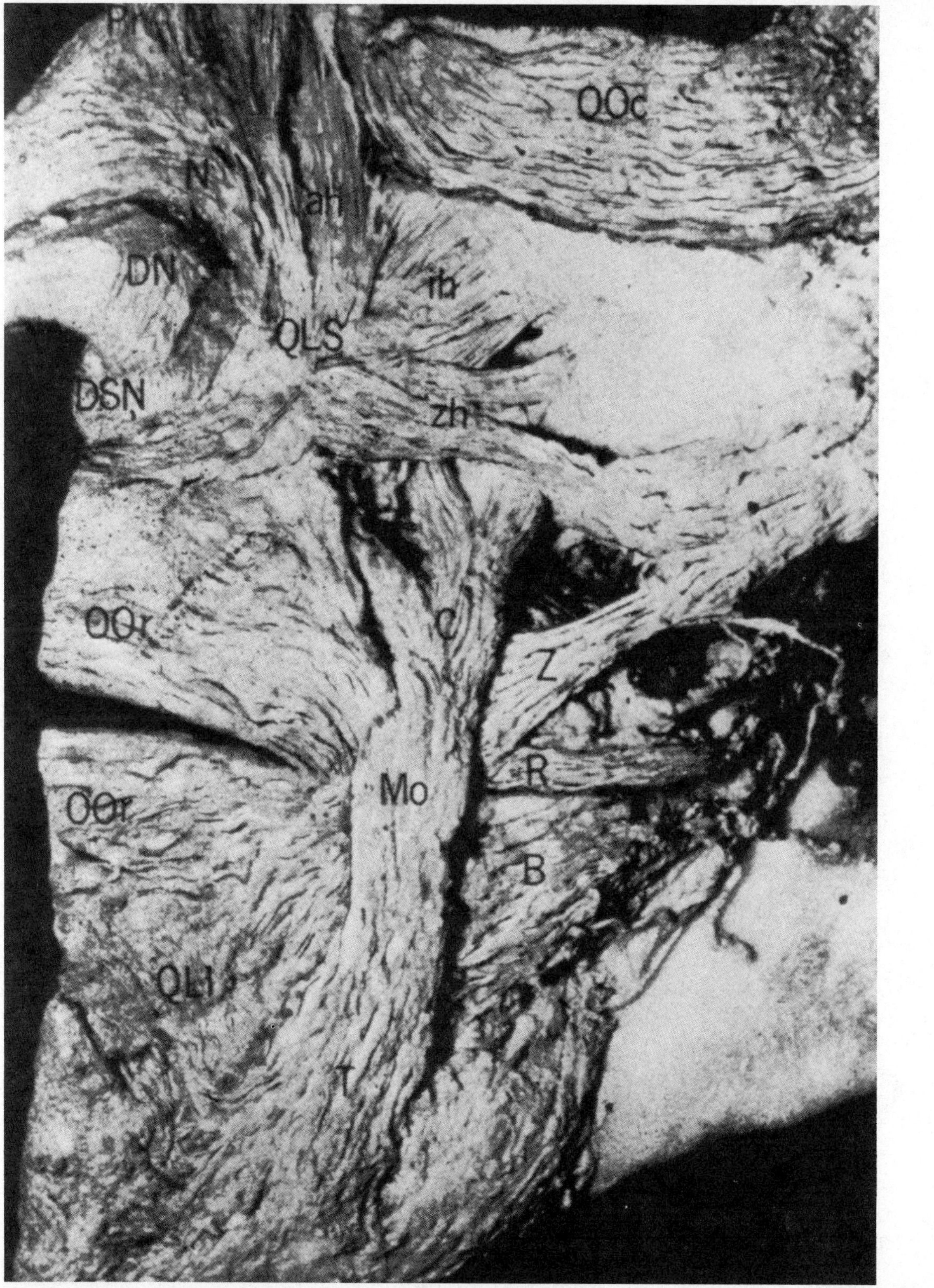

FIGURE 11–5   Dissection of facial musculature.
(OOc) orbicularis oculi muscle; (Pr) procerus muscle;
(N) nasalis muscle; (DN) dilatoris naris muscle;
(DSN) depressor septi nasi muscle; three parts of
(QLS) levator labii superior muscle: (ah) levator labii
superior alaeque nasi, (ih) infraorbital head,
(zh) zygomaticus minor muscle; (Z) zygomaticus major
muscle; (C) levator anguli oris muscle; (OOr) or-
bicularis oris; (QLI) depressor labii inferior muscle;
(Mo) modiolus; (T) depressor anguli oris muscle;
(R) risorius muscle; (B) buccinator muscle. (Courtesy of
A.L. Martone and L.F. Edwards, "Anatomy of the
Mouth and Related Structures: Part II, Musculature of
Expression," in *Journal of Prosthetic Dentistry* 12,
No. 1, 1962, p. 18.)

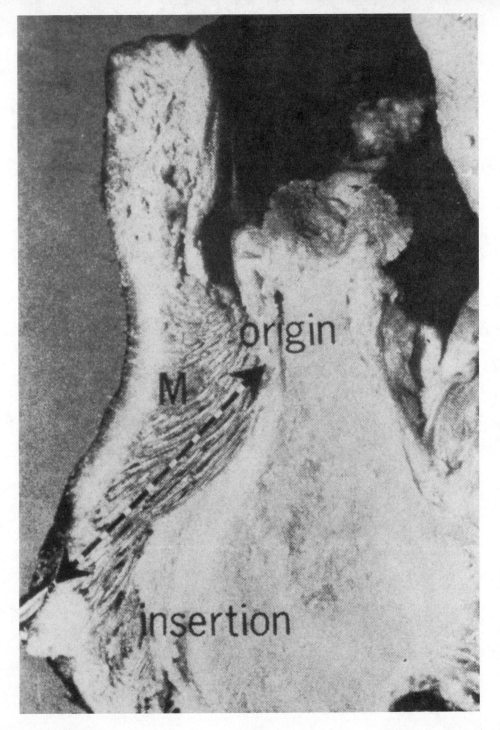

FIGURE 11–6 Sagittal section of mandible and lower lip illustrating origin and insertion of (M) mentalis muscle. The two-headed arrow approximates the direction of active muscular forces. (Courtesy of Alexander L. Martone, "Anatomy of Facial Expression and its Prosthetic Significance," in *Journal of Prosthetic Dentistry* 12, No. 6, 1962, p. 1032.)

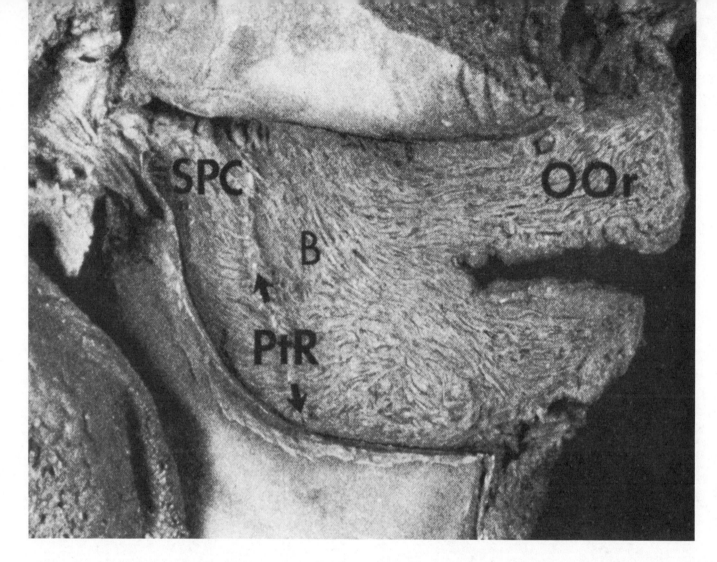

FIGURE 11–7   Lingual view of dissection showing the continuous bands of muscle fibers forming wall of pharynx, cheek, and lip. (OOr) orbicularis oris superior muscle, (B) buccinator muscle, (SPC) superior pharyngeal constrictor muscle, (PtR) pterygomandibular raphe. This preparation illustrates the difficulty in dividing the labial muscle fibers into discrete muscles. (Courtesy of Alexander L. Martone, "Anatomy of Facial Expression and its Prosthetic Significance," in *Journal of Prosthetic Dentistry* 12, No. 6, 1962, p. 1034.)

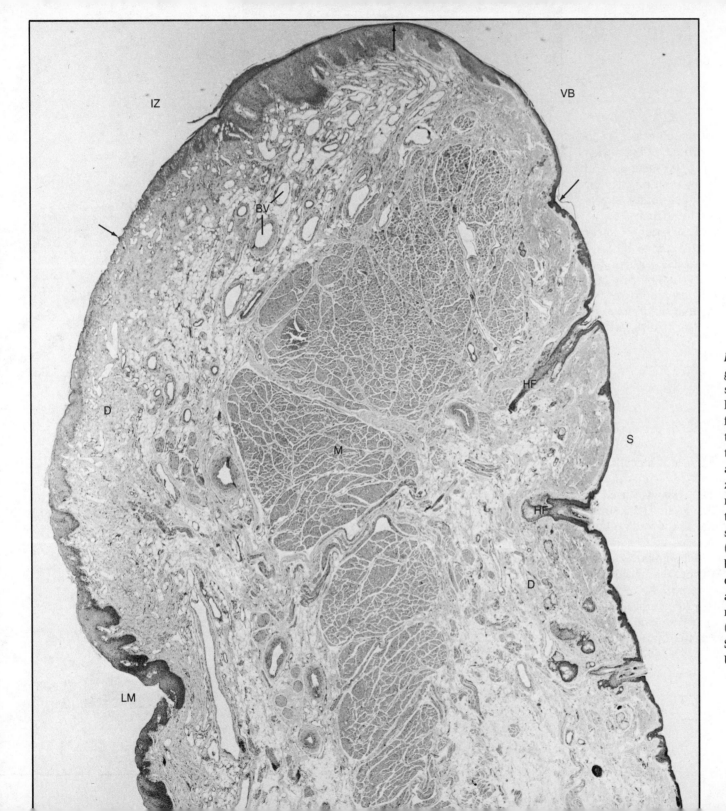

FIGURE 11–8 Photomicrograph of near-midline sagittal section of adult human lower lip. The (S) skin is separated from the (LM) labial mucosa of the oral cavity by two zones, the (VB) vermilion border and a thicker (IZ) intermediate zone. The characteristic redness of these regions is due to the numerous (BV) blood vessels below the (D) dermis. The (M) muscular tissue is probably most related to orbicularis oris inferior. (HF) hair follicles are present in the skin. (Magnification × 2.25, H & E stain.) (Courtesy of Christopher A. Squier, College of Dentistry, University of Iowa, Iowa City.)

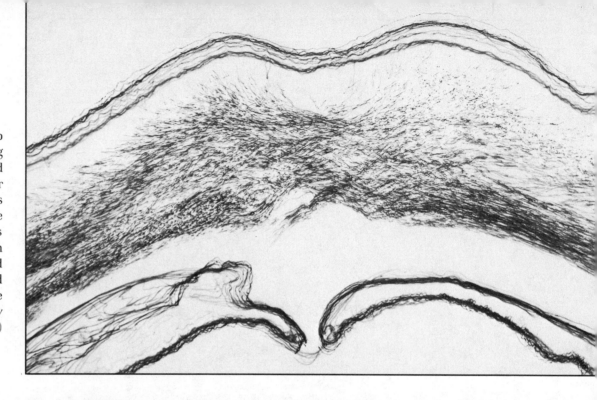

FIGURE 11-9 Horizontal reconstruction of upper lip of a human fetus. This figure was produced by cutting 15-μm sections of the lip, staining the sections, and then tracing the visible muscle fibers in every other section onto clear plastic. About 100 plastic sheets were superimposed to illustrate the patterns of the muscle fibers. In this figure note decussation of fibers in the midline and the insertion of fibers into the skin lateral to the philtrum. (Courtesy of R.A. Latham and T.G. Deaton, "The Structural Basis of the Philtrum and the Contour of the Vermilion Border: A Study of the Musculature of the Upper Lip," in *Journal of Anatomy* 121, No. 1, 1976, p. 157.)

FIGURE 11-10 Reconstruction of upper lip of a human fetus in coronal plane. The reconstruction technique explained in Figure 11-9 was also used to produce this figure. Note that (LLS) levator labii superior muscle fibers are inserting into the vermilion border. The tubercle of the lip is produced by eversion of the (PM) pars marginalis of the orbicularis oris superior muscle. Fibers from the (MN) nasalis muscle are evident at the columellar base. (Courtesy of R.A. Latham and T.G. Deaton, "The Structural Basis of the Philtrum and the Contour of the Vermilion Border: A Study of the Musculature of the Upper Lip," in *Journal of Anatomy* 121, No. 1, 1976, p. 156.)

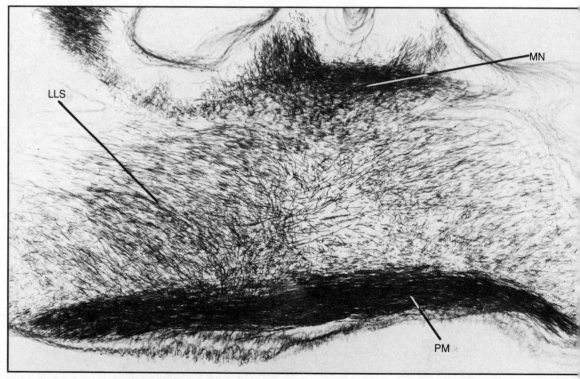

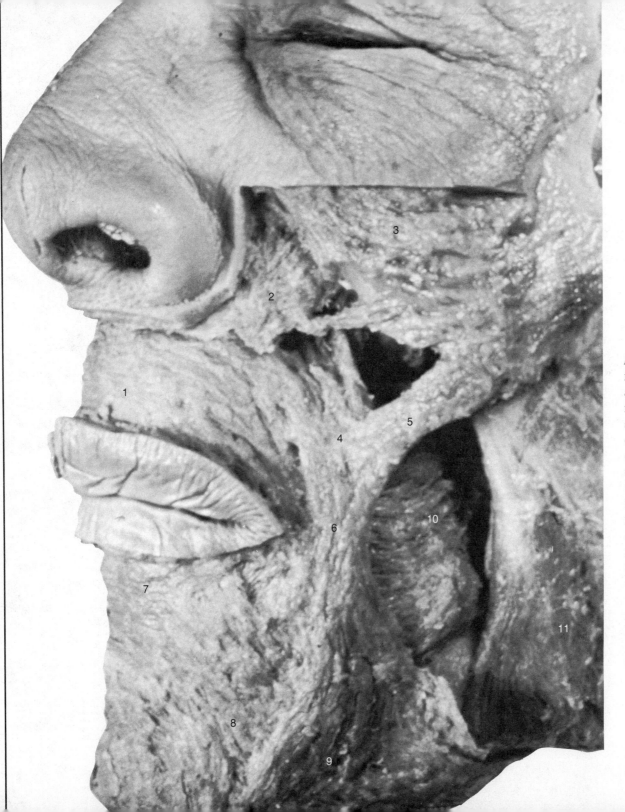

FIGURE 11–11 Dissection of right facial muscles of older adult. (1) orbicularis oris superior muscle, (2) levator labii superior muscle, (3) orbicularis oculi muscle, (4) levator aguli oris muscle, (5) zygomaticus major muscle, (6) modiolus, (7) orbicularis oris inferior muscle, (8) depressor labii inferior muscle, (9) depressor anguli oris muscle, (10) buccinator muscle, (11) masseter muscle. Note the difficulty of dividing the muscle fibers of the lower lip into discrete muscles. (Courtesy of Jesse G. Kennedy III, Department of Communicative Disorders, University of Wisconsin, Madison.)

FIGURE 11–12 Directions of muscle fibers in lower face. These figures were produced by photographing dissected cadaveric material, then tracing the muscle fibers identifiable on the photographic projection. Although it is often difficult to identify discrete labial muscles, the muscle fibers shown may be most related to (1) orbicularis oris superior muscle, (2) levator labii superior muscle, (3) orbicularis oculi muscle, (4) levator anguli oris muscle, (5) zygomatic major muscle, (6) modiolus, (7) orbicularis oris inferior muscle, (8) depressor labii inferior muscle, (9) depressor anguli oris muscle, (10) buccinator muscle, (11) masseter muscle, (12) platysma muscle, (13) risorius muscle. Specimen (A) is the same specimen photographed in Figure 11–11, age and sex unknown; (B) is the other side of this specimen, included to demonstrate typical assymmetries; (C) is an 86-year-old male; (D) is a 92-year-old male. (From J.G. Kennedy III and J.H. Abbs, "Anatomic Studies of the Perioral Motor System: Foundations for Studies in Speech Physiology," in N. Lass (Ed.), *Speech and Language: Advances in Basic Research and Practice*, Vol. 1. New York: Academic Press, 1979.)

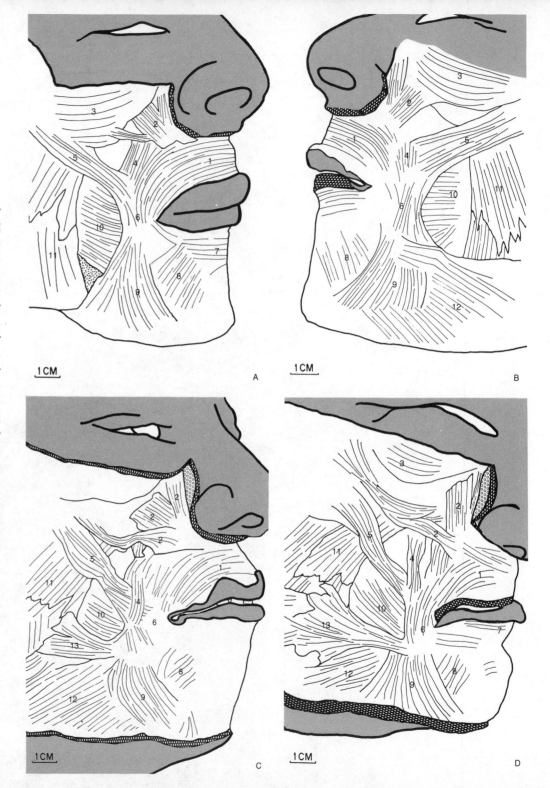

II

THE AUDITORY SYSTEM

Part II covers The Auditory System. Part II contains six chapters which describe the major portions of the auditory system, exclusive of the central auditory pathways which are described in Part III on the nervous system.

Many of the anatomical figures in this part of the Atlas are drawn from research using animals (guinea pigs, chinchillas, monkeys, and cats). The inner ears of these animals are similar in many respects to that of humans. Their contribution in research has been significant; they have enabled study of anatomy and physiology of the auditory system using techniques that are either impractical or impossible to use with human material. This point is illustrated in the electron microscopy studies. The detail in these figures was made possible because special preservation techniques and laboratory processing could be employed with fresh (physiologically vital) specimens that cannot be done on cadaver specimens. The results are visually striking micrographs which provide extraordinary structural detail.

Chapter 12, "The Temporal Bone," reviews the morphology of the temporal bone. Structural features are pointed out on human temporal bones.

Chapter 13 is "The Outer, Middle, and Inner Ear Shown Together." This short chapter orients the reader to the anatomical relationships among the three divisions of the peripheral auditory system. Specifics regarding each of these major divisions are found in subsequent chapters.

Chapter 14, "The Outer Ear," summarizes the morphologic features of the auricle and external auditory canal. The ligaments and muscles of the auricle are described, and structural landmarks are identified.

Chapter 15 discusses "The Tympanic Membrane and the Middle Ear." Detailed morphology of the tympanic membrane is presented from gross dissection, microscopic anatomy, and otoscopic views. The structure of the middle ear (tympanic) cavity is reviewed through dissections. The geometry and boundaries of the middle ear space are reviewed in detail.

Chapter 16, "The Inner Ear," is introduced via illustrations of the membranes and osseus labyrinths. This is followed by a general description of the anatomy of the cochlea which is presented via microdissection and histological sections, and supplemented by a description of the blood supply to the cochlea. (The Organ of Corti is not presented here in detail, but left to the next chapter.) The anatomy of the vestibular system (semicircular canals, maculae, and cristae ampularis) conclude the chapter. The vestibular system provides information used in regulating balance and posture; although not directly related to hearing, its anatomy is an inextricable part of the inner ear.

Chapter 17 presents details of "The Scala Media and the Organ of Corti." The presentation begins with cross-sections of the scala media to show the topographic relationships among the structures. This is followed by micrographs and illustrations of the microanatomy and ultrastructure of the organ of Corti and its hair cells.

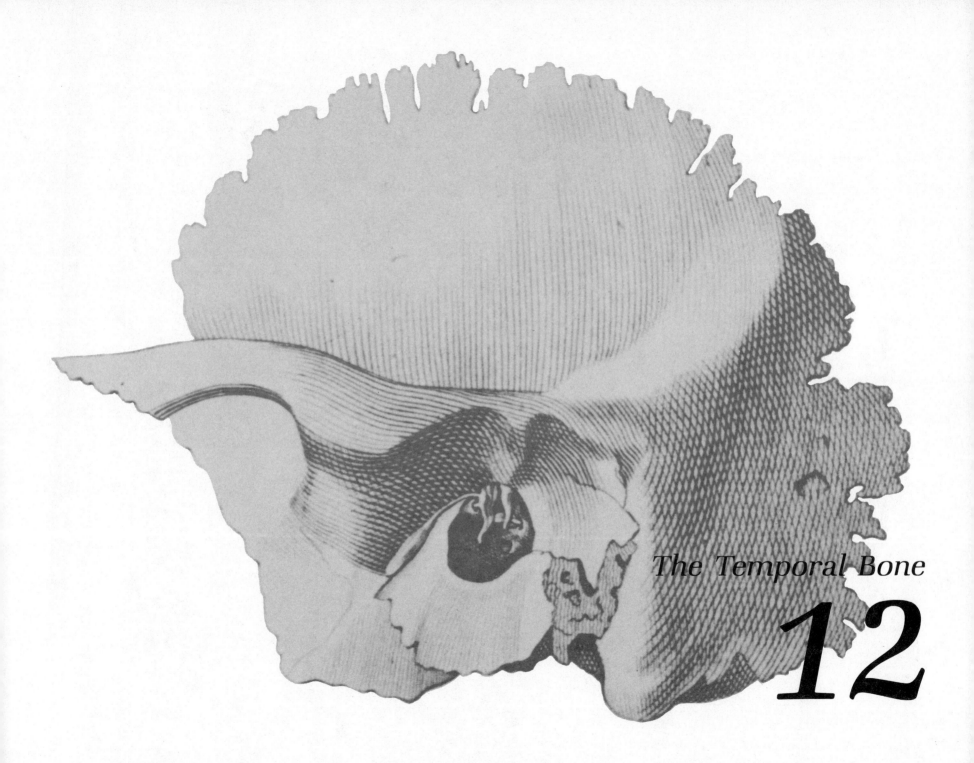

The Temporal Bone

12

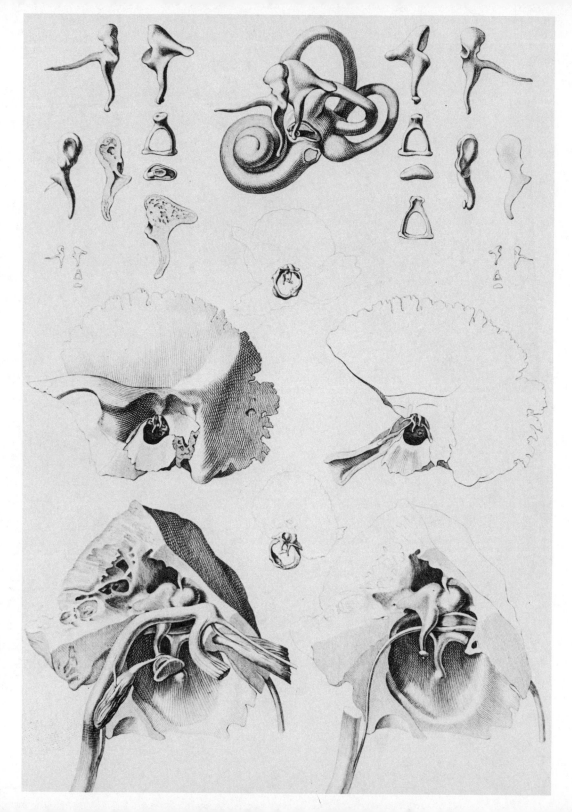

FIGURE 12–1   (From Samuel Thomas von Soemmer-
ring, *Abbildungen des Menschlichen Anges*. Frankfurt
Am. Main: Varrentrapp and Wenner, 1801.)

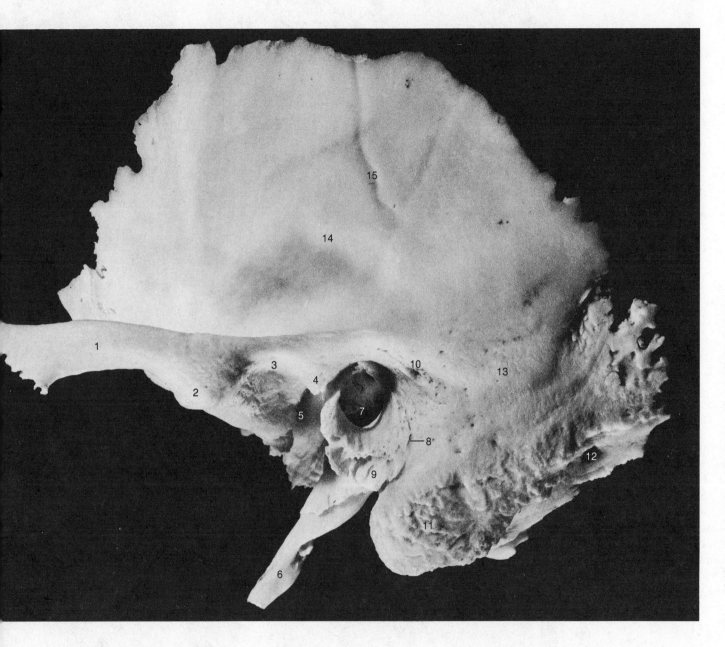

FIGURE 12–2 Lateral view of left temporal bone. (1) zygomatic process, (2) articular tubercle, (3) glenoid (mandibular) fossa, (4) postglenoid tubercle, (5) petrotympanic fissure (exit of chorda tympani nerve, a branch of 7th nerve), (6) styloid process, (7) external auditory meatus, (8) tympanomatoid fissure, (9) tympanic plate, (10) suprameatal spine, (11) mastoid process, (12) mastoid foramen, (13) temporal line, (14) temporal squama, (15) sulcus for middle temporal artery. (Photo by Paul Reimann, Department of Anatomy, University of Iowa.)

THE TEMPORAL BONE

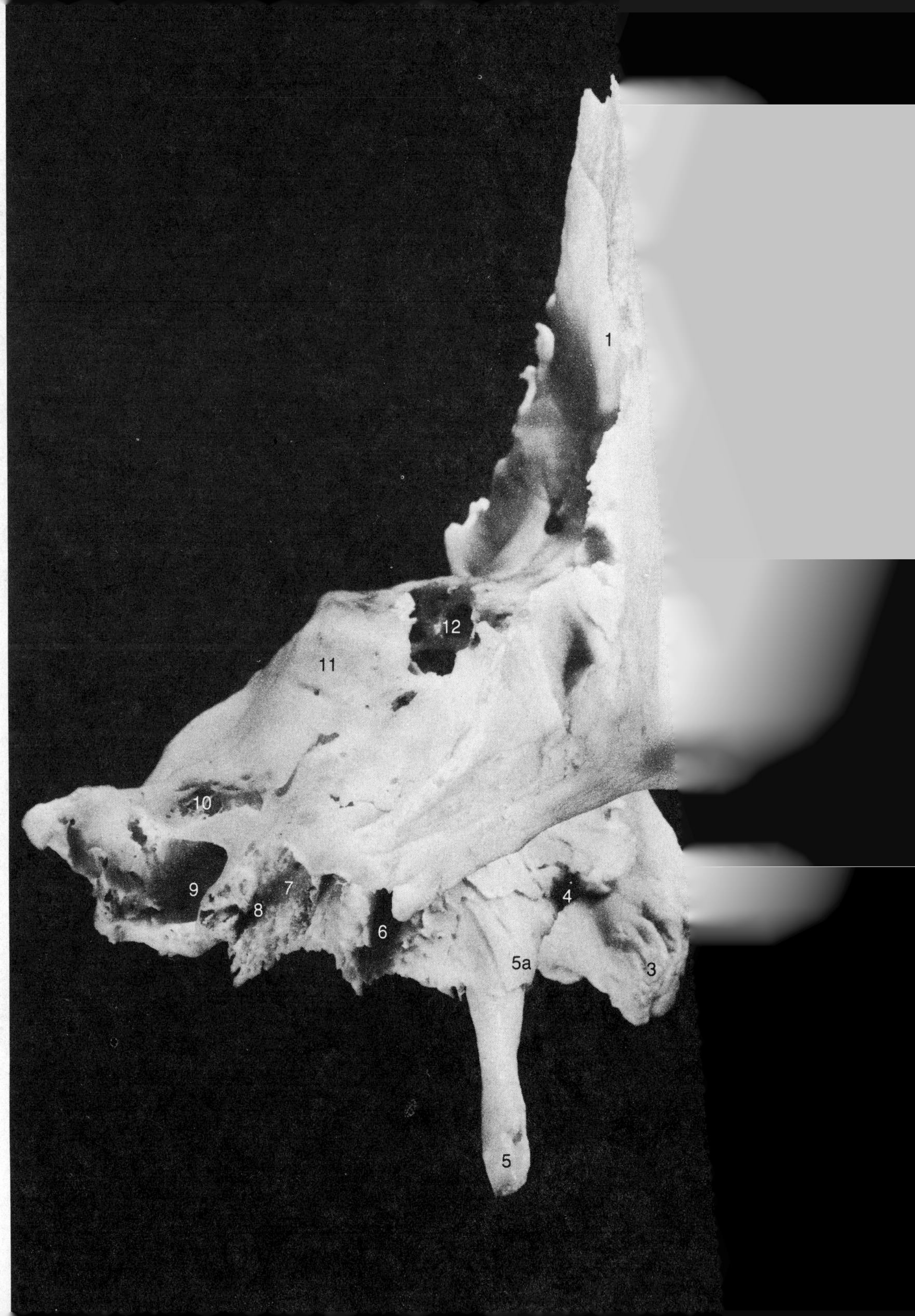

FIGURE 12–3 Anterior view of left temporal bone. (1) squama, (2) zygomatic process, (3) mastoid process, (4) part of jugular fossa, (5) styloid process, (5a) styloid sheath, (6) carotid canal, (7) semicanal for tensor tympani muscle, (8) semicanal containing osseus portion of auditory tube, (9) internal carotid foramen, (10) hiatus of facial canal (for entrance of 7th nerve), (11) arcuate eminence, (12) tegman tympani (most of which is perforated in this specimen). (Photo by Paul Reimann, Department of Anatomy, University of Iowa.)

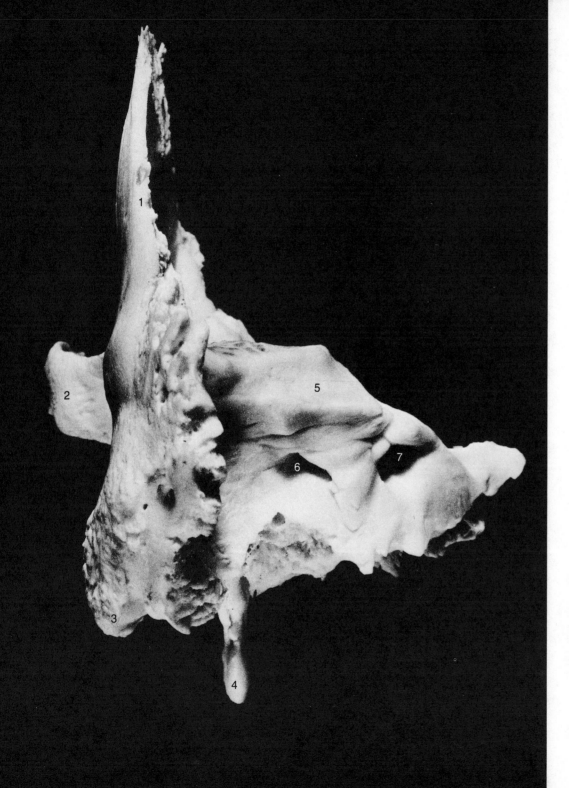

FIGURE 12–4 Posterior view of left temporal bone.
(1) temporal (external) surface of squama, (2) zygomatic process, (3) mastoid process, (4) styloid process,
(5) petrous portion, (6) external aperture of vestibular
aqueduct, (7) opening into internal auditory meatus.
(Photo by Paul Reimann, Department of Anatomy,
University of Iowa.)

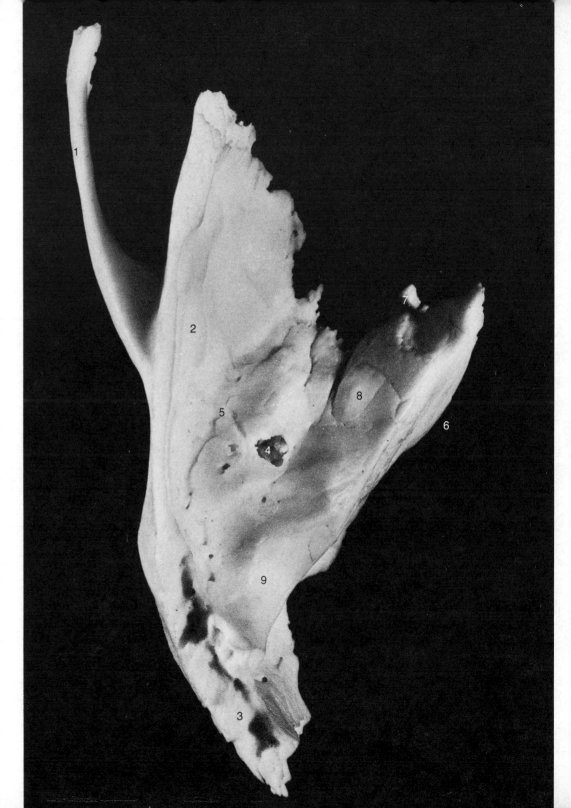

FIGURE 12–5   Superior view of left temporal bone.
(1) zygomatic process, (2) cerebral surface of squama,
(3) mastoid portion, (4) tegman tympani (there is a
perforation in the thin wall of this bone), (5) petro-
squamosal fissure, (6) petrous portion, (7) internal
auditory meatus, (8) arcuate eminence, (9) anterior
surface of the pyramid. (Photo by Paul Reimann, Department of Anatomy, University of Iowa.)

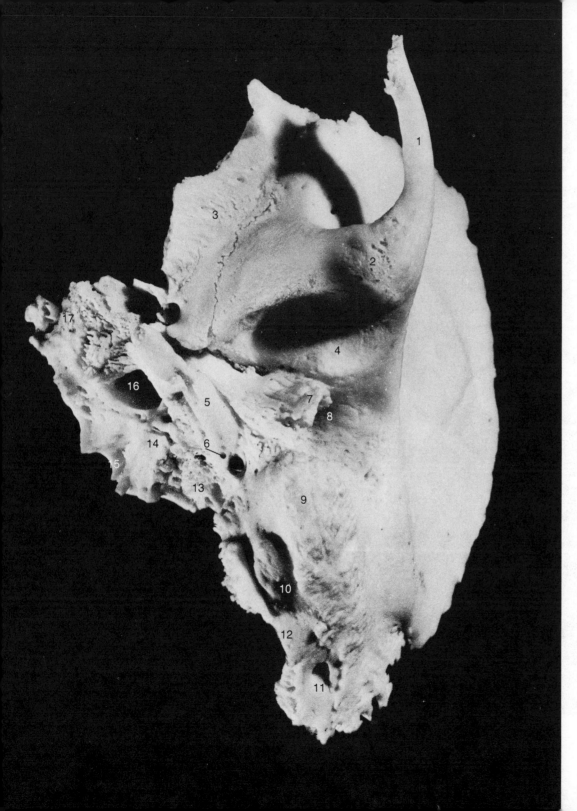

FIGURE 12–6 Inferior view (tilted slightly laterally) of left temporal bone. (1) zygomatic process, (2) articular tubercle, (3) portion of greater wing of sphenoid bone, (4) glenoid (mandibular) fossa, (5) styloid process, (6) stylomastoid foramen (exit of 7th nerve), (7) postglenoid process, (8) external auditory meatus, (9) mastoid process, (10) mastoid (digastric) notch, (11) squama, (12) sigmoid sulcus, (13) area in sigmoid sulcus and medial aspect of petrous portion dissected away, (14) jugular fossa, (15) internal auditory meatus, (16) carotid canal, (17) internal carotid foramen. (Photo by Paul Reimann, Department of Anatomy, University of Iowa.)

THE TEMPORAL BONE

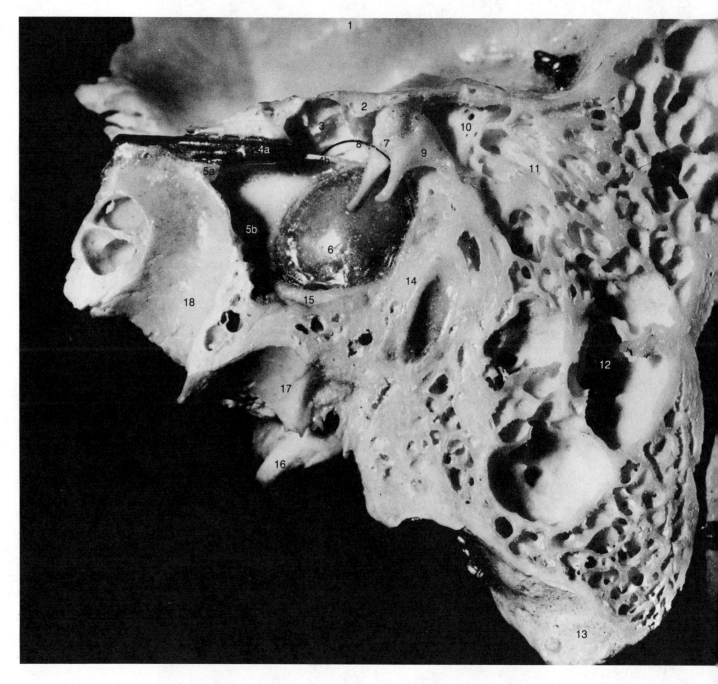

FIGURE 12–7 Dissection of temporal bone illustrating structures in tympanic and mastoid cavities. (1) middle cranial fossa, (2) tegman tympani, (3) epitympanic recess, (4a) tensor tympani muscle and its (4b) tendon, (5a) osseus portion of auditory (Eustachian) tube (partially dissected), (5b) osteum of auditory tube, (6) tympanic membrane, (7) malleus, (8) chorda tympani nerve (branch of 7th nerve), (9) incus, (10) epitympanic recess, (11) aditus to tympanic cavity, (12) mastoid air cells, (13) mastoid process, (14) facial canal in medial wall of tympanic cavity, (15) floor of tympanic cavity, (16) styloid process, (17) jugular foramen, (18) carotid canal. (Photo by Paul Reimann, Department of Anatomy, University of Iowa.)

FIGURE 12–8 Dissection of temporal bone showing structures in middle, posterior, and anterior walls of tympanic cavity. (1) petrous portion, (2) internal auditory meatus, (3) boney labyrinth of cochlea, (4) carotid canal, (5) portion of jugular fossa, (6) promontory, (7) oval window, (8) round window niche, (9) head of stapes, (10) prominence of lateral semicircular canal, (11) prominence of facial canal, (12) stapedius muscle tendon attaching to head of stapes, (13) pyramidal process, (14) stylomastoid foramen, (15) mastoid air cells. (N) bristle represents glossopharyngeal nerve fibers (9th nerve) forming tympanic plexus in mucosa overlaying the (6) promontory, giving branches to the sympathetic nerve plexus of the carotid artery in the (4) carotid canal and passing across the superior surface of the apex of the petrous portion in the form of the lesser and greater superior petorosal nerves. (Photo by Paul Reimann, Department of Anatomy, University of Iowa.)

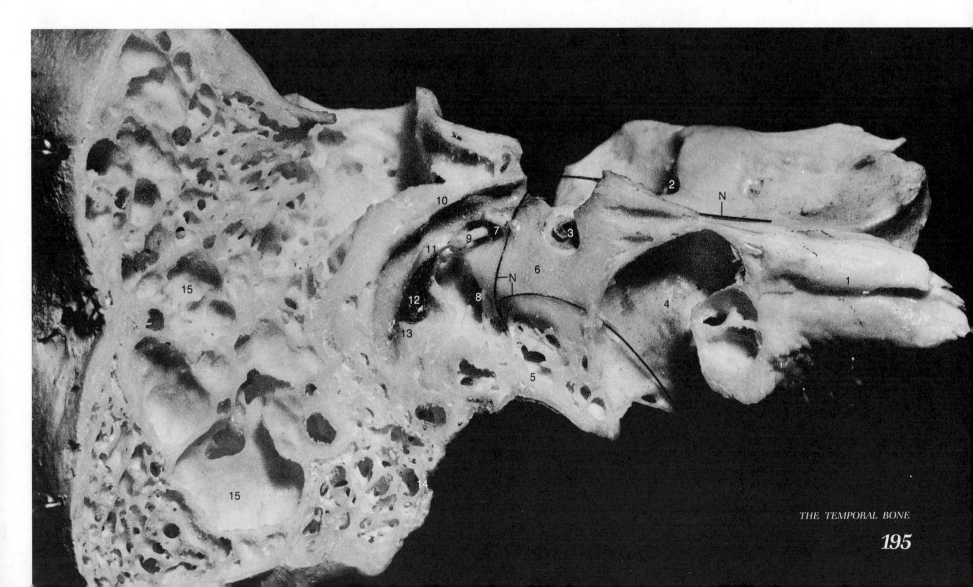

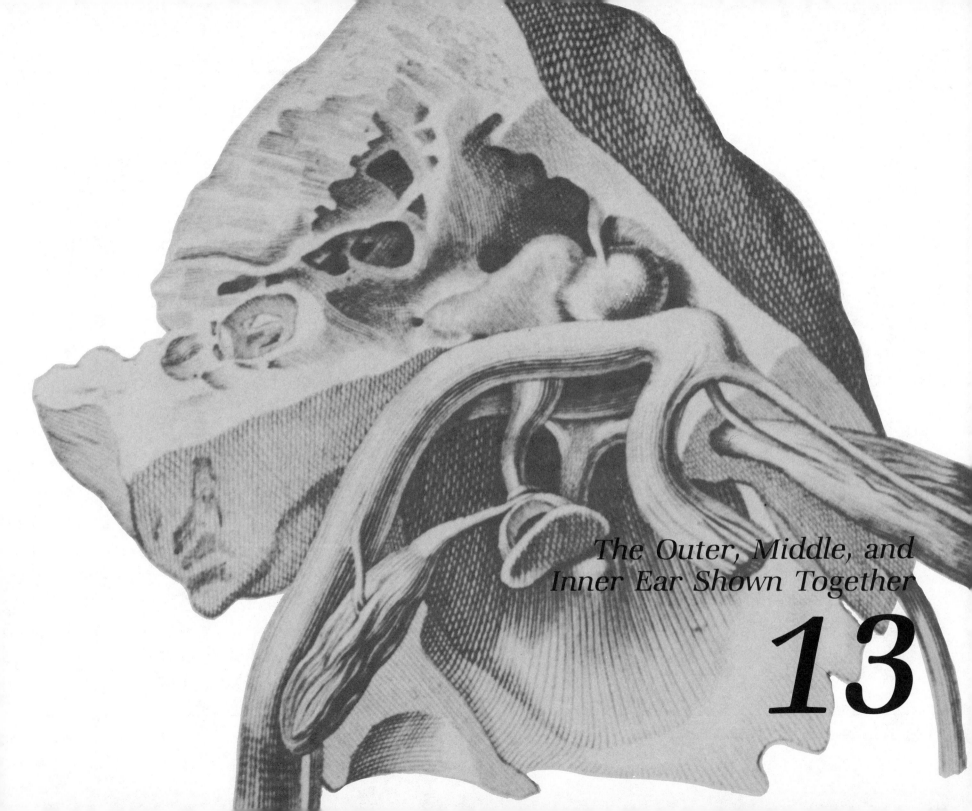

The Outer, Middle, and
Inner Ear Shown Together

13

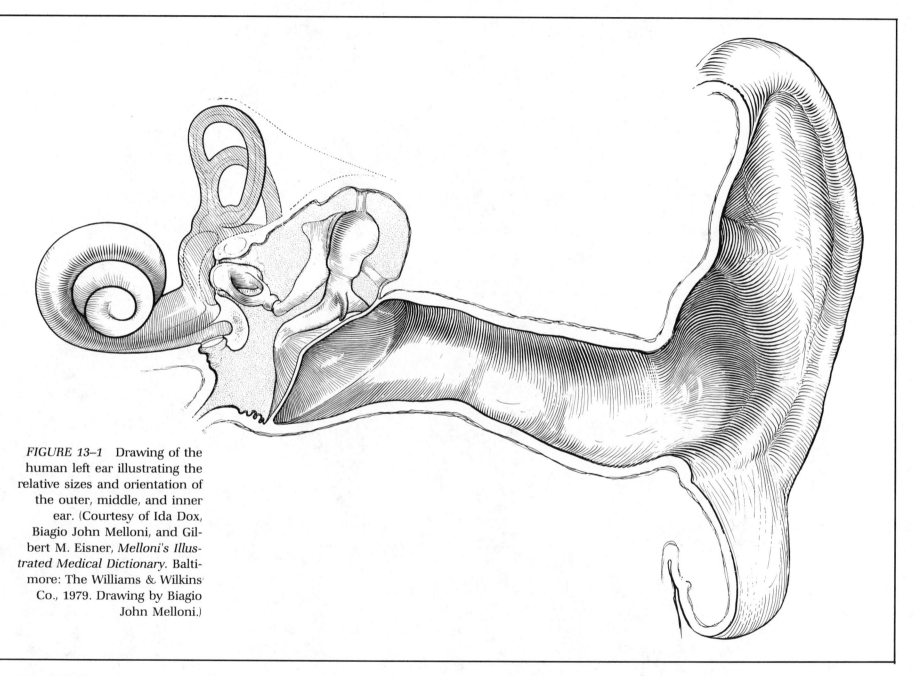

FIGURE 13–1 Drawing of the human left ear illustrating the relative sizes and orientation of the outer, middle, and inner ear. (Courtesy of Ida Dox, Biagio John Melloni, and Gilbert M. Eisner, *Melloni's Illustrated Medical Dictionary*. Baltimore: The Williams & Wilkins Co., 1979. Drawing by Biagio John Melloni.)

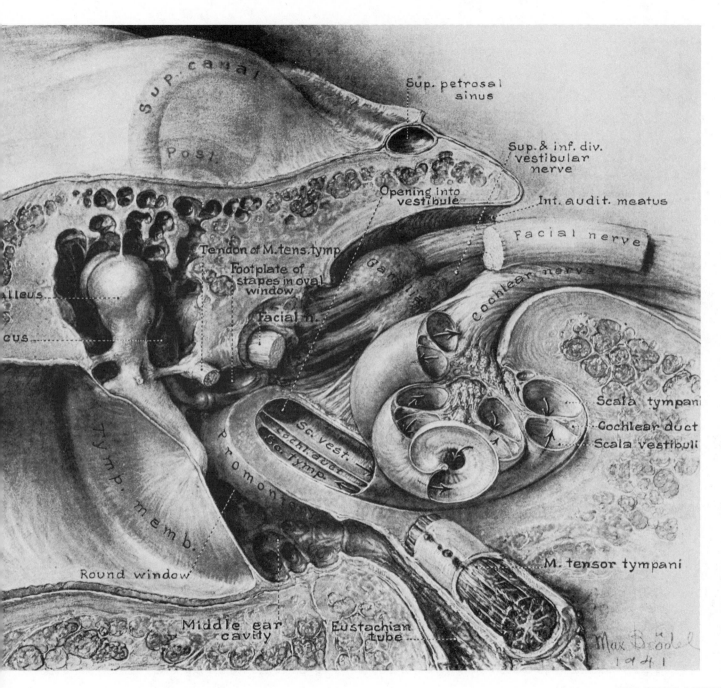

FIGURE 13–2 Classic Drawing of internal, middle, and external ear by Max Brödel. (Courtesy of W.B. Saunders Company. Max Brödel, with P. Malone, S. Guild, and S. Crowe, *Three Unpublished Drawings of the Anatomy of the Human Ear.* Philadelphia, 1946.)

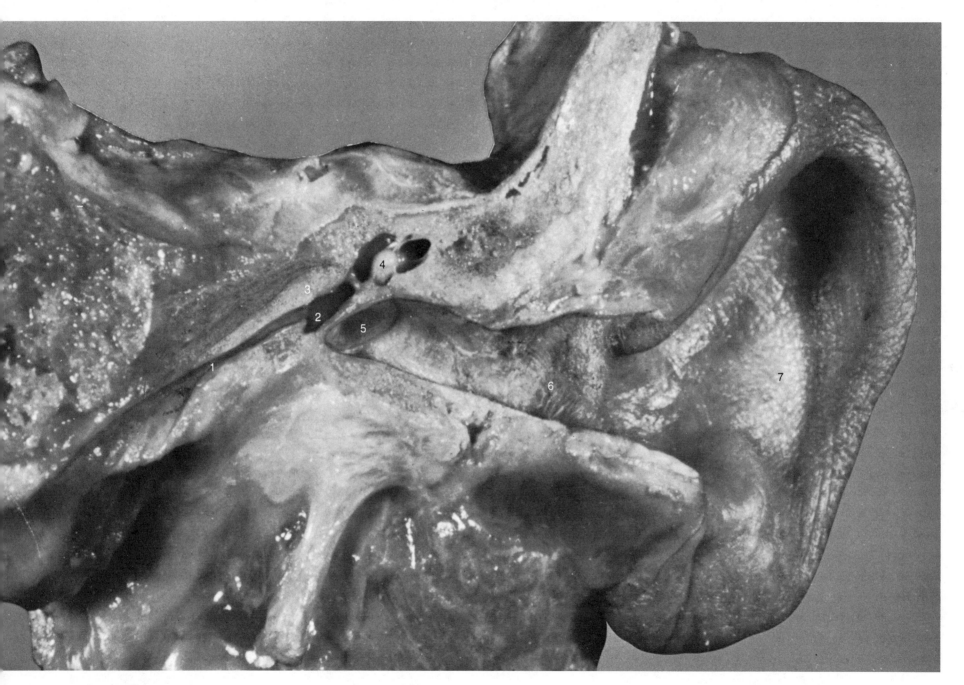

FIGURE 13–3 Anterior view of temporal bone sectioned in coronal plane. (1) auditory tube, (2) tympanic cavity, (3) tensor tympany, (4) malleus, (5) tympanic membrane, (6) external auditory meatus, (7) auricle. (Courtesy of Chihiro Yokochi and Johannes W. Rohen, *Photographic Anatomy of the Human Body*, 2nd Ed. Tokyo: Igaku-Shoin, Ltd., 1978.)

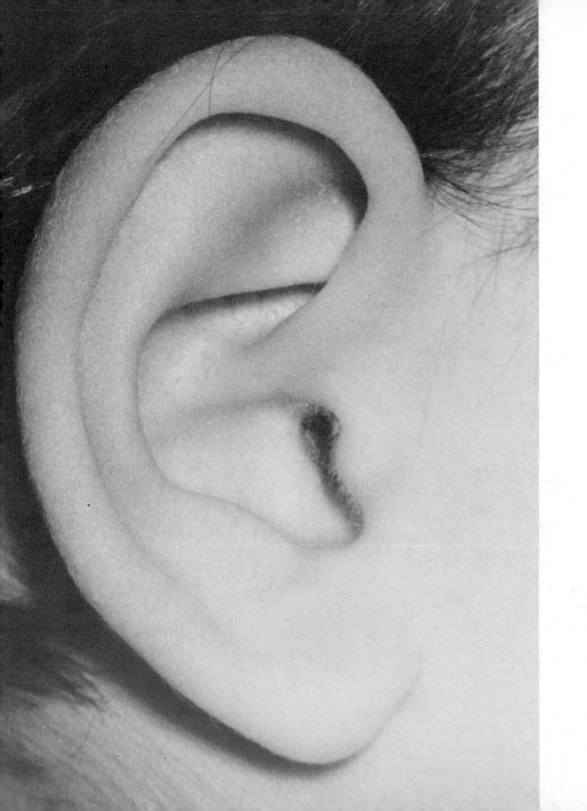

The Outer Ear

14

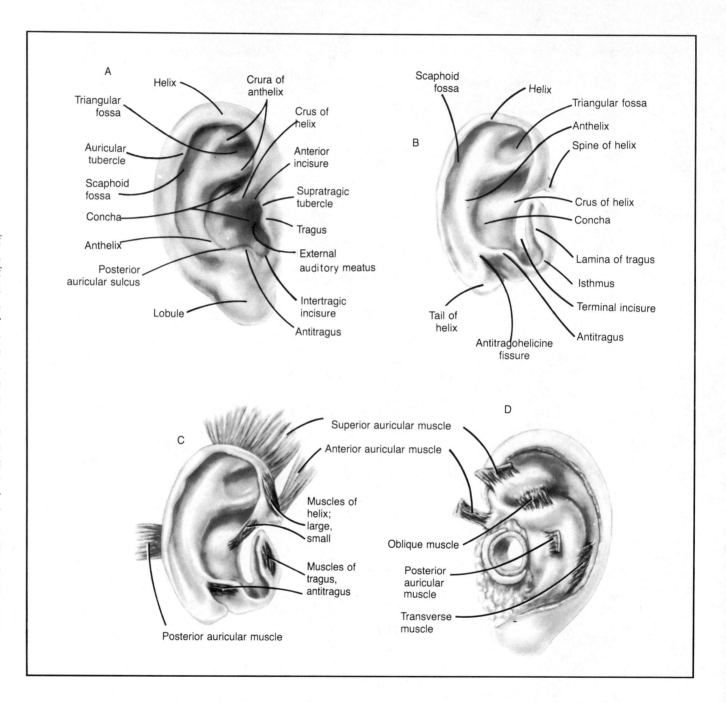

FIGURE 14–1 Drawings of auricle, auricular cartilages, and muscles. (A) lateral view of the auricle, or pinna, (B) lateral view of the auricular cartilages, (C) lateral view of the auricular cartilages with muscles attached, (D) medial view of the auricular cartilage with muscles attached. There are three extrinsic auricular muscles: the posterior, superior, and anterior auricular muscles. The other six muscles in the figure are intrinsic auricular muscles; however, they are poorly represented in the human ear and, when present vary greatly in degree of development. (Courtesy of Barry J. Anson and James A. Donaldson, *Surgical Anatomy of the Temporal Bone*, 3rd Ed. Philadelphia: W. B. Saunders Company, 1981.)

A

Helix

Triangular fossa

Auricular tubercle

Scaphoid fossa

Concha

Anthelix

Posterior auricular sulcus

Lobule

Crura of anthelix

Crus of helix

Anterior incisure

Supratragic tubercle

Tragus

External auditory meatus

Intertragic incisure

Antitragus

B

Scaphoid fossa

Helix

Triangular fossa

Anthelix

Spine of helix

Crus of helix

Concha

Lamina of tragus

Isthmus

Terminal incisure

Antitragus

Tail of helix

Antitragohelicine fissure

C

Superior auricular muscle

Anterior auricular muscle

Muscles of helix; large, small

Muscles of tragus, antitragus

Posterior auricular muscle

D

Oblique muscle

Posterior auricular muscle

Transverse muscle

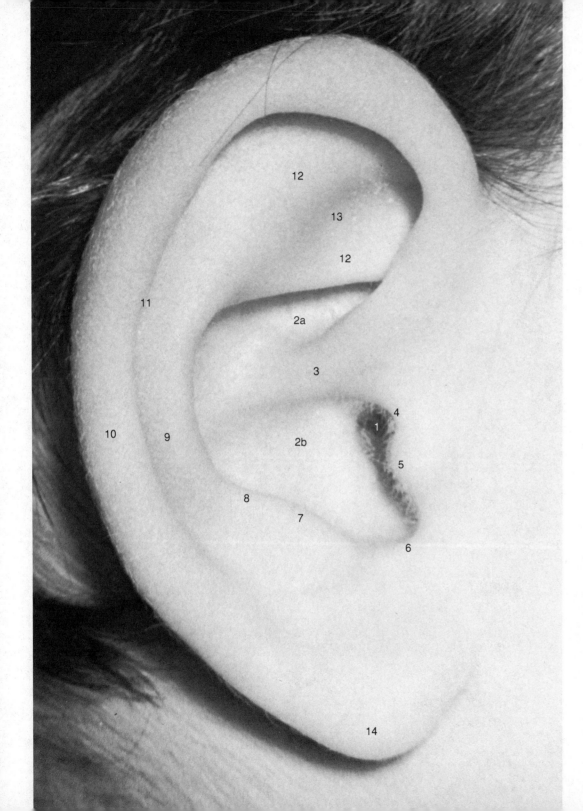

FIGURE 14–2 Right auricle of a young child. (1) entrance into external auditory meatus (note small downy hairs on skin surrounding this orifice), (2a) cymba conchae, (2b) cavum conchae, (3) crus of helix, (4) anterior incisure, (5) tragus, (6) intertragic incisure, (7) antitragus, (8) posterior auricular sulcus, (9) anthelix, (10) helix, (11) scaphoid fossa, (12) crura of anthelix, (13) triangular fossa, (14) lobule.

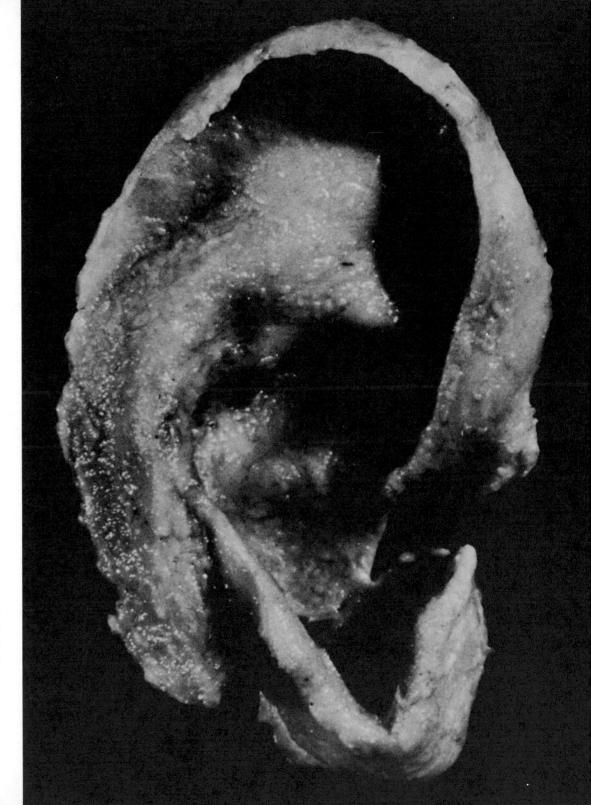

FIGURE 14–3   Photograph of cartilage removed from human auricle (pinna). (Courtesy of Chihiro Yokochi and Johannes W. Rohen, *Photographic Anatomy of the Human Body*, 2nd Ed. Tokyo: Igaku-Shoin, Ltd., 1978.)

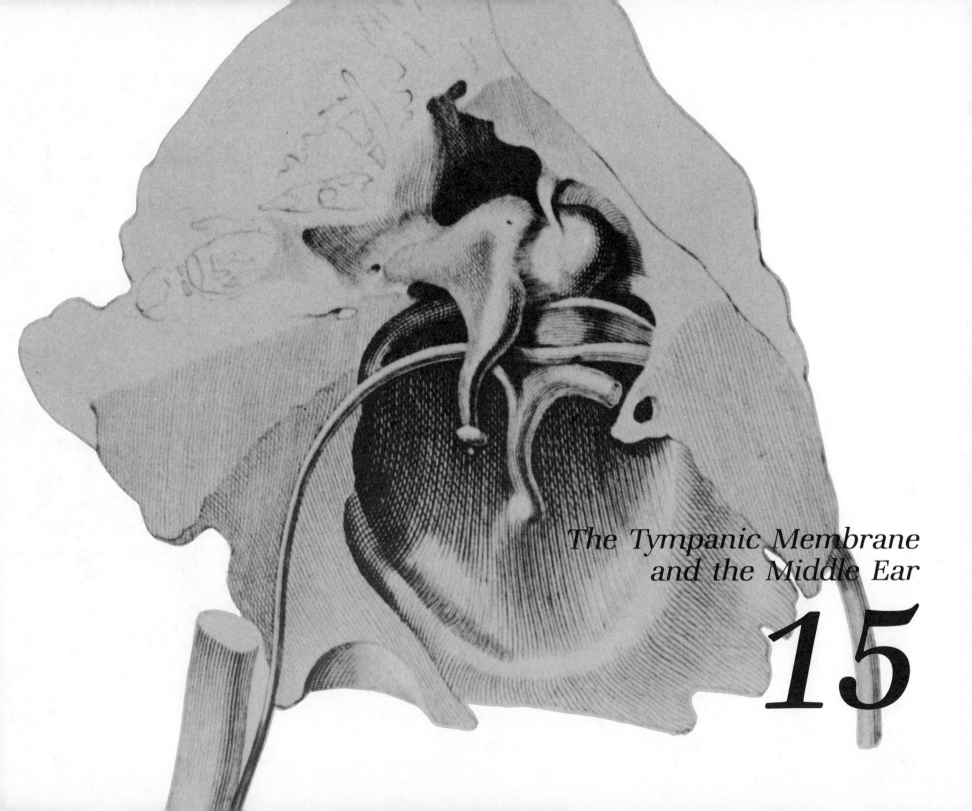

The Tympanic Membrane
and the Middle Ear

15

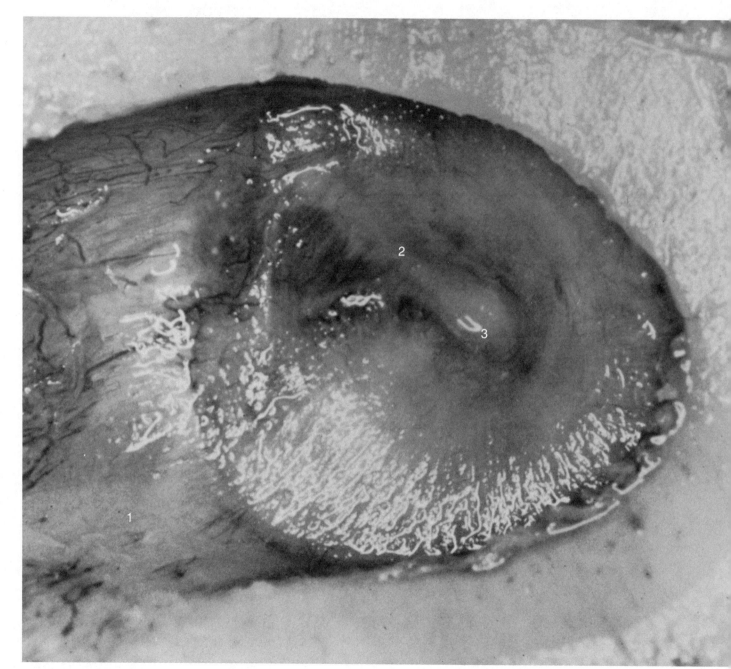

FIGURE 15–1 Part of (1) external auditory meatus has been removed in this dissection to provide a view of the tympanic membrane. The (2) manubrium of the malleus is visible through the translucent tympanic membrane. The (3) umbo is at the center of the tympanic membrane. (Courtesy of Chihiro Yokochi and Johannes W. Rohen, *Photographic Anatomy of Human Body*, 2nd Ed. Tokyo: Igaku-Shoin, Ltd., 1978.)

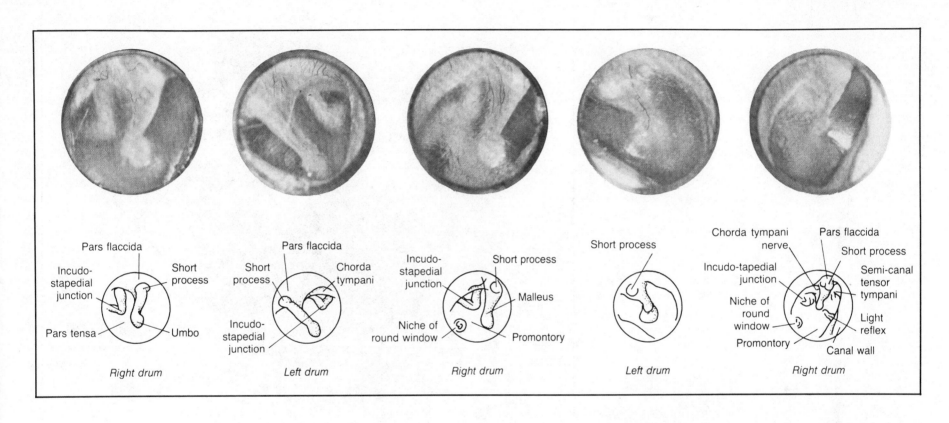

Pars flaccida

Incudo-stapedial junction

Short process

Pars tensa

Umbo

Right drum

Short process

Pars flaccida

Chorda tympani

Incudo-stapedial junction

Left drum

Incudo-stapedial junction

Short process

Malleus

Niche of round window

Promontory

Right drum

Short process

Left drum

Chorda tympani nerve

Pars flaccida

Incudo-tapedial junction

Short process

Semi-canal tensor tympani

Niche of round window

Light reflex

Promontory

Canal wall

Right drum

FIGURE 15–2 Otoscopic view of tympanic membrane. The line drawings mark structures which can be identified in the photograph above. Note the clarity with which structures can be seen through the translucent tympanic membrane. (Photos by Richard A. Buckingham, as shown in "Some Pathologic Conditions of the Eye, Ear, and Throat," courtesy of Abbott Laboratories, Chicago.)

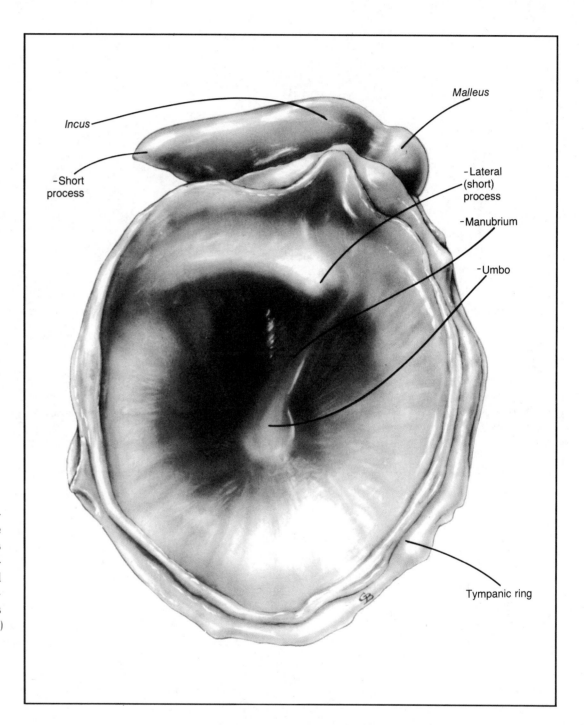

FIGURE 15–3 Tympanic ring and tympanic membrane from a specimen excised in one piece with the auditory ossicles from an unembalmed specimen. This figure shows the lateral aspect viewed from the external auditory meatus. (Courtesy of Barry J. Anson and James A. Donaldson, *Surgical Anatomy of the Temporal Bone*, 3rd Ed. Philadelphia: W.B. Saunders Company, 1981.)

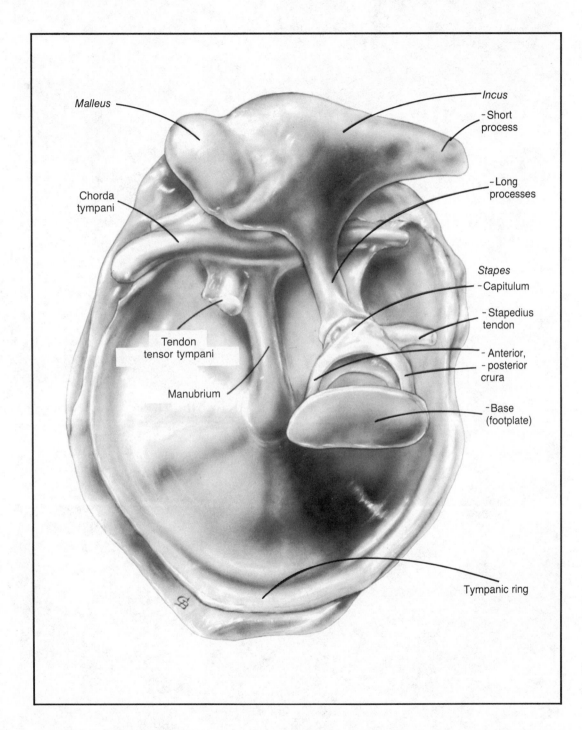

Malleus

Incus
- Short process

Chorda tympani

- Long processes

Stapes
- Capitulum

Tendon tensor tympani

- Stapedius tendon

- Anterior,
- posterior crura

Manubrium

- Base (footplate)

Tympanic ring

FIGURE 15–4 The same preparation illustrated in figure 15–2, except viewed from the medial aspect. (Courtesy of Barry J. Anson and James A. Donaldson, *Surgical Anatomy of the Temporal Bone*, 3rd Ed. Philadelphia: W.B. Saunders Company, 1981.)

FIGURE 15–5   The insert is a dissected human tympanic membrane. (A) scanning electron micrograph showing the irregularly arranged elastic and collagen fibers in the pars flaccida. (B) transmission electron micrograph of the pars tensa. The major component of the pars tensa is formed by the elastic (square) fibers. The collagen fibers are round. In (C) the fiber arrangement of the pars tensa is illustrated with a scanning electron micrograph. (Courtesy of David J. Lim, "Scanning Electron Microscopic Morphology of the Ear," in Donald A. Schumrick and Michael M. Paprella (Eds.), *Otolaryngology*, Vol. 1, 2nd Ed. Philadelphia: W.B. Saunders Company, 1980.)

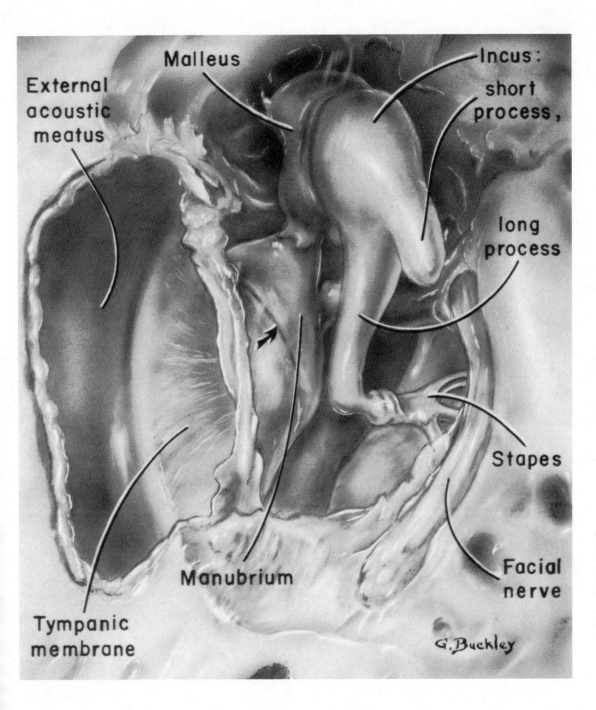

External
acoustic
meatus

Malleus

Incus:
short
process,

long
process

Stapes

Facial
nerve

Manubrium

Tympanic
membrane

G.Buckley

FIGURE 15–6 Dissection of an unembalmed specimen showing the external auditory meatus, tympanic membrane, and tympanic cavity. The tympanic ring is intact with the freed margin toward the viewer. (Courtesy of Barry J. Anson and James A. Donaldson, *Surgical Anatomy of the Temporal Bone*, 3rd Ed. Philadelphia: W.B. Saunders Company, 1981.)

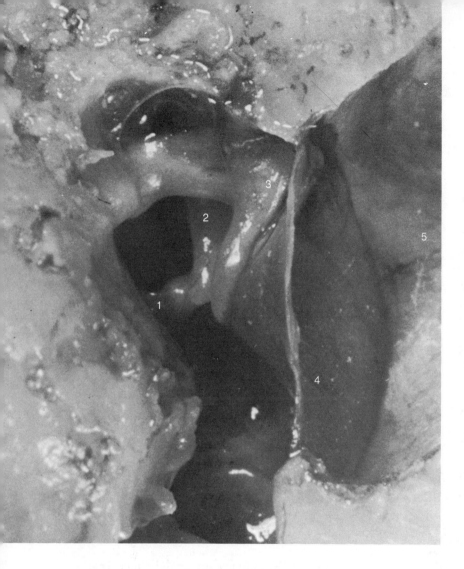

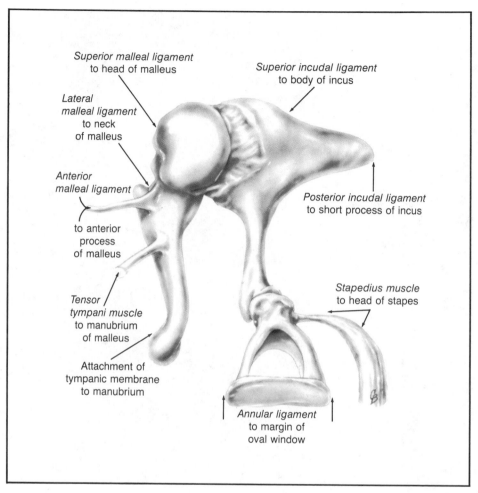

FIGURE 15–7   Anterior view of temporal bone sectioned in coronal plane. (1) stapes, (2) incus, (3) malleus, (4) tympanic membrane, (5) external auditory meatus. (Courtesy of Chihiro Yokochi and Johannes W. Rohen, *Photographic Anatomy of the Human Body*, 2nd Ed. Tokyo: Igaku-Shoin, Ltd., 1978.)

FIGURE 15–8   Auditory ossicles with the insertions of attached ligaments and muscles, viewed from the medial aspect. (Courtesy of Barry J. Anson and James A. Donaldson, *Surgical Anatomy of the Temporal Bone*, 3rd Ed. Philadelphia: W.B. Saunders Company, 1981.)

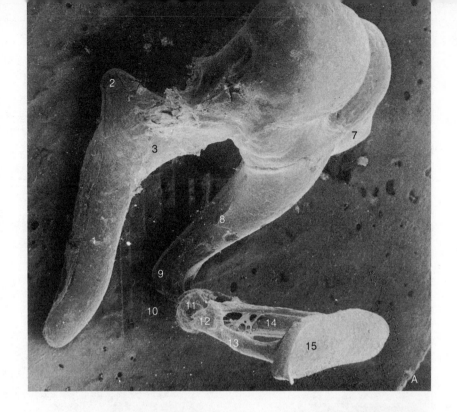

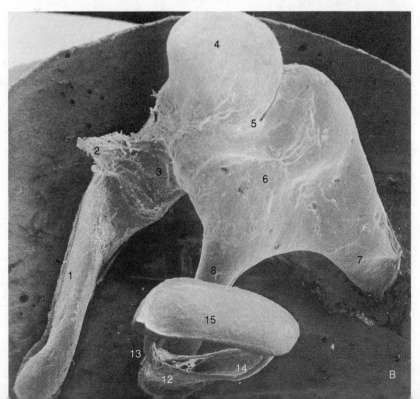

FIGURE 15–9 Scanning electron micrographs of middle-ear ossicles viewed from (A) the anterior aspect (front) and (B) the medial aspect (as if looking from within the inner ear). Parts of the malleus are (1) manubrium, (2) anterior process, (3) neck, (4) head. Parts of the incus are (6) body, (7) short process, (8) long process, (9) lenticular process. Parts of the stapes are (11) head, (12) neck, (13) anterior crus, (14) posterior crus, (15) footplate. Also shown are (5) incudomalleal articulation and (10) incudostapedial articulation. (Courtesy of Ivan Hunter-Duvar, as shown in William A. Yost and Donald W. Nielsen, *Fundamentals of Hearing: An Introduction.* New York: CBS College Publishing, 1977.)

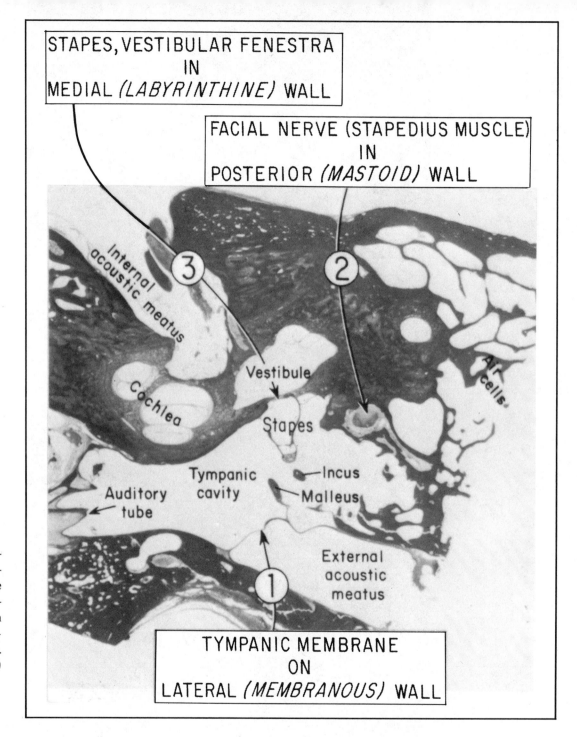

STAPES, VESTIBULAR FENESTRA
IN
MEDIAL *(LABYRINTHINE)* WALL

FACIAL NERVE (STAPEDIUS MUSCLE)
IN
POSTERIOR *(MASTOID)* WALL

Internal acoustic meatus

Cochlea

Vestibule

Stapes

Air cells

Tympanic cavity

Incus

Malleus

Auditory tube

External acoustic meatus

TYMPANIC MEMBRANE
ON
LATERAL *(MEMBRANOUS)* WALL

FIGURE 15–10 Photomicrograph of a horizontal section through the temporal bone of a 55-year-old female. The tympanic cavity, its walls, and contents are illustrated. (Magnification × 4; H. & E. stain.) (Courtesy of the Iowa Otological Collection, as shown in Barry J. Anson and James A. Donaldson, *Surgical Anatomy of the Temporal Bone*, 3rd Ed. Philadelphia: W.B. Saunders Company, 1981.)

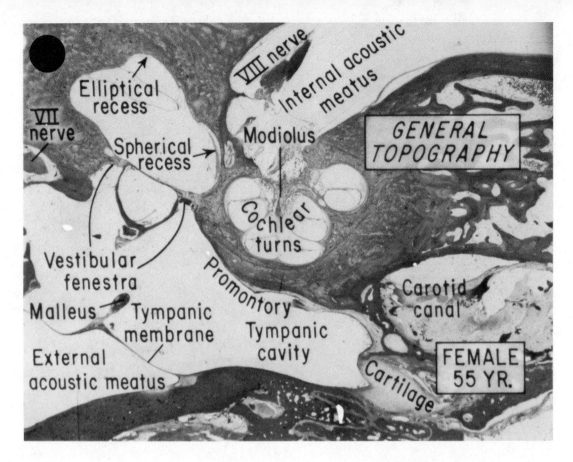

Labels on figure: VII nerve · Elliptical recess · VIII nerve · Internal acoustic meatus · Modiolus · Spherical recess · GENERAL TOPOGRAPHY · Cochlear turns · Vestibular fenestra · Promontory · Carotid canal · Malleus · Tympanic membrane · Tympanic cavity · External acoustic meatus · Cartilage · FEMALE 55 YR.

FIGURE 15–11 Photomicrograph of a horizontal section through the temporal bone. This section was taken from the same specimen as shown in Figure 15–10. (Magnification × 6; H. & E. stain.) (Courtesy of the Iowa Otological Collection, as shown in Barry J. Anson and James A. Donaldson, *Surgical Anatomy of the Temporal Bone*, 3rd Ed. Philadelphia: W.B. Saunders Company, 1981.)

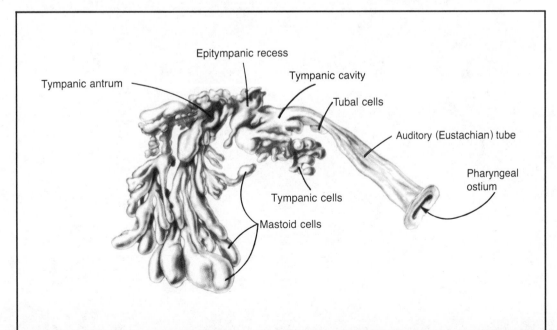

Labels on figure: Tympanic antrum · Epitympanic recess · Tympanic cavity · Tubal cells · Auditory (Eustachian) tube · Tympanic cells · Mastoid cells · Pharyngeal ostium

FIGURE 15–12 Model made by filling the tympanic cavity, cavities in the mastoid part of the temporal bone, and air cell outpocketings and extensions along the auditory tube. Air cells of the petrous part of the temporal bone are not included in the model. (Courtesy of Barry J. Anson and James A. Donaldson, *Surgical Anatomy of the Temporal Bone*, 3rd Ed. Philadelphia: W.B. Saunders Company, 1981.)

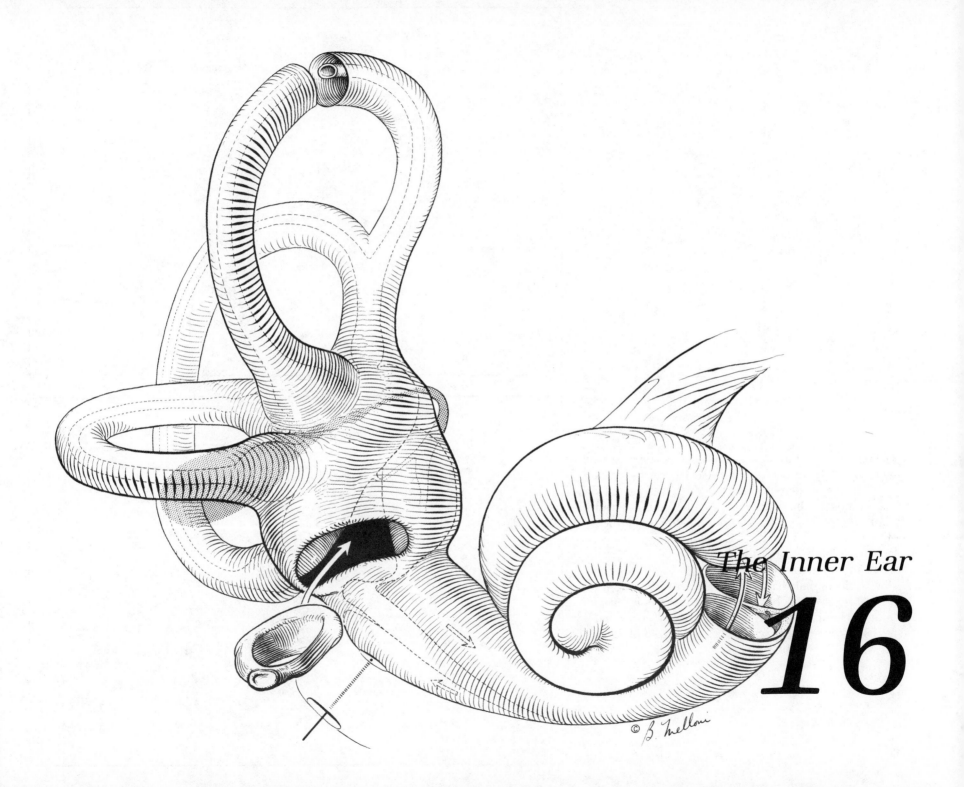

The Inner Ear

16

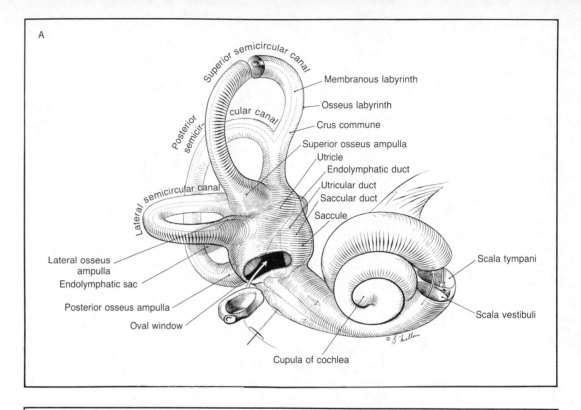

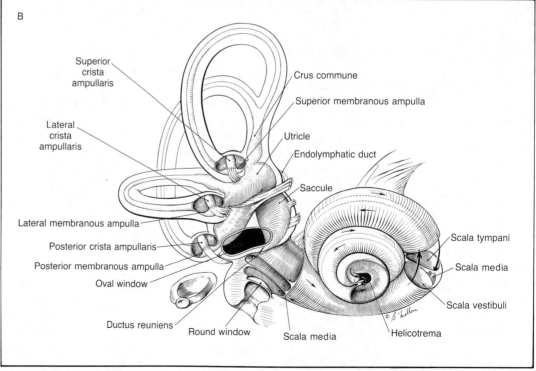

FIGURE 16–1 Membranous and osseous labyrinths of inner ear. (A) highlights the osseous labyrinths, within which the membranous labyrinth is depicted by dashed lines. (B) highlights the membranous labyrinth within the osseous labyrinth. (C) illustrates the membranous labyrinth with the osseous labyrinth removed and with the nerves of the inner ear illustrated relative to the membranous labyrinth. (D) shows how the nerve fibers exit the osseous labyrinth to unite into the vestibular or cochlear nerves. (Drawings by Biagio John Melloni, as shown in *Some Pathological Conditions of the Eye, Ear, and Throat*, courtesy of Abbott Laboratories, North Chicago, Illinois.)

THE AUDITORY SYSTEM

C

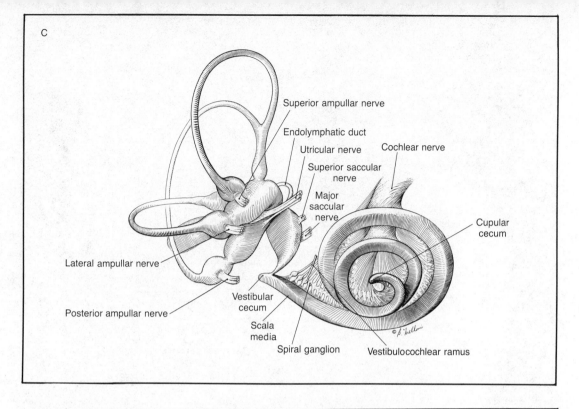

Superior ampullar nerve

Endolymphatic duct

Utricular nerve

Cochlear nerve

Superior saccular nerve

Major saccular nerve

Cupular cecum

Lateral ampullar nerve

Posterior ampullar nerve

Vestibular cecum

Scala media

Spiral ganglion

Vestibulocochlear ramus

D

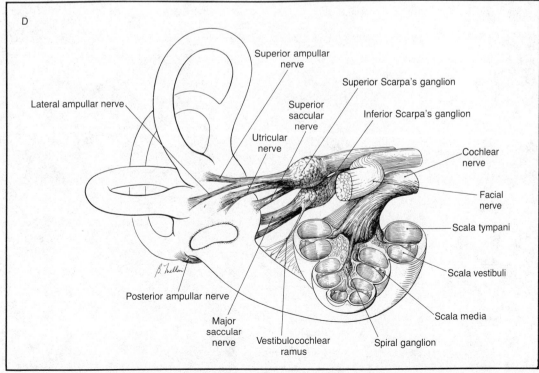

Superior ampullar nerve

Superior Scarpa's ganglion

Lateral ampullar nerve

Superior saccular nerve

Inferior Scarpa's ganglion

Utricular nerve

Cochlear nerve

Facial nerve

Scala tympani

Scala vestibuli

Posterior ampullar nerve

Scala media

Major saccular nerve

Vestibulocochlear ramus

Spiral ganglion

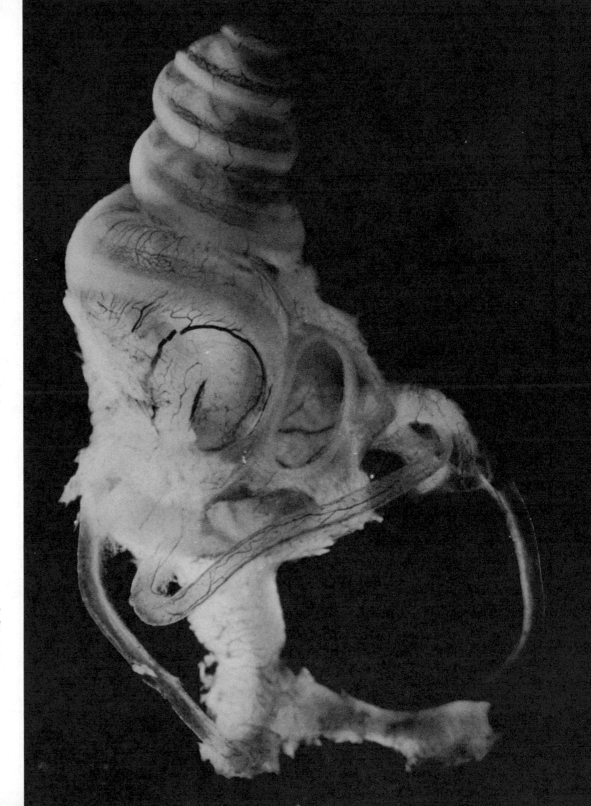

FIGURE 16–2 Microdissection of labyrinth. (Courtesy of H. Engström and B. Engström, *The Structure and Function of the Inner Ear: Part I, The Organ of Corti.* Copenhagen: Tøpholm and Westermann I/S, 1976.)

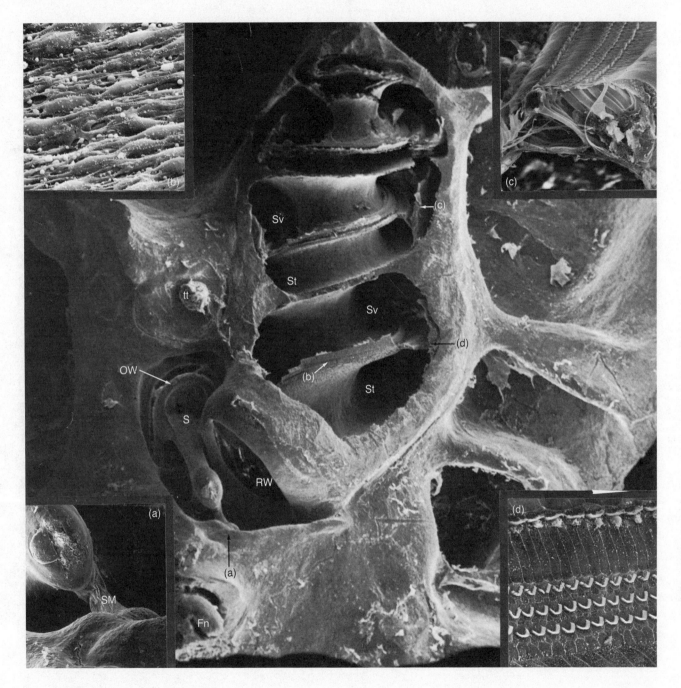

FIGURE 16–3 Scanning electron micrograph showing the coiling of the chincilla cochlea ($3\frac{3}{4}$ turns): (S) stapes, (OW) oval window, (RW) round window. The inserts show details at the points indicated on the central photograph. In (a), (SM) stapedial muscle. (b) tympanic layer below the basilar membrane. (c) cross section of the organ of Corti. (d) hairs of the inner and outer hair cells: (Sv) scala vestibuli, (St) scala tympani, (tt) attachment of tensor tympani, (Fn) facial nerve. (Courtesy of Ivan Hunter-Duvar, as shown in William A. Yost and Donald W. Nielsen, *Fundamentals of Hearing: An Introduction.* New York: CBS College Publishing, 1977.)

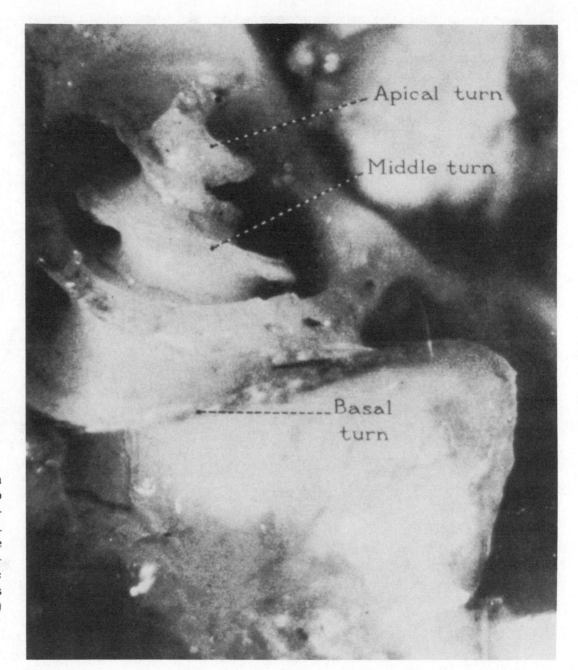

FIGURE 16–4   Dissection of the osseous spiral lamina of the left cochlea viewed from the ventral aspect to show the basal, middle, and apical turns. (Magnification × 15.) This material is from a cat. (From C.N. Woolsey and E.N. Walzl, "Topical Projection of Nerve Fibers from Local Regions of the Cochlea to the Cerebral Cortex of the Cat," in *Bulletin of the Johns Hopkins Hospital* 71:315–344. Baltimore: The Johns Hopkins University Press, 1942.)

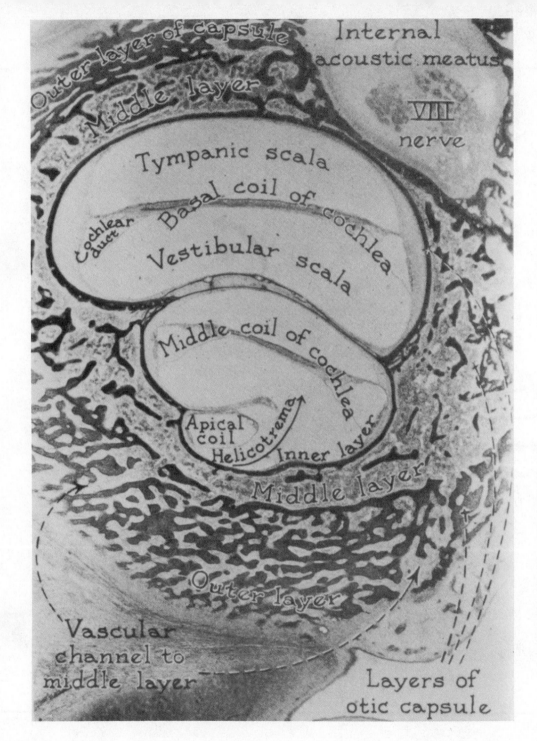

FIGURE 16–5 Photomicrograph of a section through the cochlea, parallel to but away from the mid-modiolar axis. In addition to cochlear structures, the inner, middle, and outer layers of the otic capsule, vascular channel to the middle layer of the otic capsule, and the 8th nerve in the internal auditory (acoustic) meatus are labelled. Material from a 6-month human fetus in the Wisconsin otological collection. (Magnification × 17.) (Courtesy of B.J. Anson, T.R. Winch, R. Warpeha, and J. Donaldson, "The Blood Supply of the Otic Capsule of the Human Ear with Special Reference to That of the Cochlea," in *Annals of Otology, Rhinology, and Larynogology* 75, No. 4, 1966, p. 936.)

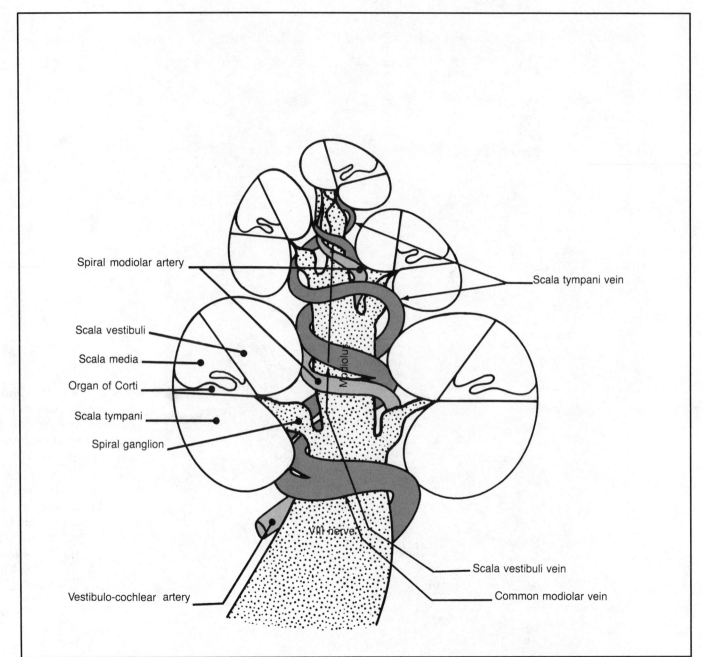

FIGURE 16–6 Schematic of a radial section through the modiolus to show the vascular anatomy of the human cochlea. The basal half of the basal turn is supplied by the vestibulocochlear artery; the rest of the cochlea is supplied by the spiral modiolar artery. (Courtesy of A.G. Axelsson, "The Vascular Anatomy of the Cochlea in the Guinea Pig and Man," in *Acta Otolaryngologica*, Supplementum 243, 1968, p. 40.)

Spiral modiolar artery

Scala tympani vein

Scala vestibuli

Scala media

Organ of Corti

Scala tympani

Spiral ganglion

Modiolus

VIII nerve

Scala vestibuli vein

Vestibulo-cochlear artery

Common modiolar vein

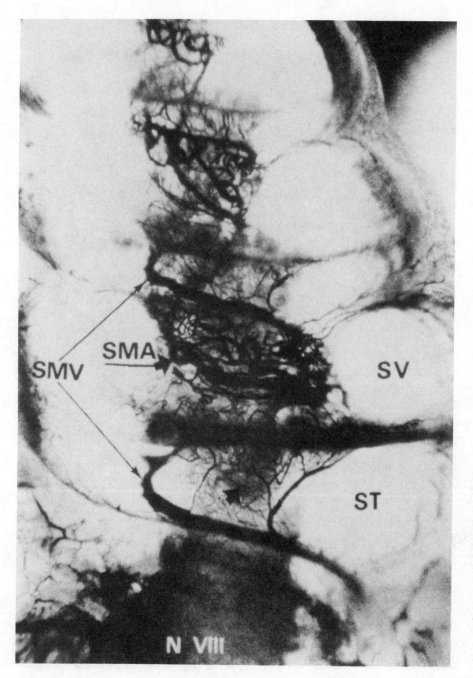

FIGURE 16–7 Photomicrograph of a radial section through the cochlea. (SMA) spiral modiolar artery, (SMV) spiral modiolar vein (after perfusion of the vascular system with a contrast medium), (SV) scala vestibuli, (ST) scala tympani, (8th nerve) cochlear nerve. The arrow points to the capillary net in the modiolus wall. This material is from a guinea pig. (Magnification × 32.5.) (Courtesy of A.G. Axelsson, "The Vascular Anatomy of the Cochlea in the Guinea Pig and Man," in *Acta Otolaryngologica*, Supplementum 243, 1968, p. 32.)

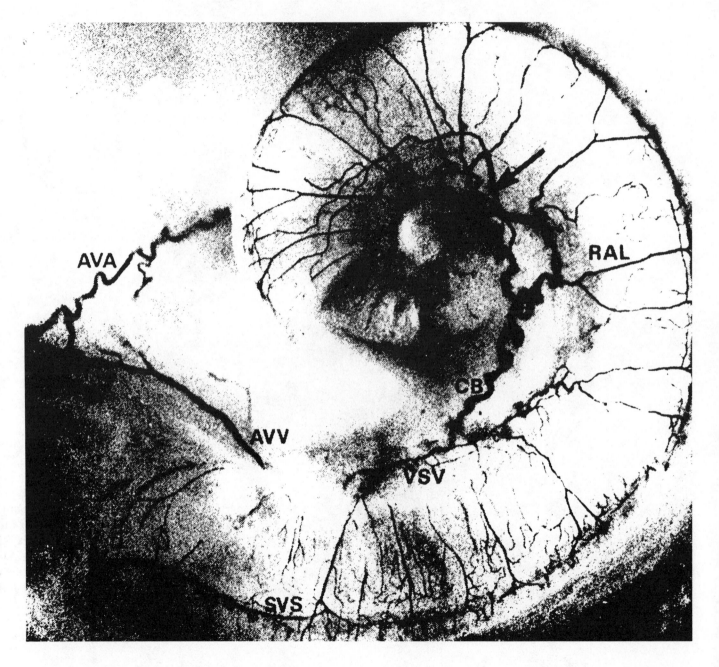

FIGURE 16–8 Photomicrograph of a transverse section of the basal turn of the human cochlea. The vascular system has been perfused with a contrast medium. (AVA) anterior vestibular artery, (AVV) anterior vestibular vein, (CB) cochlear branch of the vestibulocochlear artery giving off (RAL) radiating arterioles over the scala vestibuli, (VSV) vein of the scala vestibuli, (SVS) stria vascularis at the basal end. The arrow shows the region where the spiral modiolar artery arrives in the cochlea. (Magnification × 12.) (Courtesy of A.G. Axelsson, "The Vascular Anatomy of the Cochlea in the Guinea Pig and Man," in *Acta Otolaryngologica*, Supplementum 243, 1968, p. 41.)

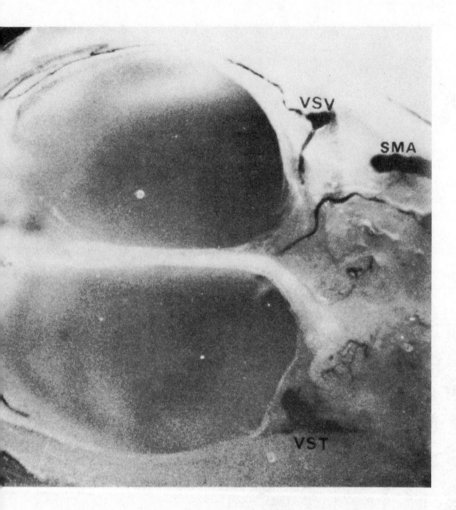

FIGURE 16–9 Photomicrograph of a radial cut through the basal turn of the human cochlea after perfusion of the vascular system with a contrast medium. (SMA) spiral modiolar artery, (VSV) vein of the scala vestibuli, (VST) vein of the scala tympani draining the spiral ganglion and external wall. (Magnification × 30.) (Courtesy of A.G. Axelsson, "The Vascular Anatomy of the Cochlea in the Guinea Pig and Man," in *Acta Otolaryngologica*, Supplementum 243, 1968, p. 42.)

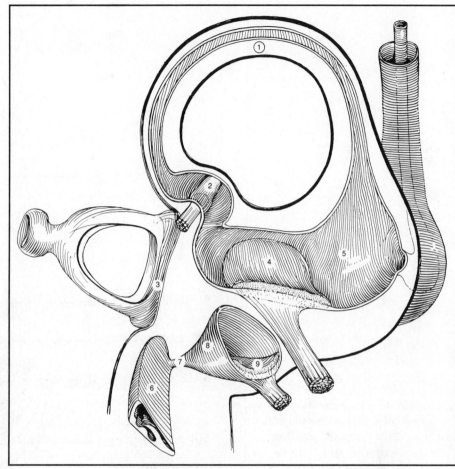

FIGURE 16–10 Drawing of the osseous and membranous labyrinths of the vestibular system sectioned in the horizontal plane and viewed from the superior aspect. (1) lateral semicircular canal, (2) lateral crista ampularis, (3) footplate of stapes in oval window, (4) macula of utricle, (5) utricle, (6) scala media, (7) ductus reuniens, (8) saccule, (9) macula of saccule. (Courtesy of Ida Dox, Biagio John Melloni, and Gilbert M. Eisner, *Melloni's Illustrated Medical Dictionary*. Baltimore: The Williams & Wilkins Co., 1979. Drawing by Melloni.)

THE INNER EAR

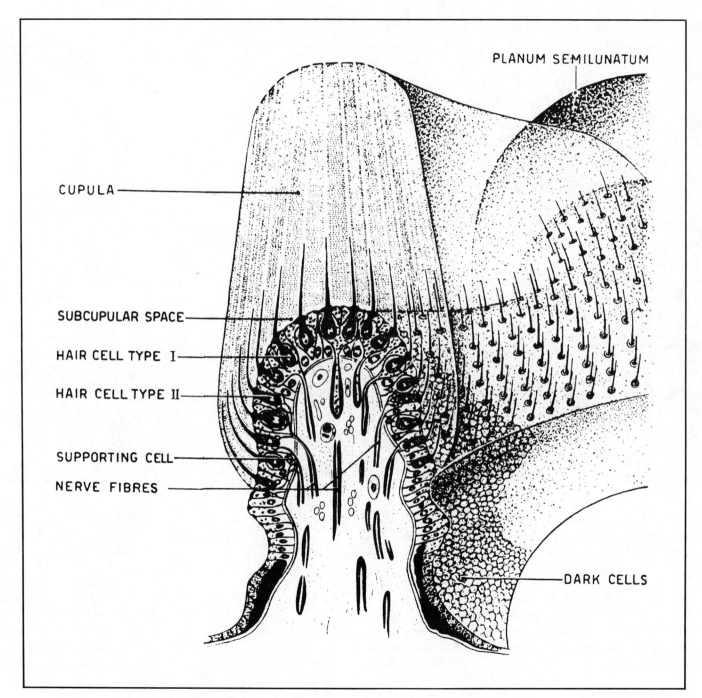

FIGURE 16–11 Schematic of one-half a crista ampularis. (Courtesy of J. Wersäll, "Studies on the Structure and Innervation of the Sensory Epithelium of the Cristae Ampullares in the Guinea Pig," in *Acta Otolaryngologica*, Supplementum 126, 1956, p. 31. As modified in Salvatore Iurato, *Submicroscopic Structure of the Inner Ear*; Oxford: Pergamon Press, Ltd., 1967.)

PLANUM SEMILUNATUM

CUPULA

SUBCUPULAR SPACE

HAIR CELL TYPE I

HAIR CELL TYPE II

SUPPORTING CELL

NERVE FIBRES

DARK CELLS

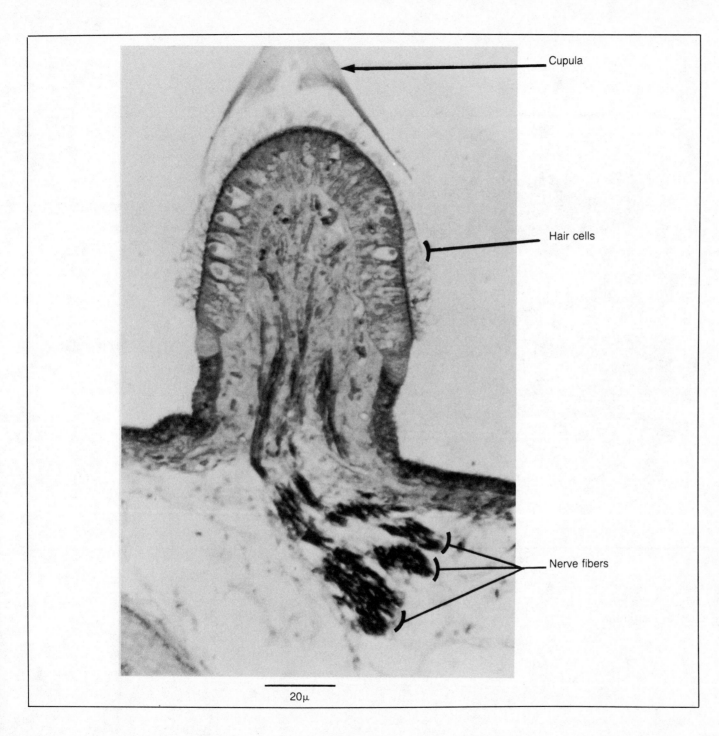

Cupula

Hair cells

Nerve fibers

20μ

FIGURE 16–12
Photomicrograph of a
cross-section through a crista
ampullaris of a guinea pig.
(Magnification × 612; iron
hematoxylin stain.) (Courtesy
of Ronald A. Bergman and
Adel K. Afifi, *Atlas of
Microscopic Anatomy:
A Companion to Histology and
Neuroanatomy.* Philadelphia:
W.B. Saunders Company, 1974.)

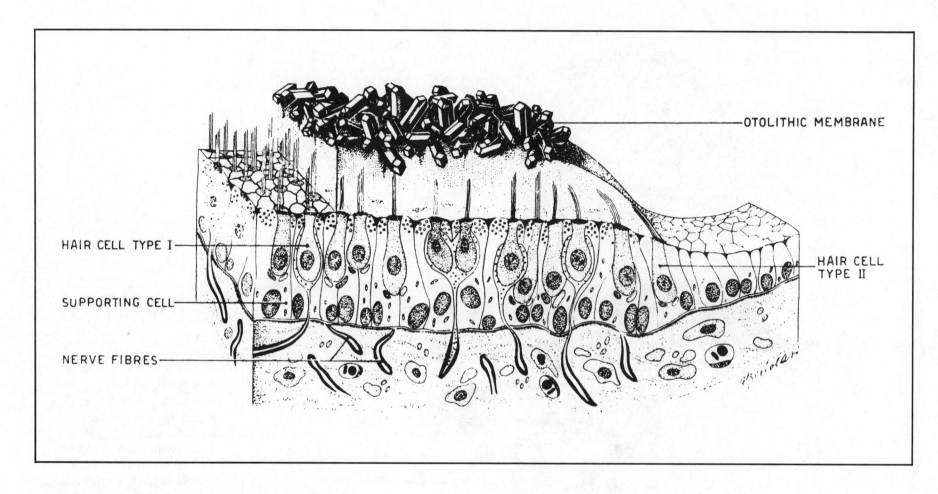

FIGURE 16–13   Schematic of a macula (from either a saccule or utricle). From Salvatore Iurato, *Submicroscopic Structure of the Inner Ear.* Oxford: Pergamon Press, Ltd., 1967.)

Labels in figure: OTOLITHIC MEMBRANE, HAIR CELL TYPE I, HAIR CELL TYPE II, SUPPORTING CELL, NERVE FIBRES

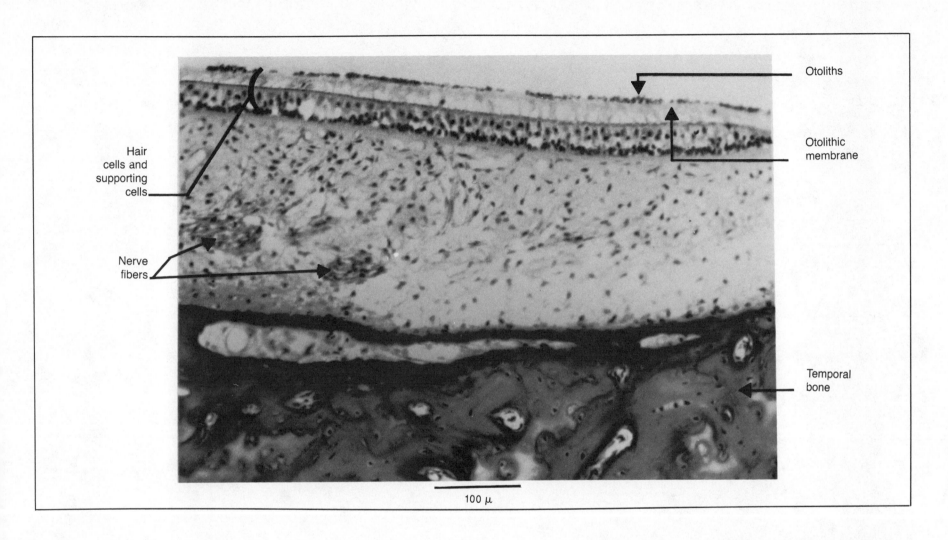

Otoliths

Otolithic
membrane

Hair
cells and
supporting
cells

Nerve
fibers

Temporal
bone

100 μ

FIGURE 16–14 Photomicrograph of the utricle of the
macula from a cat. (Magnification × 612; iron hematoxylin stain.) (Courtesy of Ronald A. Bergman and
Adel K. Afifi, *Atlas of Microscopic Anatomy: A Companion to Histology and Neuroanatomy*. Philadelphia: W.B.
Saunders Company, 1974.)

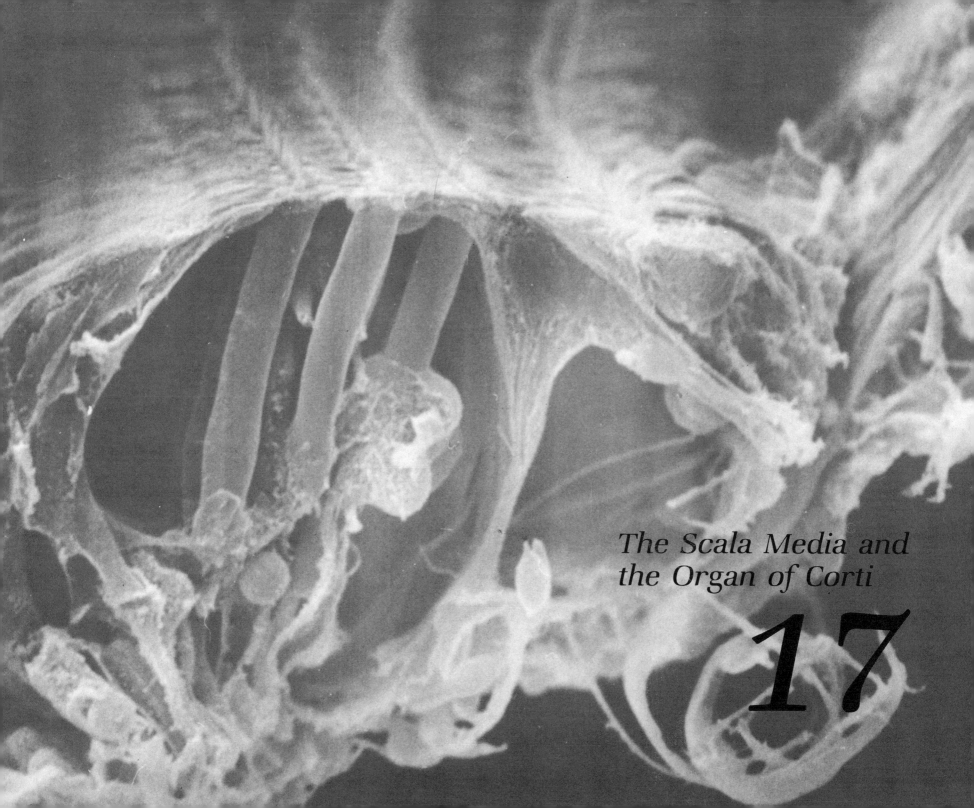

The Scala Media and
the Organ of Corti

17

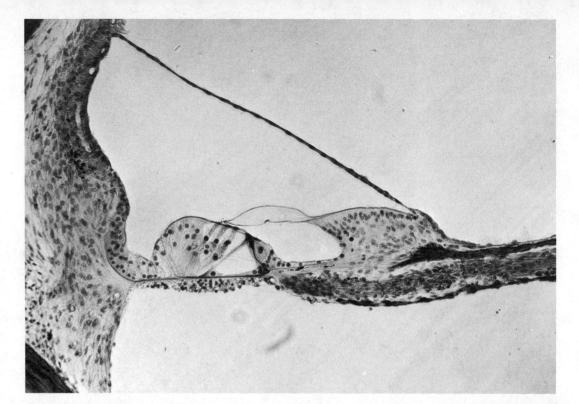

FIGURE 17–1 Photomicrograph of a radial section through the cochlea to show the structures within and around the scala media. (Courtesy of H. Engström and B. Engström, Department of Otolaryngology, Adademiska Sjukhuset, Universitet i Uppsala, Uppsala, Sweden.)

FIGURE 17–2 Photomicrograph through the basal turn of the cochlea. This material is from a cat. (Courtesy of J. Babel, A. Bischoff, and H. Spoendlin, *Ultrastructure of the Peripheral Nervous System and Sense Organs*. Stuttgart: Georg Thieme Verlag, 1970.)

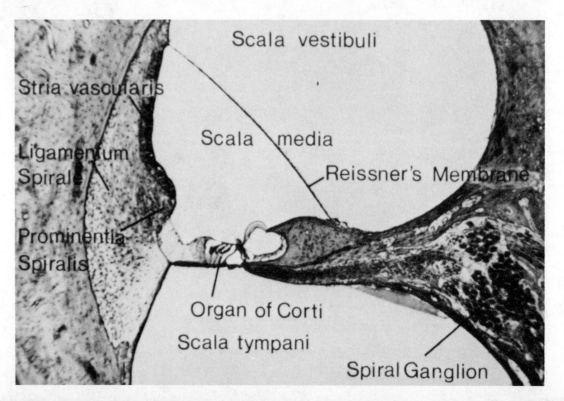

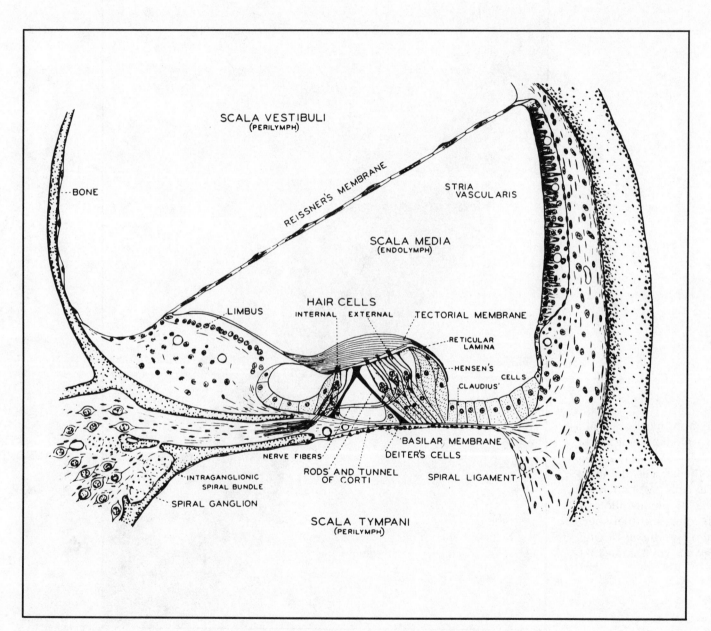

FIGURE 17–3 Schematic drawing to illustrate the structures evident in a cross-section of the scala media. (Courtesy of Hallowell Davis and Associates, "Acoustic Trauma in the Guinea Pig," in *Journal of the Acoustical Society of America* 25, No. 6, November 1953, p. 1182.)

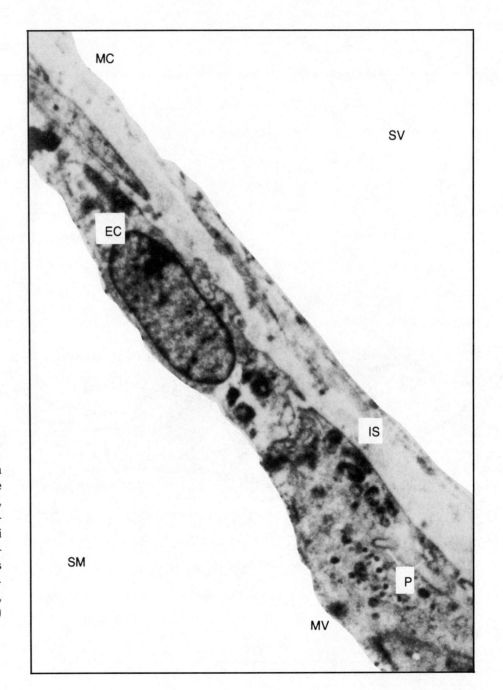

FIGURE 17–4   Transmission electron micrograph of a cross-section through Reissner's membrane from the basal turn of a 62-year-old male. (SM) scala media, (SV) scala vestibuli, (MC) mesothelial cells, (IS) intercellular substance, (EC) epithelial cells, (MV) microvilli on the surface of epithelial cells, (P) pinocytotic vesicles. (Courtesy of Lars-Göran Johnsson, "Reissner's Membrane in the Human Cochlea," in *Annals of Otology, Rhinology, and Laryngology* 80, No. 3, June 1971, p. 427.)

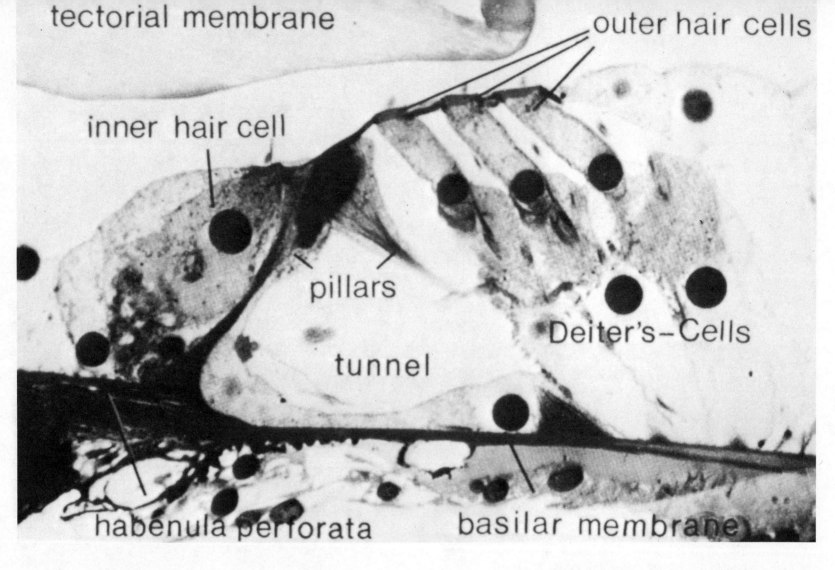

FIGURE 17–5 Photomicrograph of a cross-section through the organ of Corti in the basal turn. This material is from a guinea pig. (Courtesy of J. Babel, A. Bischoff, and H. Spoendlin, *Ultrastructure of the Peripheral Nervous System and Sense Organs.* Stuttgart: Georg Thieme Verlag, 1970.)

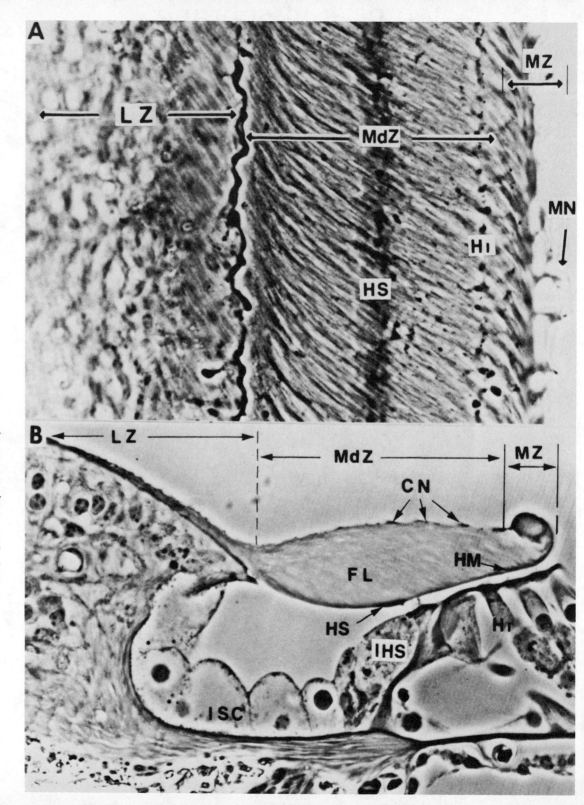

FIGURE 17–6   (A) photomicrograph of surface view of human tectorial membrane at basal coil. (LZ) limbal zone, (MdZ) middle zone, (MZ) marginal zone, (Hi) outer hair cells, (HS) Hensen's stripe, (MN) marginal net. (Magnification × 100.) (B) photomicrograph of cross-section of organ of Corti in basal coil. (LZ) limbal zone, (MdZ) middle zone, (MZ) marginal zone, (CN) cover net, (HM) Hardesty's membrane, (IHS) inner hair cells, (H₁) 1st row of outer hair cells, (SL) inner sulcus cell. (Magnification × 1201.) This material is from a guinea pig. (Courtesy of David J. Lim, "Fine Morphology of the Tectorial Membrane: Its Relationship to the Organ of Corti," in *Archives of Otolaryngology* 96, September 1972, p. 201. Copyright 1972, American Medical Association.)

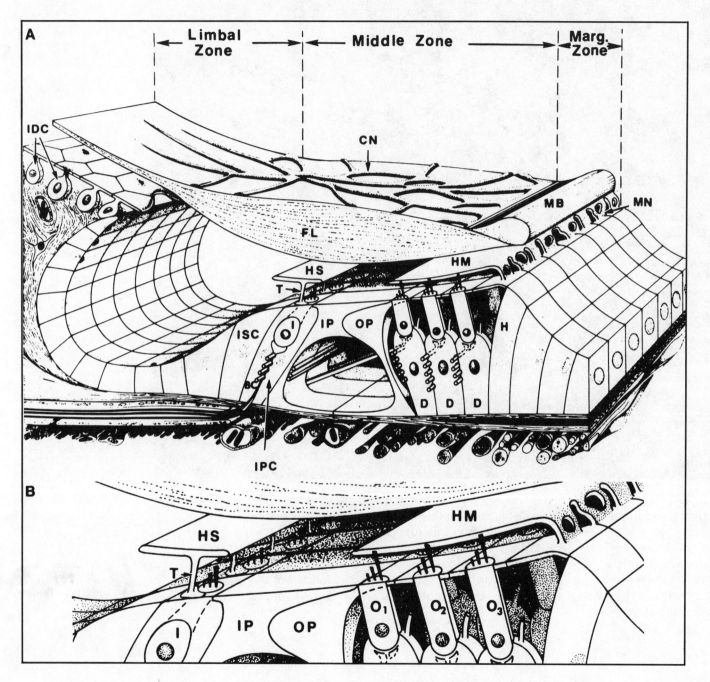

FIGURE 17-7 (A) schematic showing substructures of tectorial membrane and its relationship to organ of Corti. The tectorial membrane is anchored by (T) trabeculae of (HS) Hensen's stripe and (MN) marginal net, in addition to (HM) Hardesty's membrane, to the outer sensory hairs. (MB) marginal band, (FL) fibrous layer, (IDC) interdental cell, (ISC) inner sulcus cell, (BC) inner border cell, (IPC) inner phalangeal cell, (IP) inner pillar, (OP) outer pillar, (D) Deiters' cell, (H) Hensen's cell. (B) schematic of enlarged portion of sensory hair–tectorial membrane junction. O_1, O_2, and O_3 represent the 1st, 2nd, and 3rd outer hair cells. (Courtesy of David J. Lim, "The Fine Morphology of the Tectorial Membrane: Its Relationship to the Organ of Corti," in *Archives of Otolaryngology* 96, September 1972, p. 202. Copyright 1972, American Medical Association.)

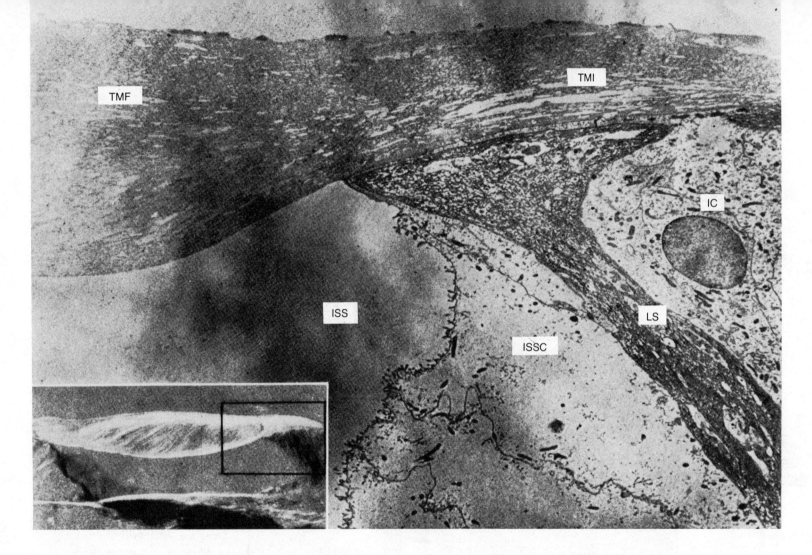

FIGURE 17–8 Transmission electron micrograph of the tectorial membrane. The transition zone is between the part inserted into the (TMI) limbus spiralis and the (TMF) main part. (ISS) inner spiral sulcus, (ISSC) inner spiral sulcus cells, (LS) limbus spiralis, (IC) interdental cells. (Magnification × 4500.) The inset is a photomicrograph of the tectorial membrane in which the zone outlined indicates the area examined with the electron microscope. (Magnification × 225.) (Courtesy of Salvatore Iurato, "Functional Implications of the Nature and Submicroscopic Structure of the Tectorial and Basilar Membranes," in *Journal of the Acoustical Society of America* 34, No. 8, 1962, p. 1389.)

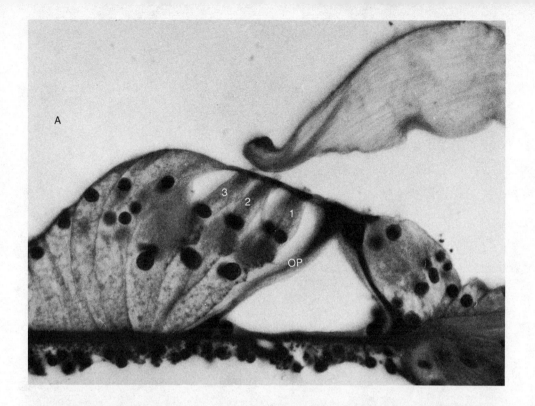

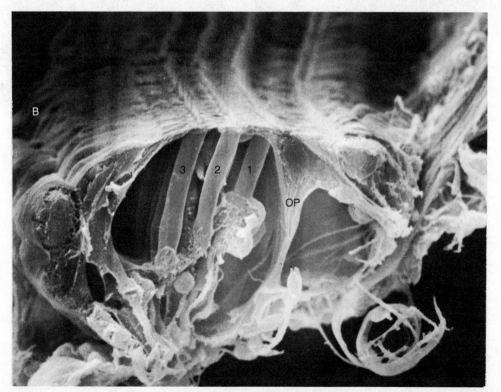

FIGURE 17–9   (A) photomicrograph and (B) scanning electron micrograph of a cross-section through the organ of Corti. (1–3) three rows of outer hair cells, (OP) outer pillar. (Part (A) courtesy of H. Engström and B. Engström, Department of Otolaryngology, Akademiska Sjukhuset, Universitet i Uppsala, Uppsala, Sweden. Part (B) courtesy of H. Engström and B. Engström, "Ultra-struktur des inneren ohres," in J. Berendes, K. Link, and F. Zöller (Eds.), *Hals-Nasen-Ohren-Heilkunde in Praxis and Klinik*, Band 5, Ohr 1; Stuttgart: Georg Thieme Verlag, 1979.)

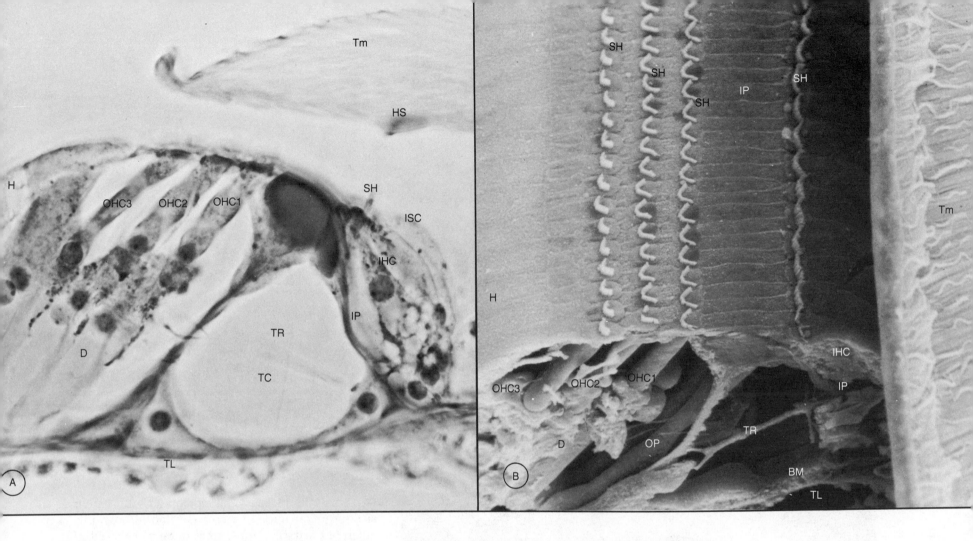

FIGURE 17–10 (A) photomicrograph of cross-section of organ of Corti; (B) scanning electron micrograph of similar area, in which tectorial membrane has been pulled back to expose sensory hairs. (IHC) inner hair cell, (OHC) three rows of outer hair cells, (OP) outer and (IP) inner pillars of Corti, (TC) tunnel of Corti, (BM) basilar membrane with underlying (TL) tympanic layer of cells, supporting cells of (D) Deiters and (H) Hensen, (TM) tectorial membrane, (HS) Hensen's stripe, (ISC) inner sulcus cells, (TR) a tunnel radial nerve fiber, (SH) sensory hairs. These materials are from a chinchilla. (Courtesy of Ivan Hunter-Duvar, as shown in William A. Yost and Donald W. Nielsen, *Fundamentals of Hearing: An Introduction.* New York: CBS College Publishing, 1977.)

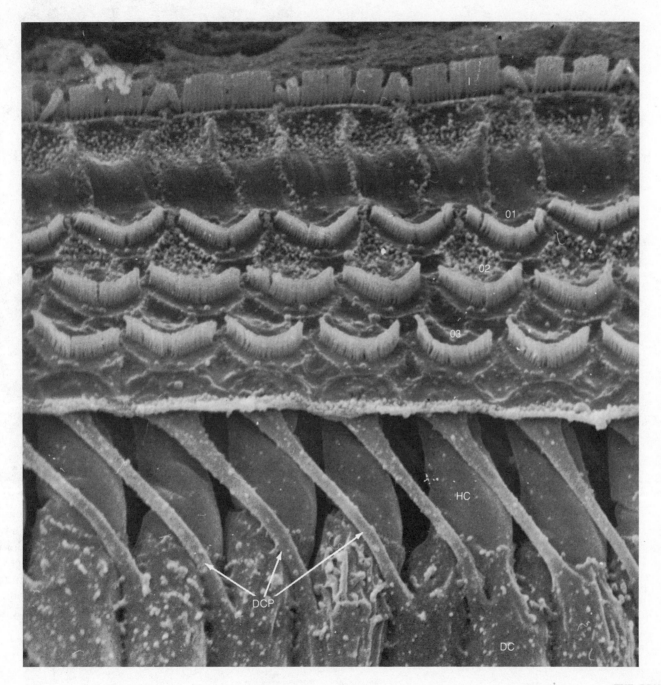

FIGURE 17–11 Scanning electron microgram of the organ of Corti sensory hairs of (I) the inner hair cells and (01, 02, and 03) three rows of outer hair cells. (HC) hair cells, (DC) Deiters' cells, (DCP) Deiters' cell process. (Modified from H. Engström and B. Engström, "Ultrastruktur des inneren ohres," in J. Berendes, K. Link, and F. Zöller (Eds.), *Hals-Nasen-Ohren-Heilkunde in Praxis und Klinik*, Band 5, Ohr I. Stuttgart: Georg Thieme Verlag, 1979.)

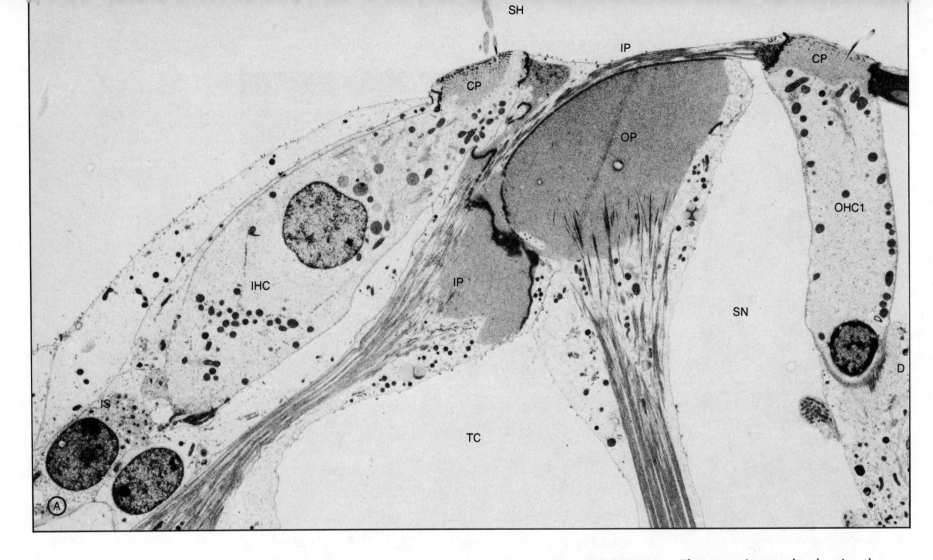

FIGURE 17–12 Electron micrographs showing the organ of Corti. (A) is a transmission electron micrograph providing a detailed view of structures not possible with other methods; (B) is a scanning electron micrograph of the same area for comparison (note the three-dimensional perspective). (SH) sensory hairs, (CP) cuticular plate, (SN) space of the nuel, (TC) tunnel

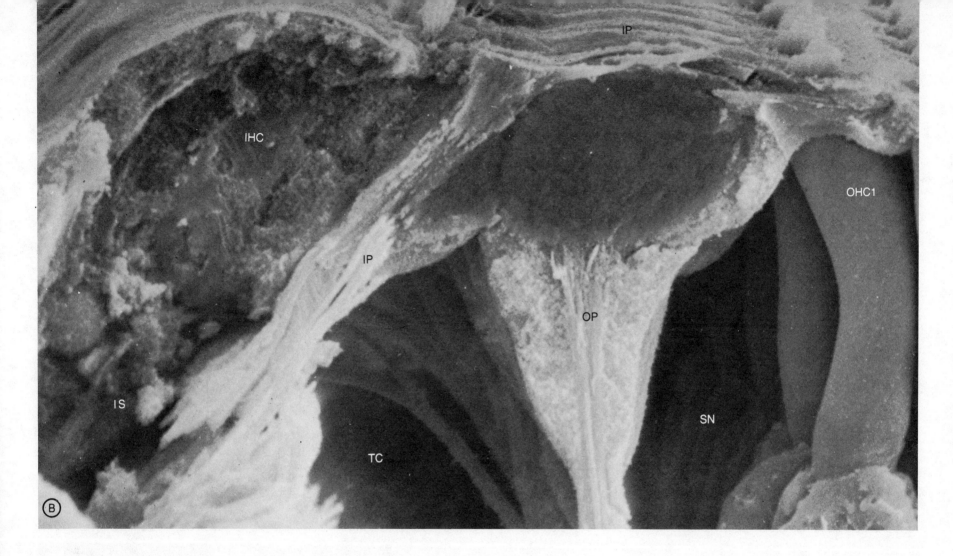

of Corti, (OP) outer pillar, (IP) inner pillar, (OHCI) 1st row, outer hair cell, (IHC) inner hair cell, (IS) inner spiral bundle, (D) Deiters' cell. These materials are from a chinchilla. (Courtesy of Ivan Hunter-Duvar, as shown in William A. Yost and Donald W. Nielsen, *Fundamentals of Hearing: An Introduction*. New York: CBS College Publishing 1977.)

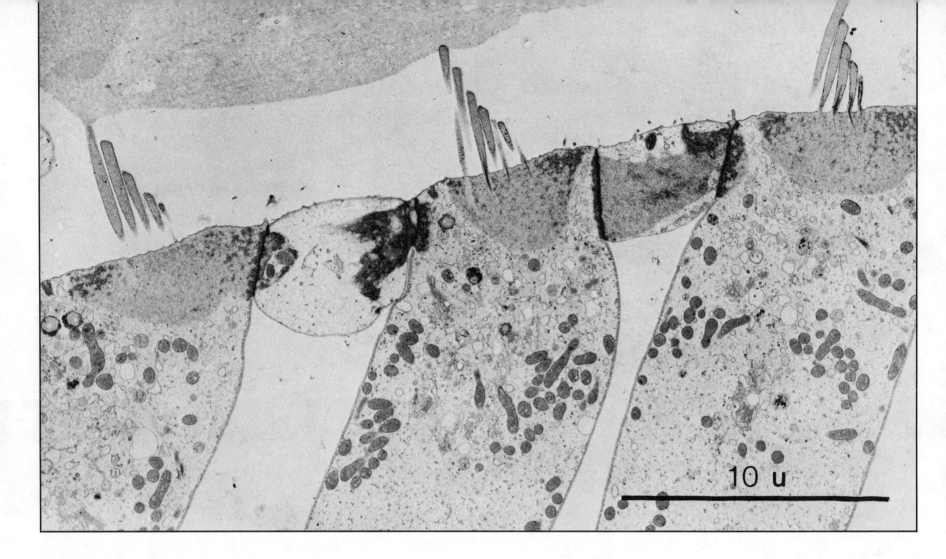

FIGURE 17–13 Transmission electron micrograph showing a longitudinal section of outer hair cells with their tall hairs touching the tectorial membrane. This material is from a squirrel monkey. (Courtesy of Robert S. Kimura, "Hairs of the Cochlear Sensory Cells and Their Attachment to the Tectorial Membrane," in *Acta Otolaryngologica* 61, No. 1, January 1966, p. 57.)

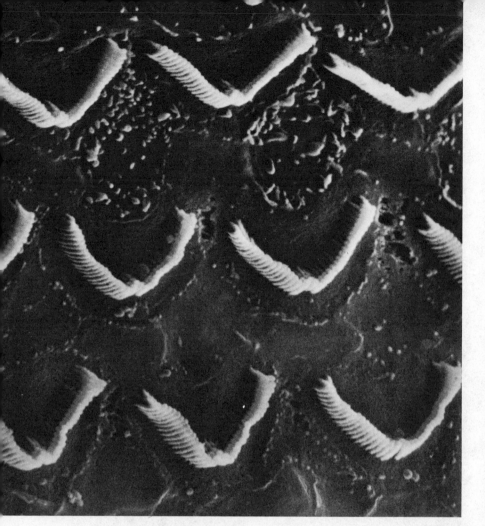

FIGURE 17–14 Scanning electron micrograph showing the sensory hairs on the outer hair cells as viewed from above. This is from the basal turn of a guinea pig cochlea. (Courtesy of H. Engström and B. Engström, "Structure of Hairs on Cochlear Sensory Cells," in *Hearing Research* 1, No. 1, October 1978, p. 53.)

FIGURE 17–15 Scanning electron micrograph of the sensory hairs on an outer hair cell as viewed from in front and above. This material is from a guinea pig. (Courtesy of H. Engström and B. Engström, "*Ultrastruktur des inneren ohres*," in J. Berendes, K. Link, and F. Zöllner (Eds.), *Hals-Nasen-Ohren-Heilkunde in Praxis and Klinik*, Band 5, Ohr I. Stuttgart: Georg Thieme Verlag, 1979.)

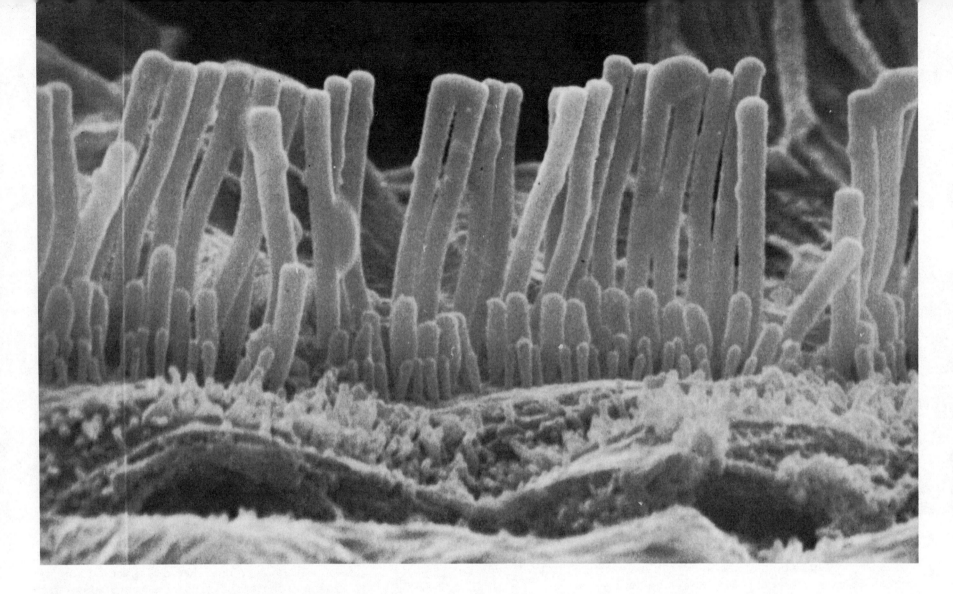

FIGURE 17–16 Scanning electron micrograph of the sensory hairs on the inner hair cells. This material is from a guinea pig. (Courtesy of H. Engström and B. Engström, Department of Otolaryngology, Adademiska Sjukhuset, Universitet i Uppsala, Uppsala, Sweden.)

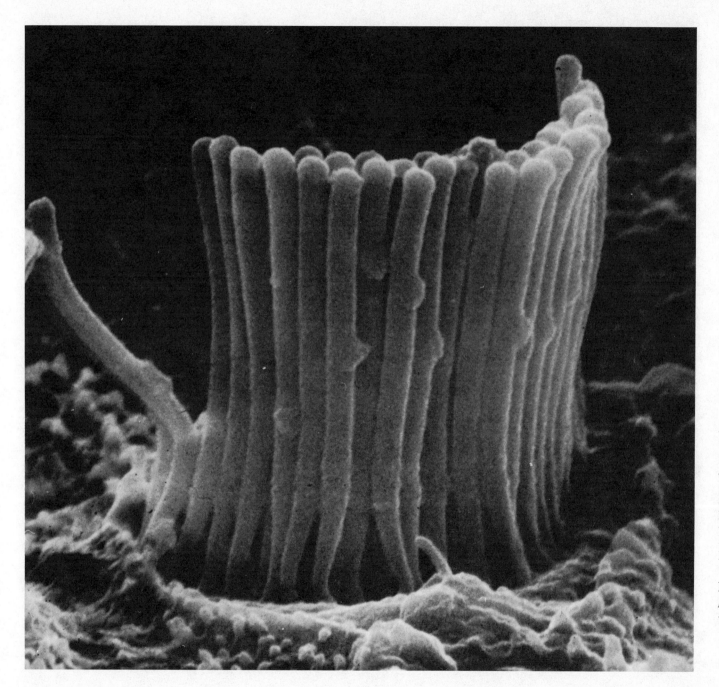

FIGURE 17–17 Scanning electron micrograph of sensory hairs on an outer hair cell as viewed from the side. Note the smooth rounded tips on the hairs and also "blebs" on some hairs. This material is from a Rhesus monkey. (Courtesy of H. Engström and B. Engström, "Structure of Hairs on Cochlear Sensory Cells," in *Hearing Research* 1, No. 1, October 1978, p. 54.)

III

THE NERVOUS SYSTEM

Part III discusses The Nervous System. Because of its pervasive influence on all aspects of speech, language, and hearing, the anatomy of the nervous system is extensively covered from a variety of approaches. These include gross dissection, sections of the brain cut in several anatomical planes, line drawings, and photographs. These approaches have permitted us to present external morphology as well as structural details in the interior of the cerebral hemispheres, brainstem, and spinal cord that otherwise would not be visible. Stains also have been used to illustrate myelinated structures within the nervous system, thus allowing tracts to be traced along the length of the nervous system or within specific neural networks or structures.

In general, the presentation of the nervous system begins rostrally and proceeds caudally. Separate chapters are devoted to the cranial nerves (Chapter 21) and the auditory nervous system (Chapter 22).

Chapter 18 describes "The Cerebral and Cerebellar Hemispheres," beginning with a review of the surface morphology of the cerebral hemispheres in which major anatomical landmarks and cortical areas are identified. This is followed by dissections of the cerebral hemispheres which illustrate commissural, association tracts, and structures beneath the cerebral cortex. The vascular supply to the cerebral hemispheres and cerebellum, along with the meningeal membranes are presented next, followed by a review of the surface morphology of the cerebellar hemispheres.

Chapter 19 presents "Coronal, Sagittal, and Horizontal Sections of the Brain." They have been prepared with a myelin stain so that fiber tracts appear dark. These sections should help the reader develop an appreciation of the structure of the nervous system in three dimensions as well as providing detailed information about specific structures.

Chapter 20 presents "The Brainstem and Spinal Cord." The reader is introduced to the general topography of the brainstem through a midsagittal section of the brain. This is followed by a review of external morphology and transverse sections of the brainstem taken at different levels along its length. The anatomy of the reticular formation in the brainstem is illustrated in a series of preparations. The chapter concludes with a review of the anatomy of the spinal cord via gross dissection and histological cross-sections.

Chapter 21 covers "The Cranial Nerves." Although general relationships are described, the emphasis of this chapter is on those cranial nerves which are of the greatest importance to speech, language, and hearing, cranial nerves V through XII. The origin of the cranial nerves in the brainstem is shown, and their course and distribution are depicted graphically.

Chapter 22, "The Auditory Nervous System," is the concluding chapter of Part III. In it the reader finds detailed information on the innervation of the cochlea, cristae, and macculae and the morphology of the postlabyrinthine auditory pathways.

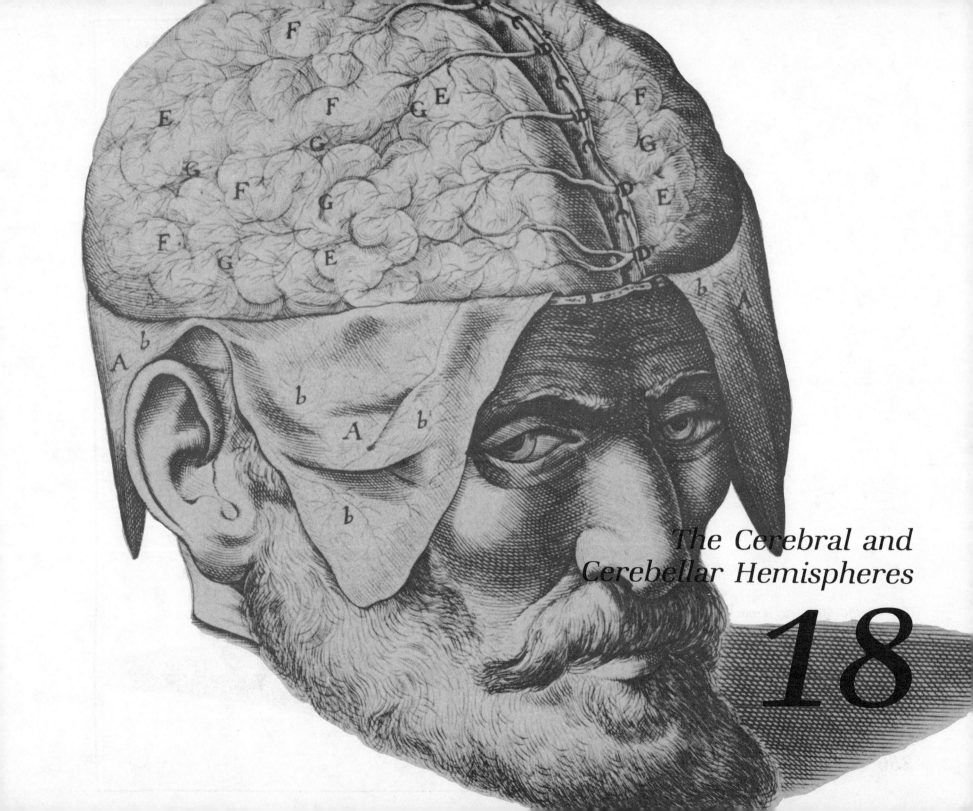

The Cerebral and
Cerebellar Hemispheres

18

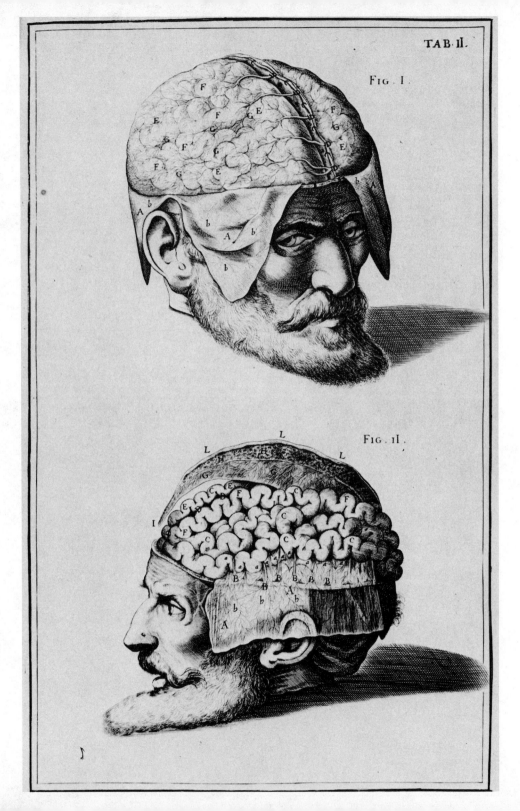

FIGURE 18-1 (From Guilio Casserio, "Tabulae Anatomicae," in Adriaan van de Spiegel (Ed.), *Opera quae Extant Omnia*. Amsterdam: Johannem Blaeu, 1645.)

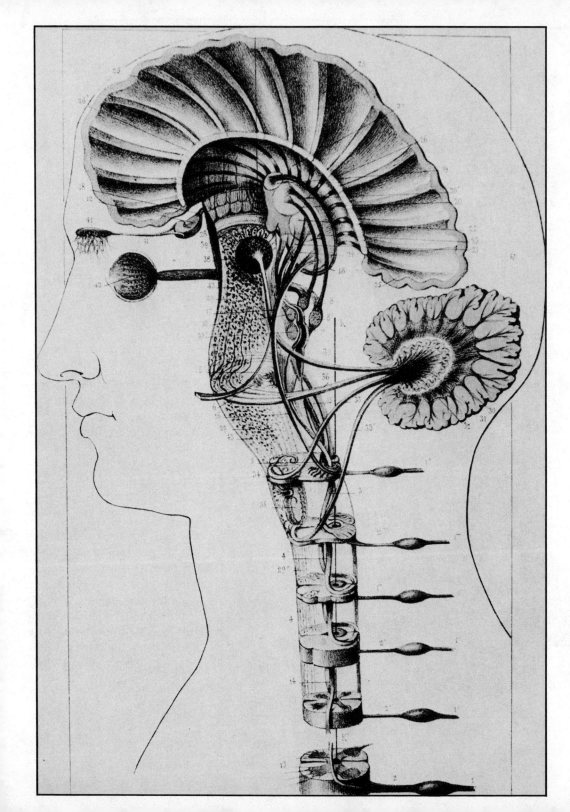

FIGURE 18–2 (From Jules Bernard Luys, *Recherches sur le systéme Nerveux Cérébrospinal, sa Structure, ses Fonctions et ses Maladies,* 2 volumes. Paris: J.-B. Bailiere, 1865.)

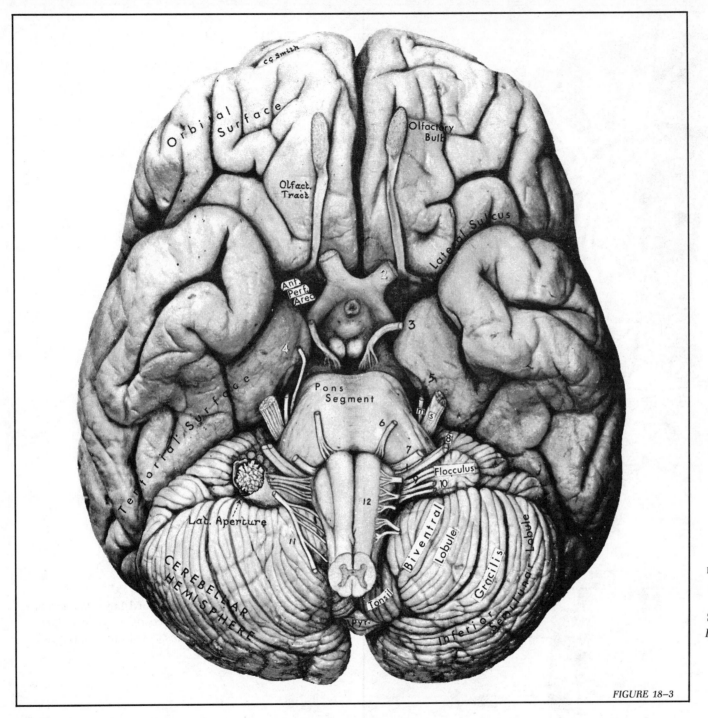

Labels on figure: Orbital Surface, Olfactory Bulb, Olfact. Track, Lateral Sulcus, Ant. Perf. Area, Pons Segment, Tentorial Surface, Flocculus, Lat. Aperture, CEREBELLAR HEMISPHERE, Biventral Lobule, Gracilis, Inferior Semilunar Lobule, Tonsil, Pyr.

FIGURE 18-3

FIGURE 18-3 Human brain viewed from below. Numerals identify the cranial nerves. (From Carlton G. Smith, *Serial Dissections of the Human Brain*. Baltimore: Urban & Schwarzenberg, 1981.)

FIGURE 18-4 Photograph of the human brain viewed from the lateral aspect showing the right cerebral hemisphere, cerebellum, pons, and medulla oblongata. (From Carlton G. Smith, *Serial Dissections of the Human Brain*. Baltimore: Urban & Schwarzenberg, 1981.)

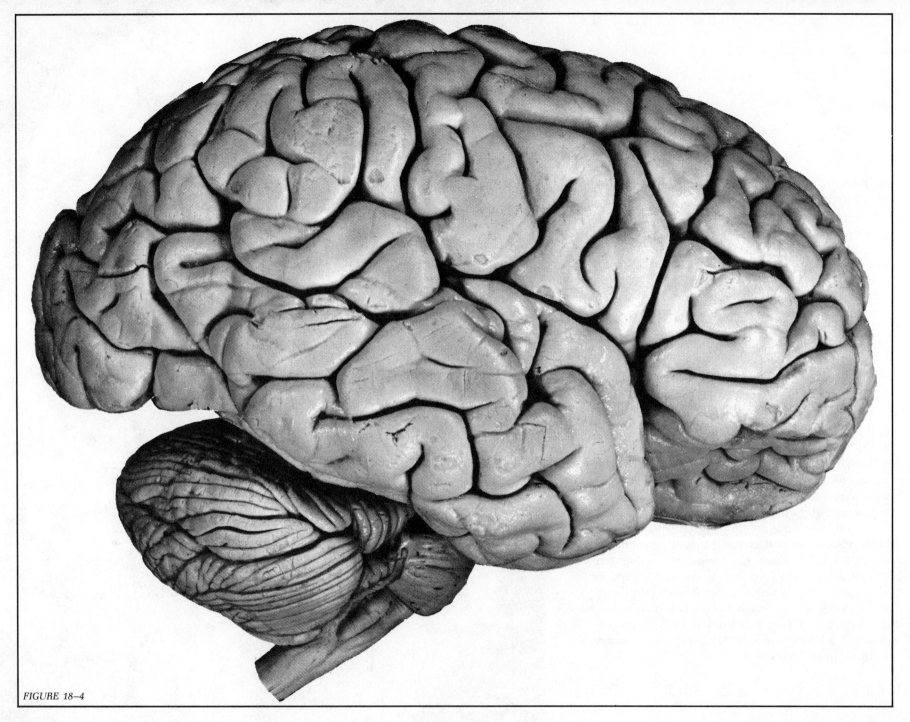

FIGURE 18–4

THE CEREBRAL AND CEREBELLAR HEMISPHERES

259

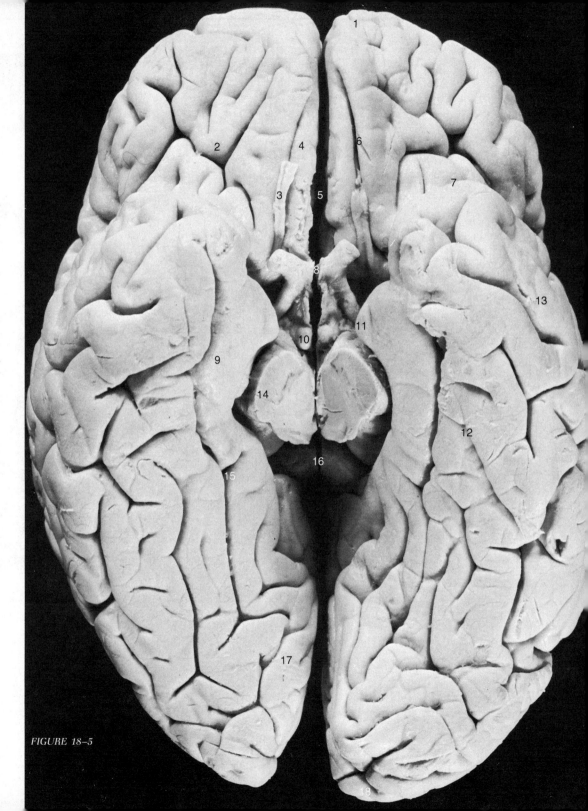

FIGURE 18–5   Right and left cerebral hemispheres with the midbrain transected viewed from the inferior aspect. This brain was sectioned in the midsagittal plane, and then the two sides were pieced together. (1) frontal pole, (2) orbital gyri, (3) olfactory tract, (4) straight gyrus, (5) interhemispheric fissure, (6) olfactory sulcus, (7) temporal pole, (8) optic chiasm (sectioned), (9) parahippocampal gyrus, (10) mammillary body, (11) uncus, (12) occipitotemporal gyri, (13) inferior temporal gyrus, (14) cerebral peduncle, (15) collateral sulcus, (16) splenium of corpus collosum, (17) lingual gyrus, (18) occipital pole. (Material courtesy of Gary van Hoesen, Department of Anatomy, University of Iowa. Photo by Paul Reimann, Department of Anatomy, University of Iowa.)

FIGURE 18–6   Right cerebral hemisphere viewed from the lateral aspect. (1) occipital pole, (2) transverse occipital gyri, (3) lateral occipital gyri, (4) angular gyrus, (5) supramarginal gyrus, (6) postcentral sulcus, (7) postcentral gyrus, (8) central sulcus, (9) precentral gyrus, (10) precentral sulcus, (11) lateral sulcus, (12) superior temporal gyrus, (13) superior temporal sulcus, (14) middle temporal gyrus, (15) middle temporal sulcus, (16) inferior temporal gyrus, (17) superior frontal gyrus, (18) middle frontal gyrus, (19) inferior frontal gyrus, (20) temporal pole, (21) frontal pole. (Material courtesy of Gary van Hoesen, Department of Anatomy, University of Iowa. Photo by Paul Reimann, Department of Anatomy, University of Iowa.)

FIGURE 18–5

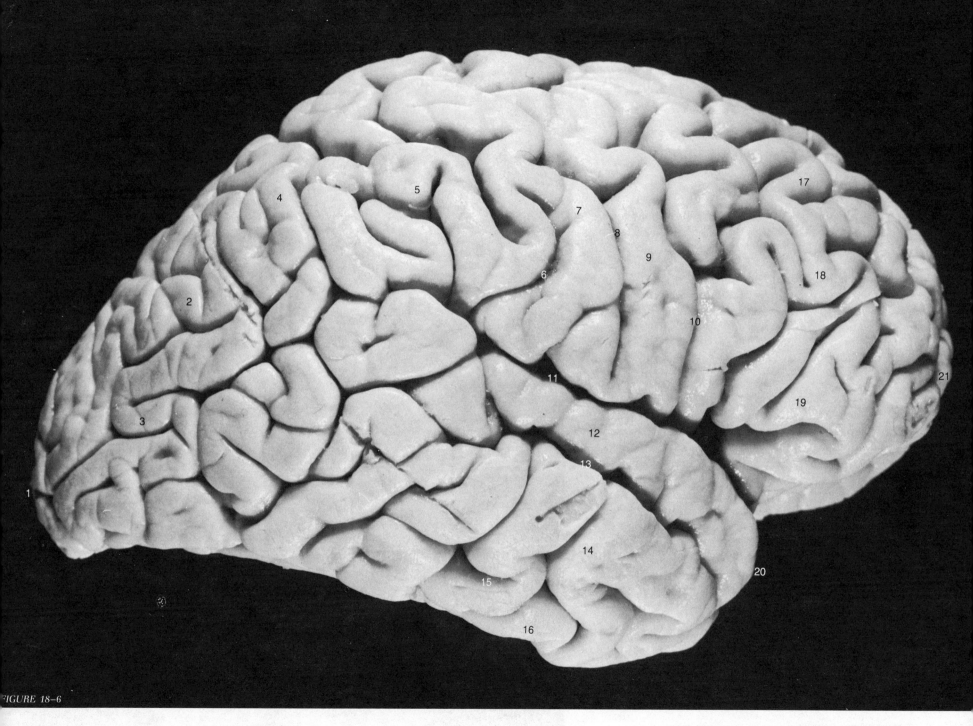

FIGURE 18–6

THE CEREBRAL AND CEREBELLAR HEMISPHERES

FIGURE 18–7 Left and right cerebral hemispheres viewed from the superior aspect. (1) frontal pole, (2) middle frontal gyrus, (3) superior frontal sulcus, (4) superior frontal gyrus, (5) interhemispheric fissure, (6) precentral sulcus, (7) precentral gyrus, (8) central sulcus, (9) postcentral gyrus, (10) postcentral sulcus, (11) superior parietal lobule, (12) occipital gyri, (13) occipital pole. (Material courtesy of Gary van Hoesen, Department of Anatomy, University of Iowa. Photo by Paul Reimann, Department of Anatomy, University of Iowa.)

FIGURE 18–8 Right cerebral hemisphere with the midbrain transected viewed from the medial aspect. (1) frontal pole, (2) superior frontal gyrus, (3) cingulate sulcus, (4) cingulate gyrus, (5) genu of corpus callosum, (6) rostrum of corpus callosum, (7) subcallosal area, (8) parolfactory gyrus, (9) straight gyrus, (10) body of corpus callosum, (11) septum pellucidum, (12) thalamus, (13) central sulcus, (14) paracentral lobule, (15) splenium of corpus callosum, (16) midbrain (transected), (17) parahippocampal gyrus, (18) collateral sulcus, (19) middle occipitotemporal gyrus, (20) precuneus, (21) calcarine sulcus, (22) parietooccipital sulcus, (23) cuneus, (24) lingual gyrus, (25) occipital pole. (Material courtesy of Gary van Hoesen, Department of Anatomy, University of Iowa. Photo by Paul Reimann, Department of Anatomy, University of Iowa.)

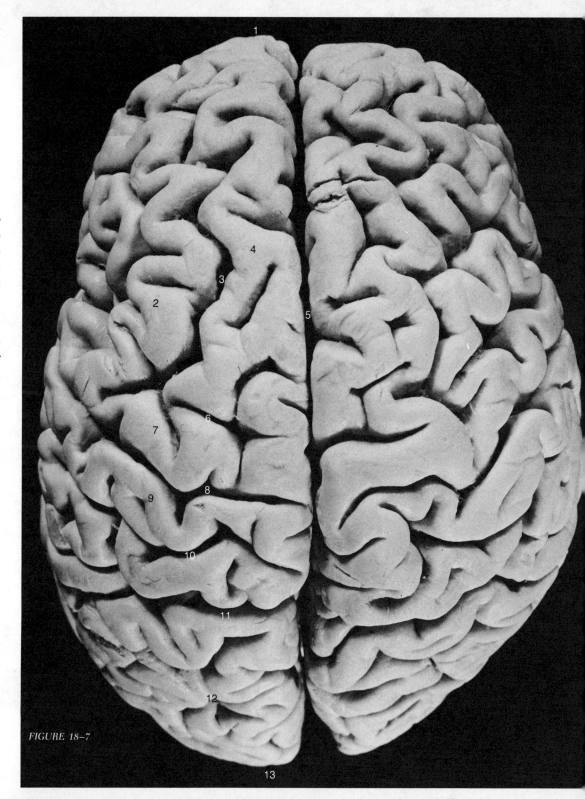

FIGURE 18–7

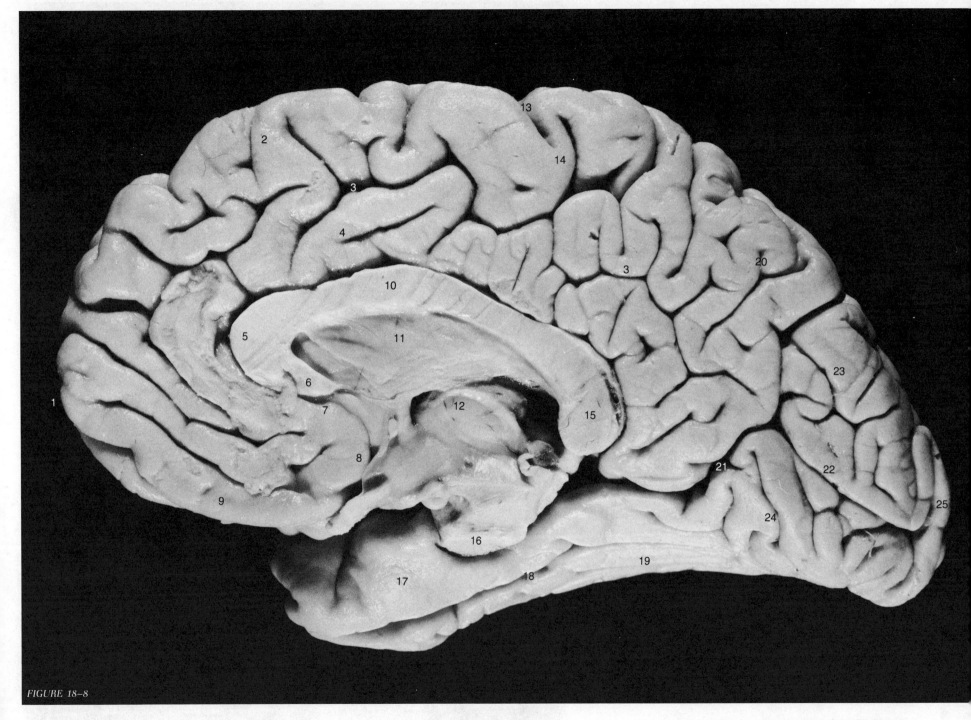

FIGURE 18–8

THE CEREBRAL AND CEREBELLAR HEMISPHERES

263

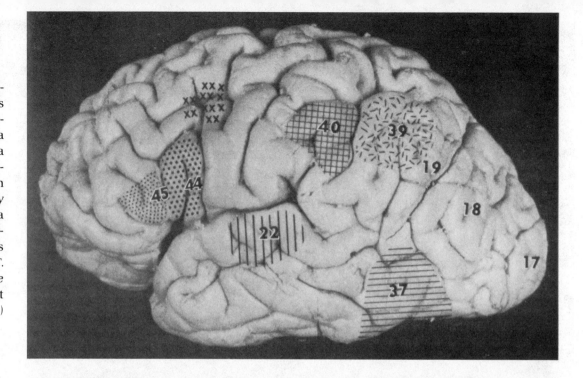

FIGURE 18–9 Lateral surface of some of the areas related to language. The numbers refer to Brodmann's cytoarchitectural divisions. Area (22) auditory association cortex, area (37) visual-auditory association, area (39) angular gyrus, area (40) supramarginal gyrus, area (45) and the adjoining part of area (44) constitute approximately Broca's area, (XXX) has traditionally been related to writing, but many other areas are certainly involved. The extent and placement of Wernicke's area is variable. It is sometimes depicted as the area between areas 22, 40, and 39; it may also be shown as including areas 22, 40, and/or 39. (From E.E. Crosby, T. Humphrey, and E. Lauer, *Correlative Anatomy of the Nervous System*. New York: Macmillan, 1962. Copyright © 1962 by Macmillan Publishing Co., Inc.)

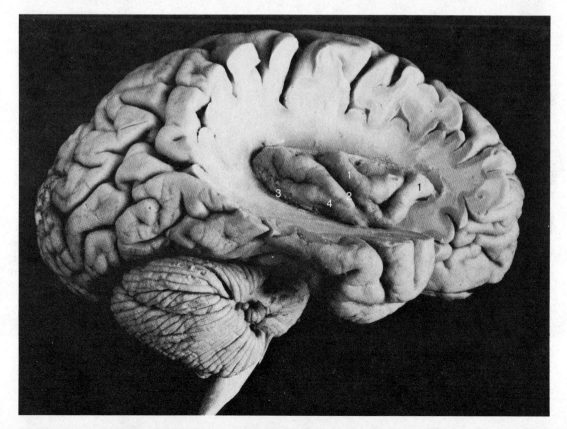

FIGURE 18–10 Dissection of the right cerebral hemisphere viewed from the lateral aspect to show the insula. The frontal, frontoparietal, and temporal opercula, which bound the lateral sulcus and its rami, have been removed. (1) short gyri of insula, (2) central sulcus of insula, (3) circular sulcus of insula, (4) long gyrus of insula. (Courtesy of Nedzad Gluhbegovic and Terence H. Williams, *The Human Brain: A Photographic Guide*. New York: Harper & Row, 1980.)

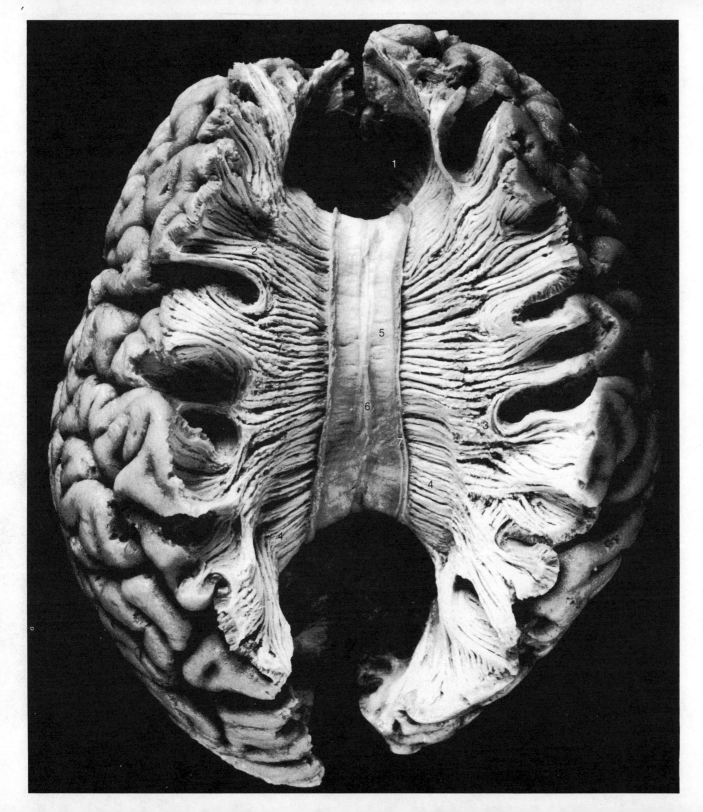

FIGURE 18–11 Dissection of
the brain viewed from above to
show the corpus callosum, its
radiation, and indusium
griseum (a thin covering over
the intermediate portion of the
corpus callosum). (1) frontal
forceps, (2) commissural cal-
losal fibers, (3) short arcuate
fibers, (4) occipital forceps,
(5) indusium griseum, (6) medial longitudinal stria, (7) lateral longitudinal stria. (Courtesy of Nedzad Gluhbegovic
and Terence H. Williams, *The
Human Brain: A Photographic
Guide*. New York: Harper &
Row, 1980.)

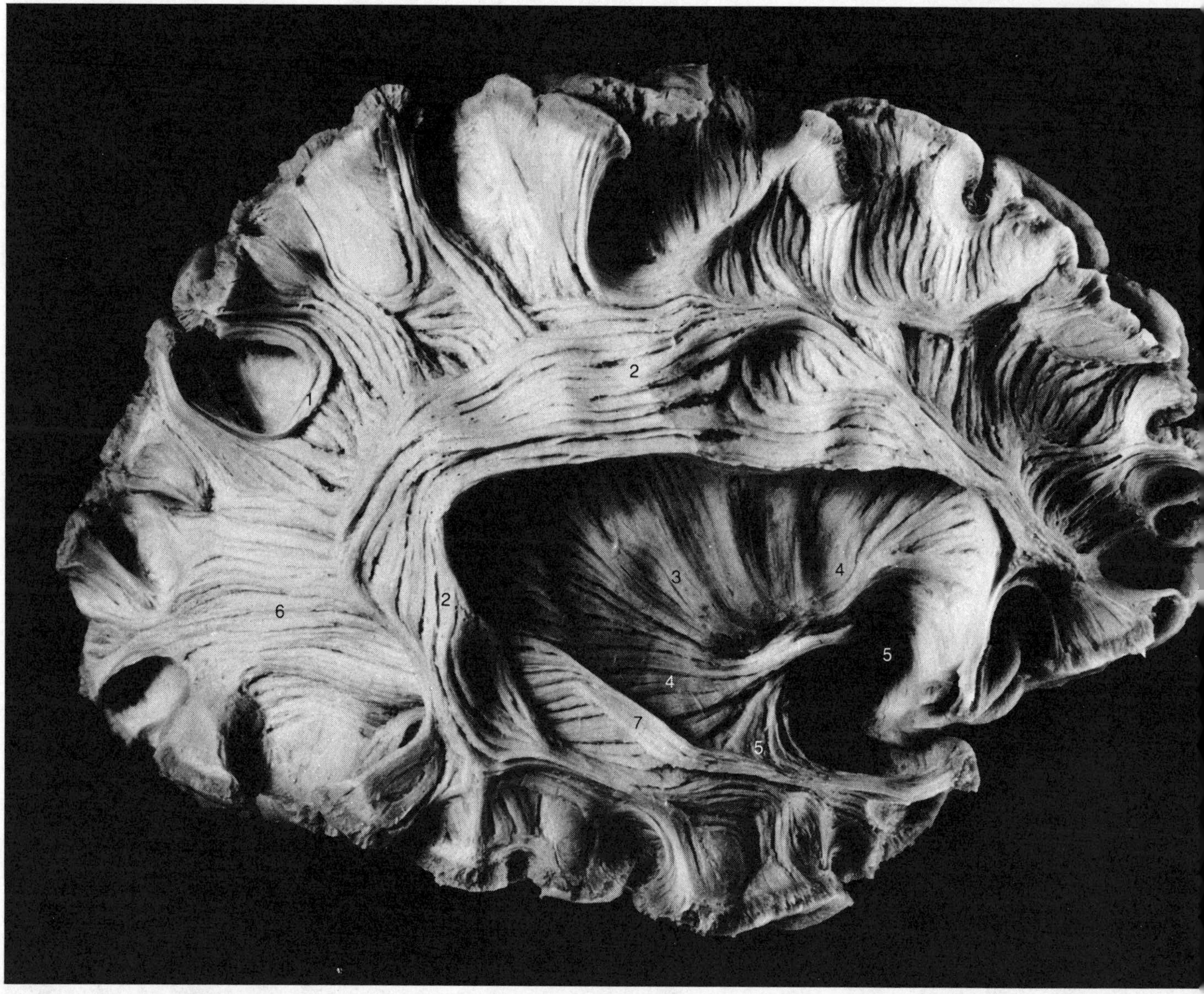

FIGURE 18–12 Dissection of the right cerebral hemisphere viewed from the lateral aspect to show the short and long association tracts. (1) short arcuate fibers, (2) superior longitudinal fascicle, (3) external capsule, (4) inferior occipitofrontal fascicle, (5) uncinate fascicle, (6) sagittal stratum, (7) inferior longitudinal fasciculus. (Courtesy of Nedzad Gluhbegovic and Terence H. Williams, *The Human Brain: A Photographic Guide*. New York: Harper and Row, 1980.)

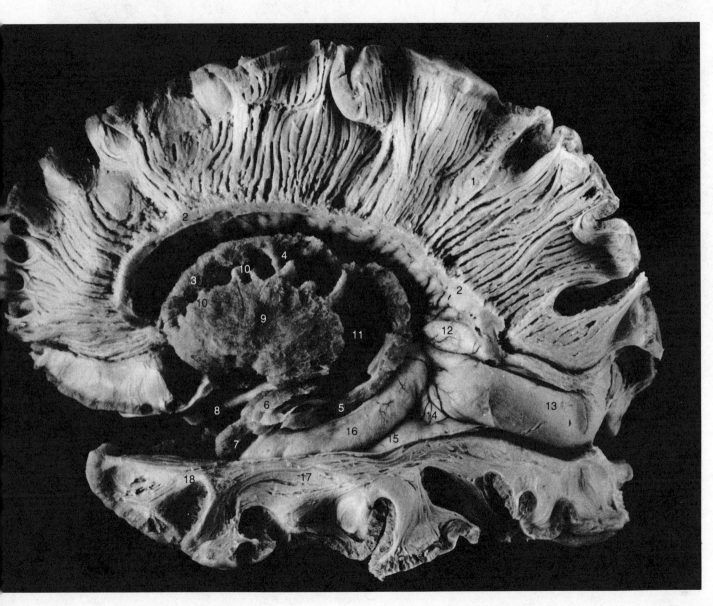

FIGURE 18–13 Dissection of the left cerebral hemisphere viewed from the lateral aspect to show the basal ganglia. The extreme, external, and internal capsules have been removed. (1) corona radiata, (2) corpus callosum, (3) head of caudate nucleus, (4) body of caudate nucleus, (5) tail of caudate nucleus, (6) "foot" of lentiform nucleus, (7) amygdaloid nuclear complex, (8) optic tract, (9) putamen, (10) gray connections between putamen and caudate nucleus, (11) pulvinar of thalamus, (12) bulb of occipital horn of lateral ventricle, (13) calcar avis, (14) collateral trigone, (15) collateral eminence, (16) hippocampus, (17) inferior longitudinal fasciculus, (18) short arcuate fibers. (Courtesy of Nedzad Gluhbegovic and Terence H. Williams, *The Human Brain: A Photographic Guide.* New York: Harper and Row, 1980.)

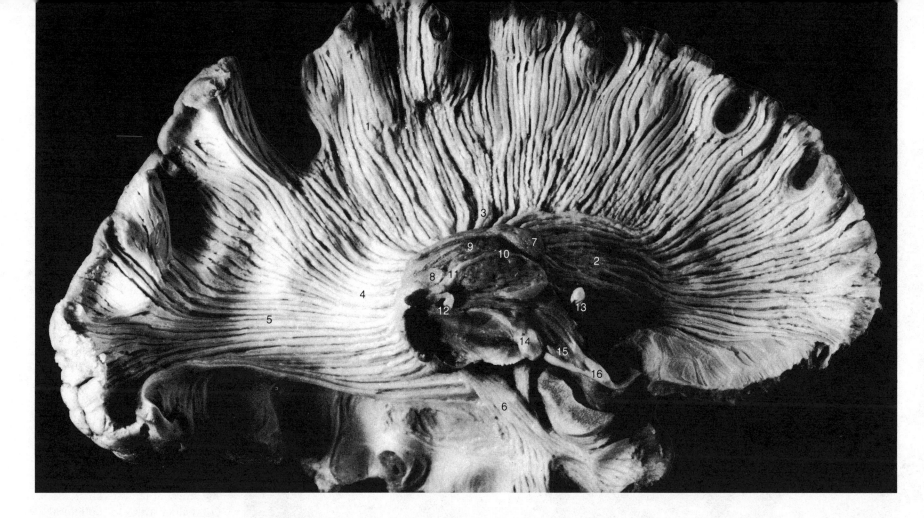

FIGURE 18–14 Dissection of the left cerebral hemisphere viewed from the medial aspect to show the cortical projection systems. The corpus callosum (except for the splenium and a small part of the body) and the medial and part of the lateral thalamic nuclei have been removed. (1) corona radiata, (2) anterior thalamic peduncle, (3) superior thalamic peduncle, (4) posterior thalamic peduncle, (5) sagittal stratum, (6) inferior (caudal) thalamic peduncle, (7) anterior thalamic nuclear group, (8) pineal body, (9) dorsomedial thalamic nucleus, (10) stria medullaris thalami, (11) habenular trigone, (12) posterior (epithalamic) commissure, (13) anterior (rostral) commissure, (14) mamillary body, (15) tuber cinereum, (16) optic chiasma. (Courtesy of Nedzad Gluhbegovic and Terence H. Williams, *The Human Brain: A Photographic Guide*. New York: Harper and Row, 1980.)

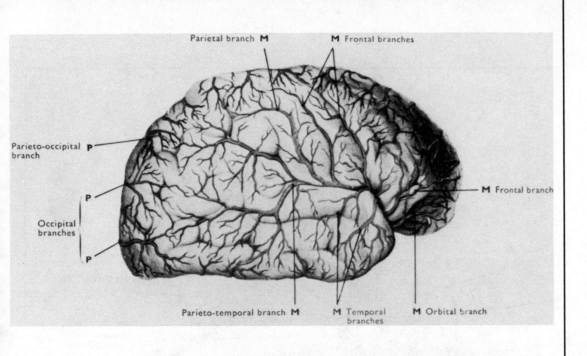

FIGURE 18–15 Right cerebral hemisphere viewed from the lateral aspect to show the branches of the (M) middle cerebral artery and (P) posterior cerebral artery. (Courtesy of John N. Walton, *Brain's Diseases of the Nervous System*, 8th Ed. Oxford: Oxford University Press, 1977.)

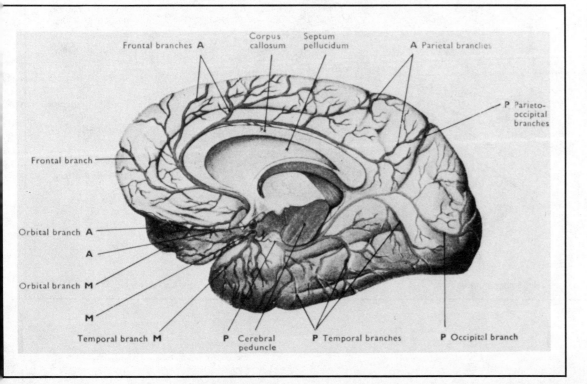

FIGURE 18–16 Right cerebral hemisphere viewed from the medial aspect to show the branches of the (A) anterior cerebral artery, (M) middle cerebral artery, and (P) posterior cerebral artery. (Courtesy of John N. Walton, *Brain's Diseases of the Nervous System*, 8th Ed. Oxford: Oxford University Press, 1977.)

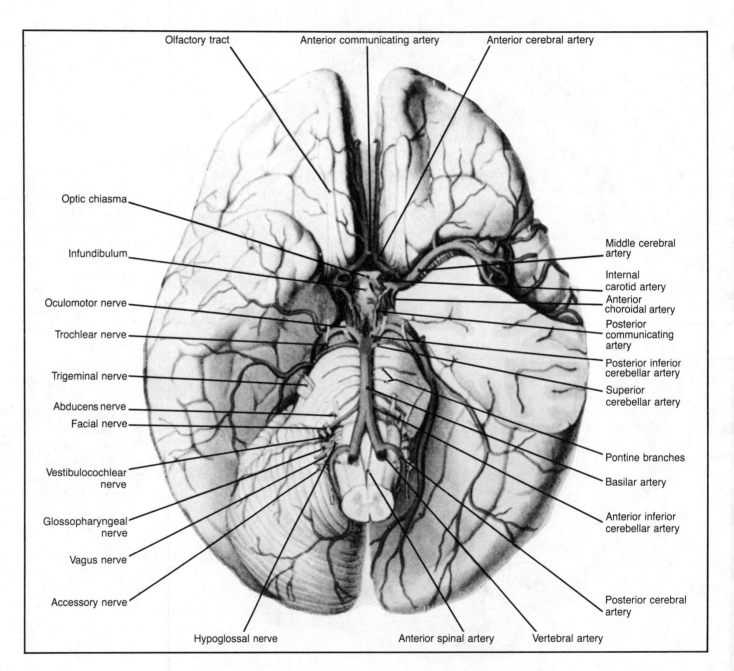

Olfactory tract

Anterior communicating artery

Anterior cerebral artery

Optic chiasma

Infundibulum

Oculomotor nerve

Trochlear nerve

Trigeminal nerve

Abducens nerve

Facial nerve

Vestibulocochlear
nerve

Glossopharyngeal
nerve

Vagus nerve

Accessory nerve

Middle cerebral
artery

Internal
carotid artery

Anterior
choroidal artery

Posterior
communicating
artery

Posterior inferior
cerebellar artery

Superior
cerebellar artery

Pontine branches

Basilar artery

Anterior inferior
cerebellar artery

Posterior cerebral
artery

Hypoglossal nerve

Anterior spinal artery

Vertebral artery

FIGURE 18–17 Brain viewed from the inferior aspect to show the major arteries. (Courtesy of John N. Walton, *Brain's Diseases of the Nervous System*, 8th Ed. Oxford: Oxford University Press, 1977.)

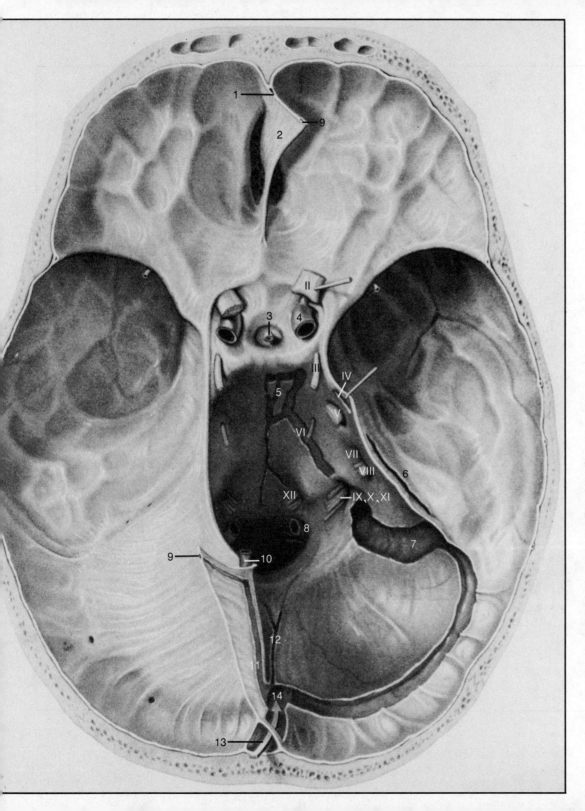

FIGURE 18–18 Dura and dural sinuses along the base of the cranial cavity as viewed from the superior aspect. The right half of the tentorium cerebelli has been removed, as well as the falx cerebri except for its anterior and posterior attachments. The dura has been trimmed from some of the sinuses. (1) superior sagittal sinus, (2) falx cerebri, (3) infundibulum, (4) internal carotid artery, (5) basilar plexus, (6) superior petrosal sinus, (7) transverse sinus, (8) vertebral artery, (9) inferior sagittal sinus, (10) vena magna, (11) sinus rectus, (12) occipital sinus, (13) superior sagittal sinus, (14) confluens sinuum. The cranial nerves are marked with their respective Roman numerals. (From G. Wolf-Heidegger, *Atlas of Systematic Human Anatomy*, Vol. 2. Basel, Switzerland: S. Karger AG, 1962 (German). New York: Hafner Publishing Company, 1962 (English).)

THE CEREBRAL AND CEREBELLAR HEMISPHERES

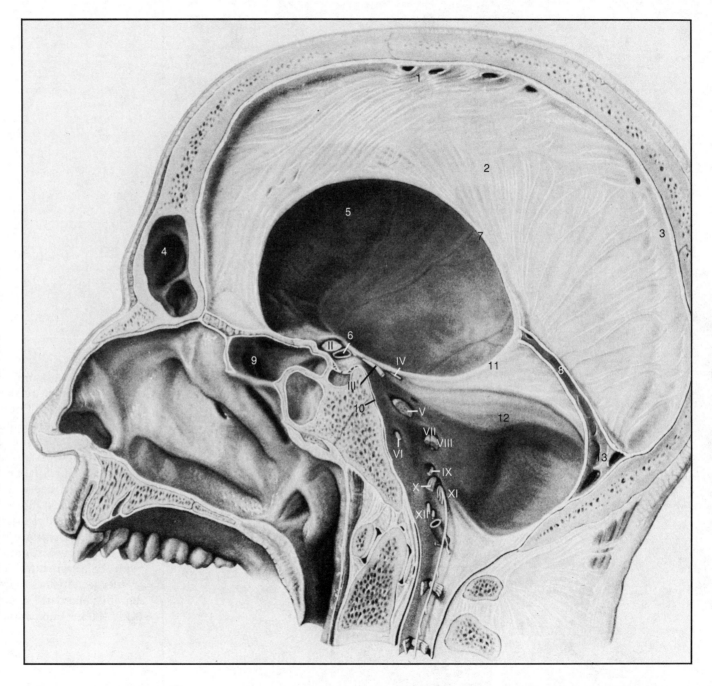

FIGURE 18–19 Head, sectioned slightly to the left of the midsagittal plane and viewed from the left to illustrate the dura and dural sinuses. (1) superior cerebral veins opening from superior cerebral sinus, (2) falx cerebri, (3) cut edge of dura, (4) frontal sinus, (5) cranial cavity, (6) internal carotid artery, (7) inferior sagittal sinus, (8) sinus rectus, (9) sphenoid sinuses, (10) basilar plexus, (11) tentorium cerebelli, (12) falx cerebelli, (13) confluens sinuum. The cranial nerves are marked with their respective Roman numerals. (From G. Wolf-Heidegger, *Atlas of Systematic Human Anatomy*, Vol. 3. Basel, Switzerland: S. Karger AG, 1962 (German). New York: Hafner Publishing Company, 1962 (English).)

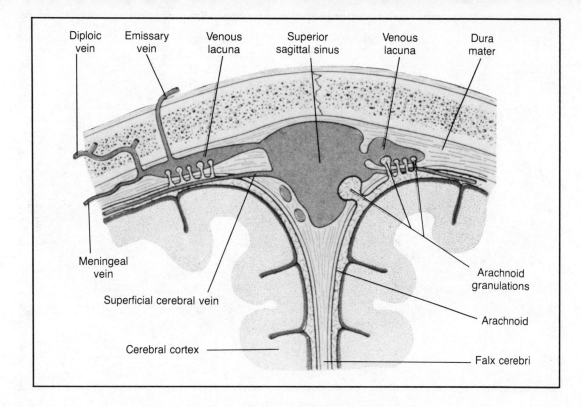

Diploic vein — Emissary vein — Venous lacuna — Superior sagittal sinus — Venous lacuna — Dura mater

Meningeal vein

Superficial cerebral vein

Cerebral cortex

Arachnoid granulations

Arachnoid

Falx cerebri

FIGURE 18–20   Coronal section through the vertex of the skull to show the arrangement of the veins and the meninges of the brain and arachnoid granulations. (Courtesy of Peter L. Williams and Roger Warwick, *Functional Neuroanatomy of Man.* Edinburgh: Longman Group, Ltd., 1975.)

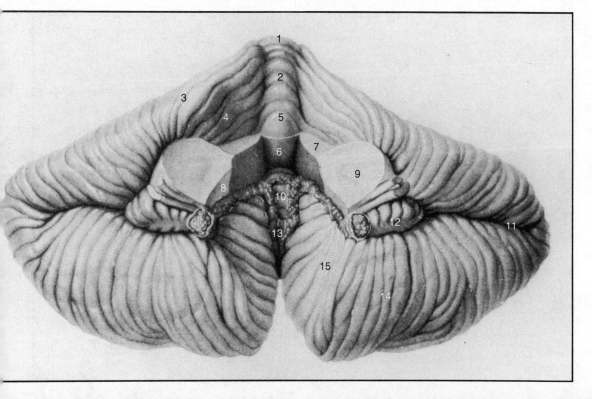

FIGURE 18–21   Cerebellum viewed from the anteroinferior aspect. The cerebellar peduncles have been cut. (1) culmen, (2) central lobule, (3) quadrangular lobule, (4) ala of central lobule, (5) lingula of vermis, (6) superior medullary velum, (7) superior cerebellar peduncle, (8) inferior cerebellar peduncle, (9) middle cerebellar peduncle, (10) nodulus, (11) horizontal fissure, (12) flocculus, (13) uvula of vermis, (14) biventral lobule, (15) tonsil. (From G. Wolf-Heidegger, *Atlas of Systematic Human Anatomy.* Basel, Switzerland: S. Karger AG, 1962 (German). New York: Hafner Publishing Company, 1962 (English).)

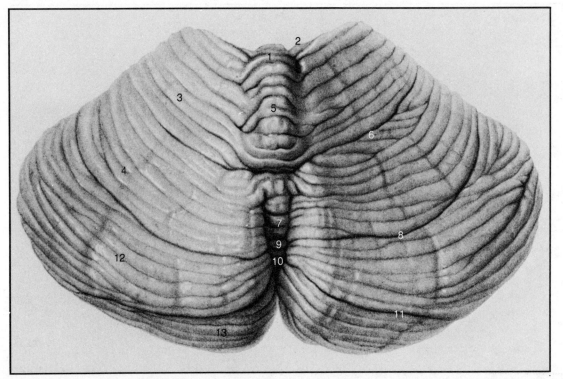

FIGURE 18–22 Cerebellum viewed from the inferior aspect. The medulla oblongata has been cut and the cerebellar tonsils have been removed. (1) inferior semilunar lobule, (2) biventral lobule, (3) pyramis of vermis, (4) uvula of vermis, (5) cut surface of cerebellar tonsil, (6) nodulus, (7) peduncle of flocculus, (8) paraflocculus, (9) flocculus, (10) medulla oblongata, (11) pons. (From G. Wolf-Heidegger, *Atlas of Systematic Human Anatomy*. Basel, Switzerland: S. Karger AG, 1962 (German). New York: Hafner Publishing Company, 1962 (English).)

FIGURE 18–23 Cerebellum viewed from posterosuperior aspect. (1) central lobule, (2) ala of central lobule, (3) anterior quadrangular lobule, (4) posterior quadrangular lobule, (5) culmen, (6) anterosuperior fissure, (7) declive, (8) posterosuperior fissure, (9) pyramis of vermis, (10) tuber of vermis, (11) horizontal fissure, (12) superior semilunar lobule, (13) inferior semilunar lobule. (From G. Wolf-Heidegger, *Atlas of Systematic Human Anatomy*. Basel, Switzerland: S. Karger AG, 1962 (German). New York: Hafner Publishing Company, 1962 (English).)

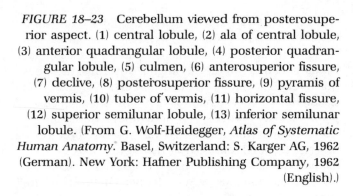

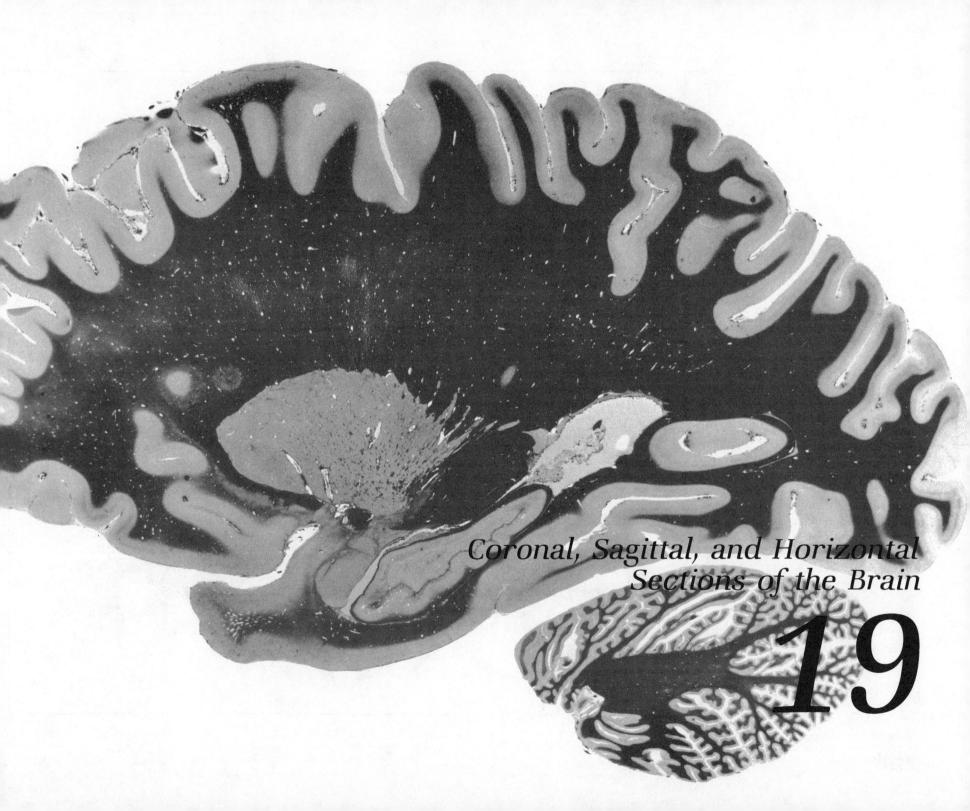

Coronal, Sagittal, and Horizontal Sections of the Brain

19

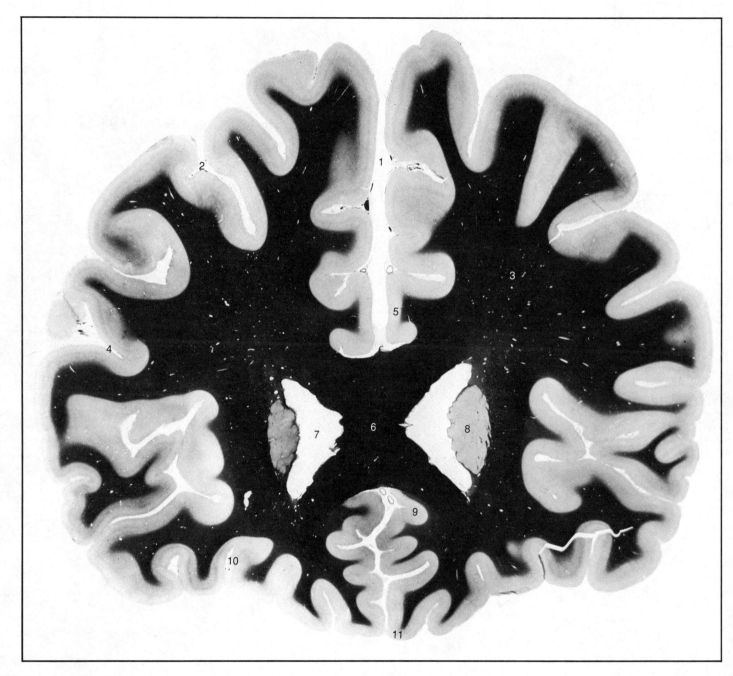

FIGURE 19–1 Photomicrograph of an adult human brain sectioned in the coronal plane. This figure is the first in a series of six figures progressing from anterior to posterior. A myelin stain has been used so that fiber tracts appear dark and cell bodies appear light. (1) interhemispheric fissure, (2) superior frontal sulcus, (3) centrum semiovale, (4) middle frontal sulcus, (5) cingulate gyrus, (6) genu of corpus callosum, (7) anterior horn of lateral ventricle, (8) caudate nucleus, (9) subcallosal area, (10) orbital gyri, (11) straight gyrus. (Courtesy of the Yakovlev Collection, NINCDS–AFIP Interagency Agreement N__ Y01–NS–7–0032–04, Armed Forces Institute of Pathology, Washington, D.C. Photo by Paul Reimann, Department of Anatomy, University of Iowa.)

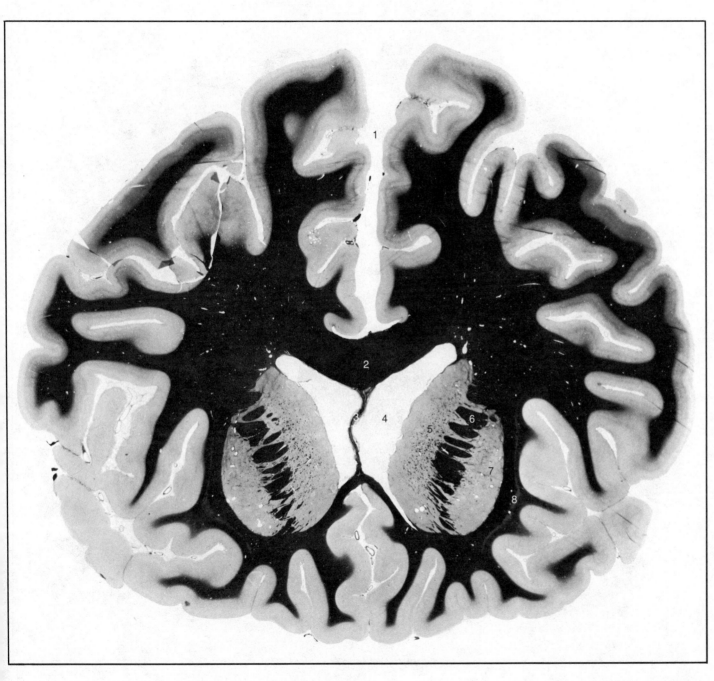

FIGURE 19–2 Photomicrograph of an adult human brain sectioned in the coronal plane. This figure is the second in a series of six figures progressing from anterior to posterior. A myelin stain has been used so that fiber tracts appear dark and cell bodies appear light. (1) interhemispheric fissure, (2) body of corpus callosum, (3) septum pellucidum, (4) lateral ventricle, (5) caudate nucleus, (6) anterior limb of internal capsule, (7) putamen, (8) claustrum. (Courtesy of the Yakovlev Collection, NINCDS–AFIP Interagency Agreement N__ Y01–NS–7–0032–04, Armed Forces Institute of Pathology, Washington, D.C. Photo by Paul Reimann, Department of Anatomy, University of Iowa.)

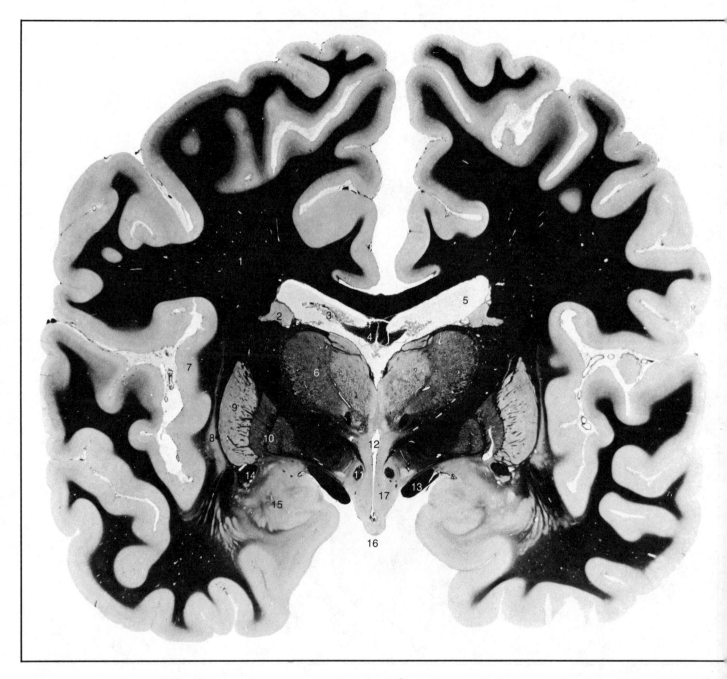

FIGURE 19–3 Photomicrograph of an adult human brain sectioned in the coronal plane. This figure is the third in a series of six figures progressing from anterior to posterior. A myelin stain has been used so that fiber tracts appear dark and cell bodies appear light. (1) corona radiata, (2) caudate nucleus, (3) choroid plexus, (4) fornix, (5) lateral ventricle, (6) thalamus, (7) insula, (8) claustrum, (9) putamen, (10) globus palladus, (11) column of fornix, (12) third ventricle, (13) optic tract, (14) anterior commissure, (15) amygdaloid body, (16) infundibulum, (17) hypothalamus. (Courtesy of the Yakovlev Collection, NINCDS–AFIP Interagency Agreement N__ Y01–NS–7–0032–04, Armed Forces Institute of Pathology, Washington, D.C. Photo by Paul Reimann, Department of Anatomy, University of Iowa.)

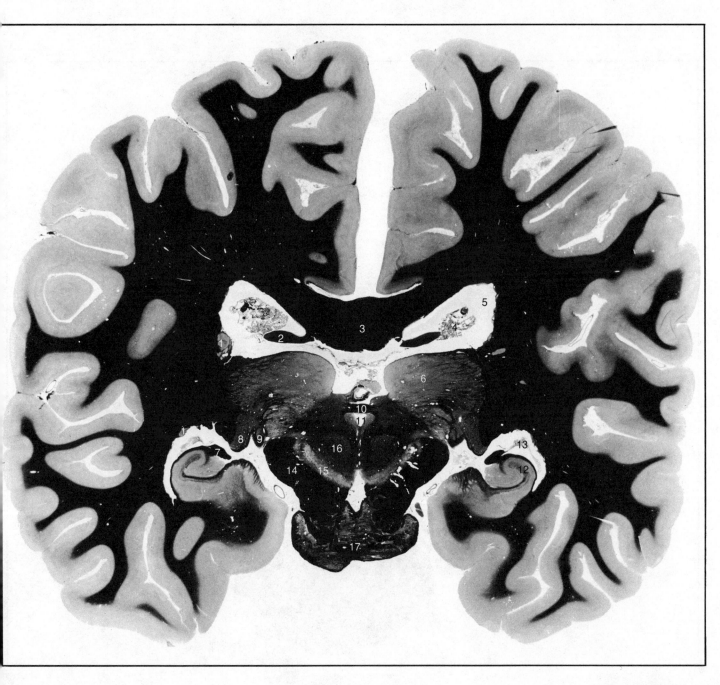

FIGURE 19–4 Photomicrograph of an adult human brain sectioned in the coronal plane. This figure is the fourth in a series of six figures progressing from anterior to posterior. A myelin stain has been used so that fiber tracts appear dark and cell bodies appear light. (1) tail of caudate nucleus, (2) fornix, (3) corpus callosum, (4) choroid plexus, (5) lateral ventricle, (6) pulvinar, (7) fimbra of fornix, (8) lateral geniculate body, (9) medial geniculate body, (10) posterior commissure, (11) cerebral aqueduct surrounded by periaqueductal gray matter, (12) hippocampus, (13) inferior horn of lateral ventricle, (14) cerebral peduncle, (15) substantia nigra, (16) red nucleus, (17) pons. (Courtesy of the Yakovlev Collection, NINCDS–AFIP Interagency Agreement N__ Y01–NS–7–0032–04, Armed Forces Institute of Pathology, Washington, D.C. Photo by Paul Reimann, Department of Anatomy, University of Iowa.)

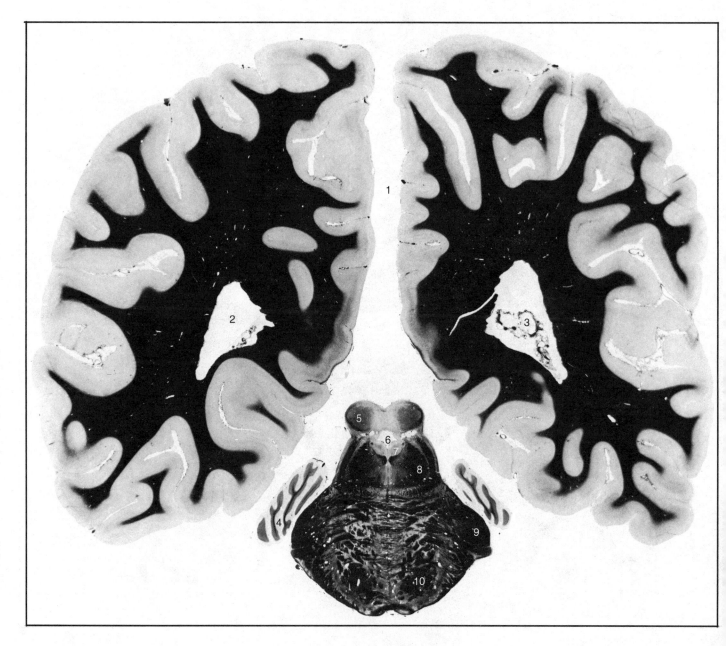

FIGURE 19–5 Photomicrograph of an adult human brain sectioned in the coronal plane. This figure is the fifth in a series of six figures progressing from anterior to posterior. A myelin stain as been used so that fiber tracts appear dark and cell bodies appear light. (1) interhemispheric fissure, (2) posterior horn of lateral ventricle, (3) choroid plexus, (4) anterior tip of cerebellar hemisphere, (5) inferior colliculus, (6) cerebral aqueduct, (7) periaqueductal gray matter, (8) superior cerebellar peduncle, (9) middle cerebellar peduncle, (10) pons. (Courtesy of the Yakovlev Collection, NINCDS–AFIP Interagency Agreement N__ Y01–NS–7–0032–04, Armed Forces Institute of Pathology, Washington, D.C. Photo by Paul Reimann, Department of Anatomy, University of Iowa.)

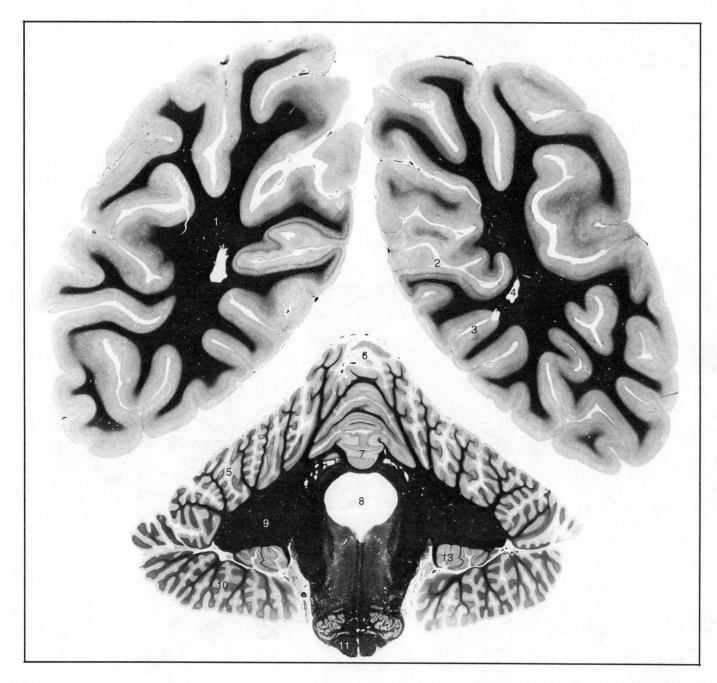

FIGURE 19–6 Photomicrograph of an adult human brain sectioned in the coronal plane. This figure is the sixth in a series of six figures progressing from anterior to posterior. A myelin stain has been used so that fiber tracts appear dark and cell bodies appear light. (1) occipital lobe, (2) calcarine fissure, (3) lingual gyrus, (4) posterior horn of lateral ventricle, (5) anterior lobe of cerebellar hemisphere, (6) vermis, (7) lingua of vermis, (8) fourth ventricle, (9) middle cerebellar peduncle, (10) posterior lobe of cerebellar hemisphere, (11) pyramid, (12) inferior olive, (13) flocculus. (Courtesy of the Yakovlev Collection, NINCDS–AFIP Interagency Agreement N__ Y01–NS–7–0032–04, Armed Forces Institute of Pathology, Washington, D.C. Photo by Paul Reimann, Department of Anatomy, University of Iowa.)

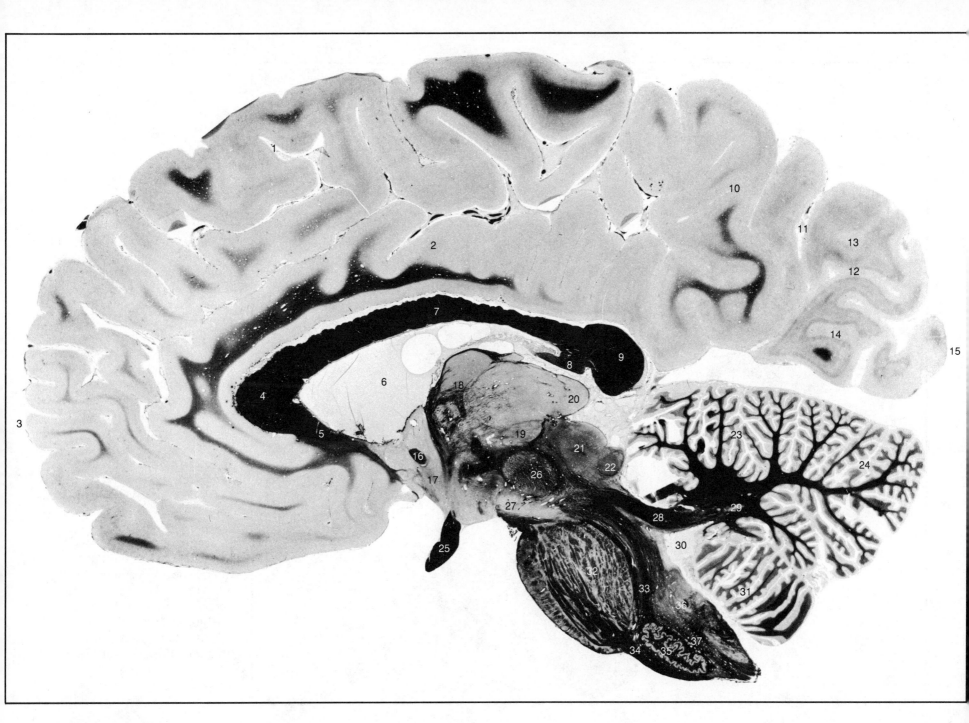

FIGURE 19–7 Photomicrograph of adult human brain sectioned in the sagittal plane. This is the first in a series of five figures progressing from medial to lateral. A myelin stain has been used so that fiber tracts appear dark and cell bodies appear light. (1) superior frontal gyrus, (2) cingulate gyrus, (3) frontal pole, (4) genu of corpus callosum, (5) rostum of corpus callosum, (6) lateral ventricle, (7) body of corpus callosum, (8) fornix, (9) splenium of corpus callosum, (10) precuneus, (11) parietooccipital sulcus, (12) calcarine sulcus, (13) cuneus, (14) lingual gyrus, (15) occipital pole, (16) anterior commissure, (17) hypothalamus, (18) thalamus, (19) subthalamic nuclei, (20) pulvinar, (21) superior colliculus, (22) inferior colliculus, (23) anterior lobe of cerebellar hemisphere, (24) posterior lobe of cerebellar hemisphere, (25) optic nerve, (26) red nucleus, (27) substantia nigra, (28) superior cerebellar peduncle, (29) central cerebellar nuclei, (30) fourth ventricle, (31) cerebellar tonsil, (32) pons, (33) medial lemniscus, (34) pyramid, (35) inferior olive, (36) nucleus gracilis, (37) medulla oblongata. (Courtesy of the Yakovlev Collection, NINCDS–AFIP Interagency Agreement N__ Y01–NS–7–0032–04, Armed Forces Institute of Pathology, Washington, D.C. Photo by Paul Reimann, Department of Anatomy, University of Iowa.)

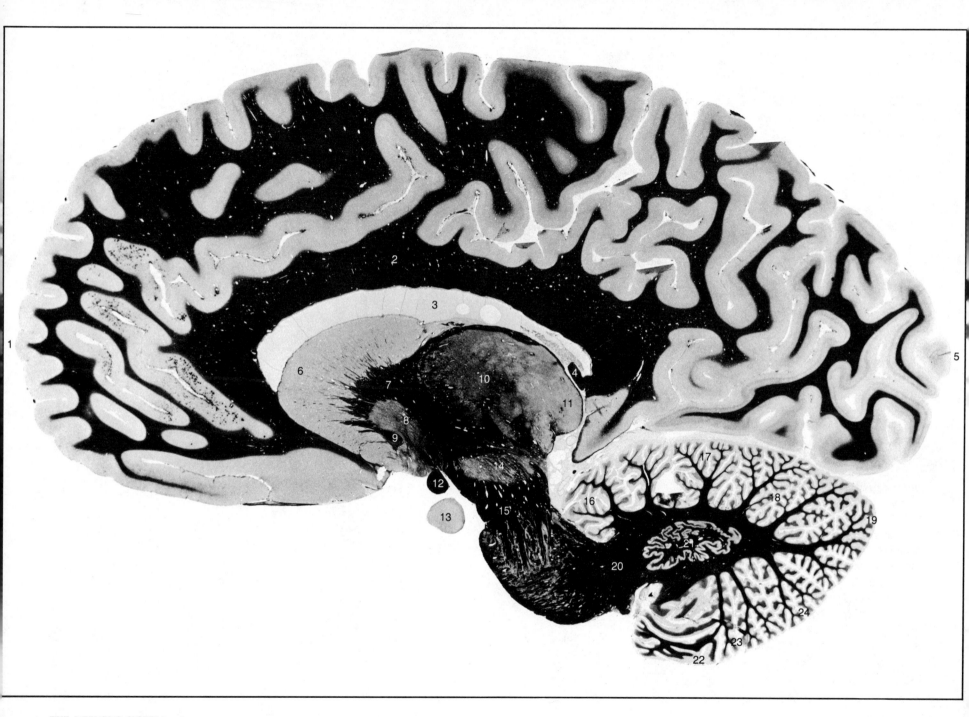

FIGURE 19–8 Photomicrograph of adult human brain sectioned in the sagittal plane. This is the second in a series of five figures progressing from medial to lateral. A myelin stain has been used so that fiber tracts appear dark and cell bodies appear light. (1) frontal pole, (2) cingulum, (3) lateral ventricle, (4) fornix, (5) occipital pole, (6) head of caudate nucleus, (7) anterior limb of internal capsule, (8) globus palladus, (9) anterior commissure, (10) thalamus, (11) pulvinar, (12) optic tract, (13) uncus, (14) substantia nigra, (15) cerebral peduncle, (16) central lobule of cerebellum, (17) quadrangular lobule of cerebellum, (18) simple lobule of cerebellum, (19) superior semilunar lobule of cerebellum, (20) middle cerebellar peduncle, (21) dentate nucleus, (22) cerebellar tonsil, (23) biventral lobule of cerebellum, (24) inferior semilunar lobule of cerebellum. (Courtesy of the Yakovlev Collection, NINCDS–AFIP Interagency Agreement N__ Y01–NS–7–0032–04, Armed Forces Institute of Pathology, Washington, D.C. Photo by Paul Reimann, Department of Anatomy, University of Iowa.)

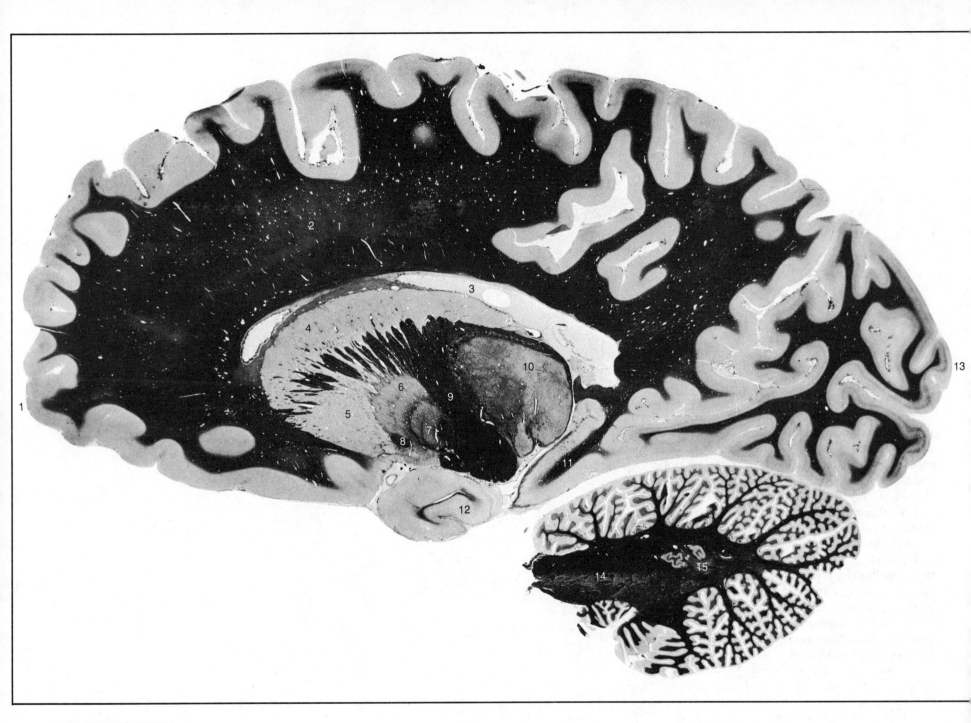

FIGURE 19–9 Photomicrograph of adult human brain sectioned in the sagittal plane. This is the third in a series of five figures progressing from medial to lateral. A myelin stain has been used so that fiber tracts appear dark and cell bodies appear light. (1) frontal pole, (2) corona radiata, (3) lateral ventricle, (4) head of caudate nucleus, (5) putamen, (6) lateral segment of globus pallidus, (7) medial segment of globus pallidus, (8) anterior commissure, (9) internal capsule, (10) pulvinar, (11) isthmus of cingulate gyrus, (12) hippocampus, (13) occipital pole, (14) middle cerebellar peduncle, (15) dentate nucleus. (Courtesy of the Yakovlev Collection, NINCDS–AFIP Interagency Agreement N__ Y01–NS–7–0032–04, Armed Forces Institute of Pathology, Washington, D.C. Photo by Paul Reimann, Department of Anatomy, University of Iowa.)

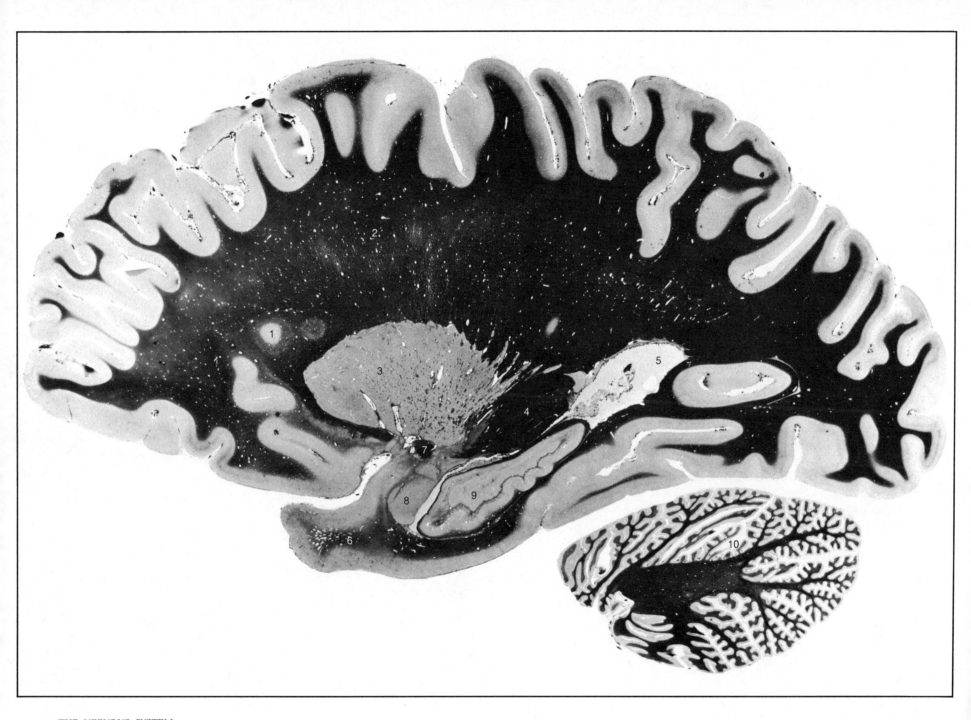

FIGURE 19–10 Photomicrograph of an adult human brain sectioned in the sagittal plane. This figure is the fourth in a series of five figures progressing from medial to lateral. A myelin stain has been used so that fiber tracts appear dark and cell bodies appear light. (1) tip of insular cortex, (2) corona radiata, (3) putamen, (4) optic radiation, (5) inferior horn of lateral ventricle, (6) temporal lobe, (7) anterior commissure, (8) amygdala, (9) hippocampus, (10) cerebellar hemisphere. (Courtesy of the Yakovlev Collection, NINCDS–AFIP Interagency Agreement N__ Y01–NS–7–0032–04, Armed Forces Institute of Pathology, Washington, D.C. Photo by Paul Reimann, Department of Anatomy, University of Iowa.)

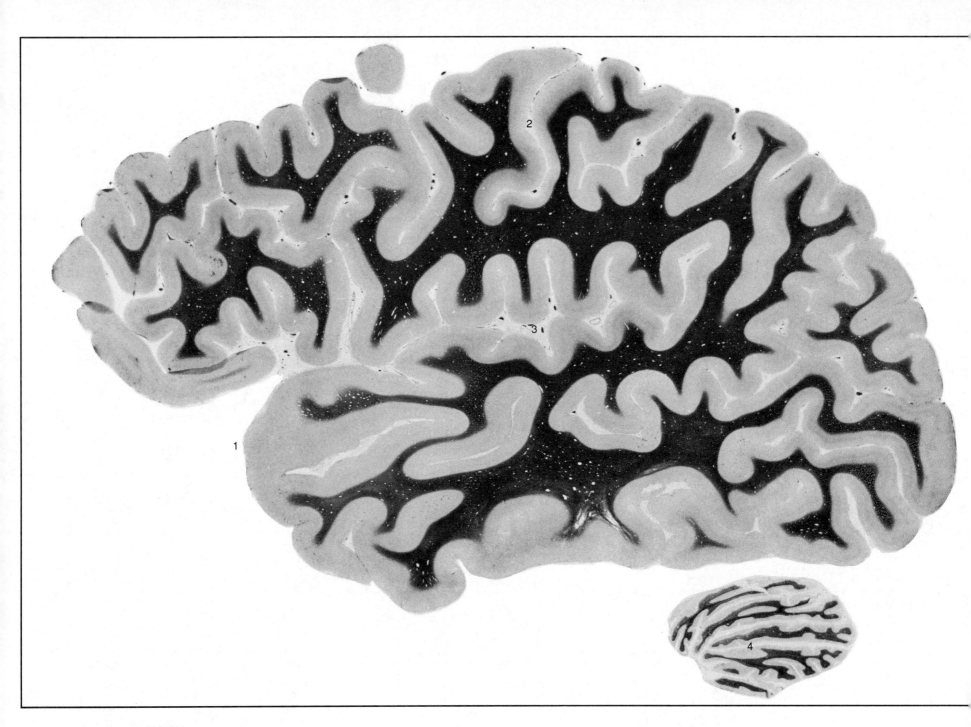

FIGURE 19–11 Photomicrograph of an adult human brain sectioned in the sagittal plane. This figure is the fifth in a series of five figures progressing from medial to lateral. A myelin stain has been used so that fiber tracts appear dark and cell bodies appear light. (1) temporal pole, (2) central sulcus, (3) lateral sulcus, (4) lateral tip of superior semilunar lobule. (Courtesy of the Yakovlev Collection, NINCDS–AFIP Interagency Agreement N__ Y01–NS–7–0032–04, Armed Forces Institute of Pathology, Washington, D.C. Photo by Paul Reimann, Department of Anatomy, University of Iowa.)

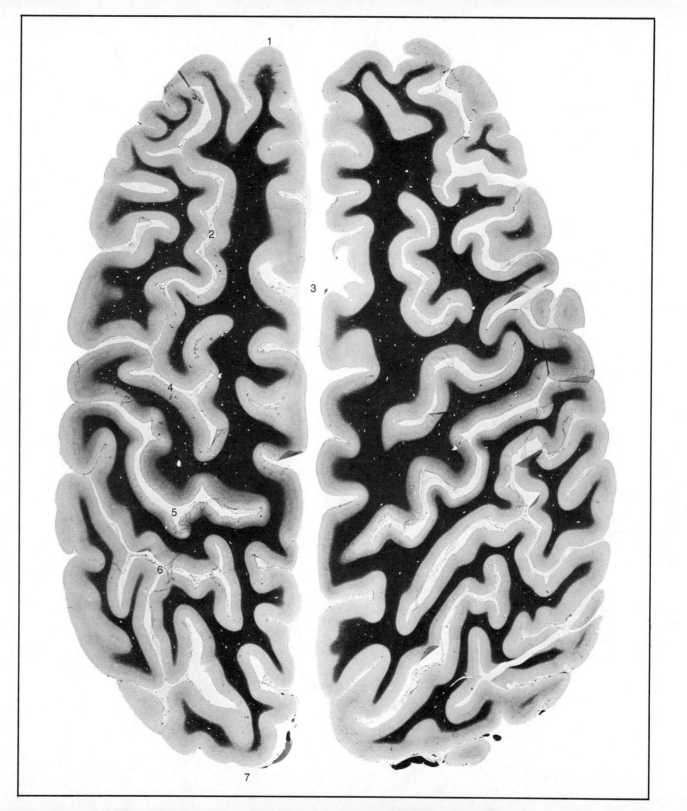

FIGURE 19–12 Photomicrograph of an adult human brain sectioned in the horizontal plane. This figure is the first in a series of seven figures progressing from superior to inferior. A myelin stain has been used so that fiber tracts appear dark and cell bodies appear light. (1) frontal pole, (2) superior frontal sulcus, (3) interhemispheric fissure, (4) precentral sulcus, (5) central sulcus, (6) postcentral sulcus, (7) occipital pole. (Courtesy of the Yakovlev Collection, NINCDS–AFIP Interagency Agreement N__ Y01–NS–7–0032–04, Armed Forces Institute of Pathology, Washington, D.C. Photo by Paul Reimann, Department of Anatomy, University of Iowa.)

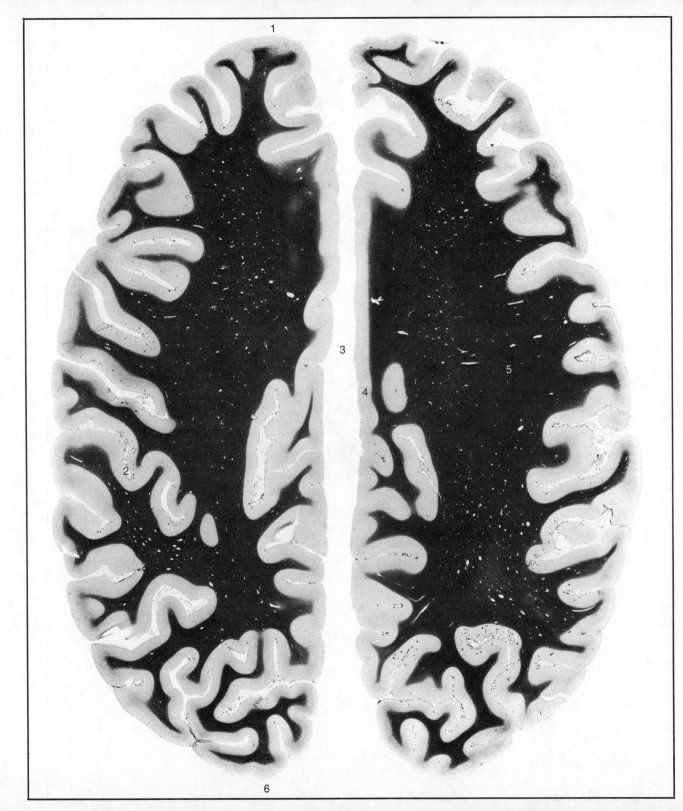

FIGURE 19–13 Photomicrograph of an adult human brain sectioned in the horizontal plane. This figure is the second in a series of seven figures progressing from superior to inferior. A myelin stain has been used so that fiber tracts appear dark and cell bodies appear light. (1) frontal pole, (2) central sulcus, (3) interhemispheric fissure, (4) cingulate gyrus, (5) centrum semiovale, (6) occipital pole. (Courtesy of the Yakovlev Collection, NINCDS–AFIP Interagency Agreement N__ Y01–NS–7–0032–04, Armed Forces Institute of Pathology, Washington, D.C. Photo by Paul Reimann, Department of Anatomy, University of Iowa.)

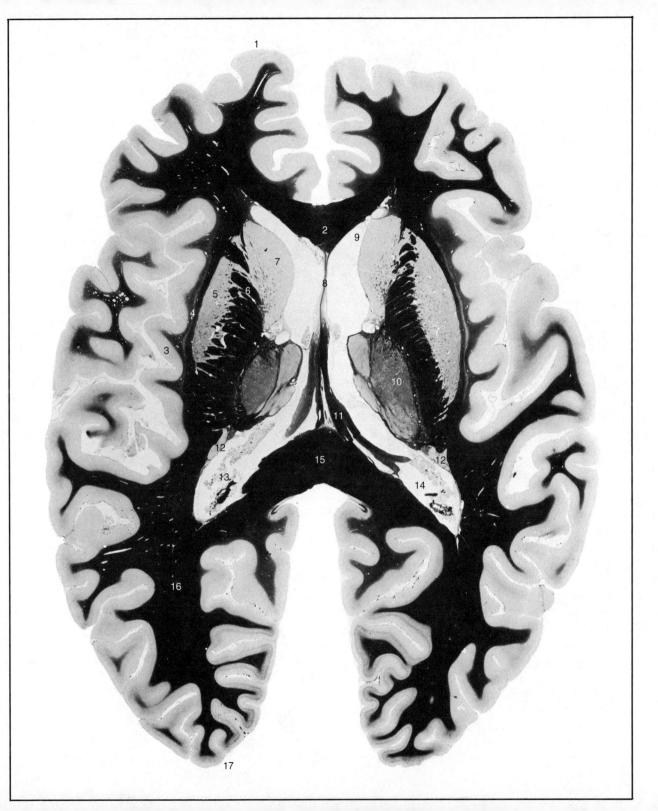

FIGURE 19–14 Photomicrograph of an adult human brain sectioned in the horizontal plane. This figure is the third in a series of seven figures progressing from superior to inferior. A myelin stain has been used so that fiber tracts appear dark and cell bodies appear light. (1) frontal pole, (2) genu of corpus callosum, (3) insula, (4) claustrum, (5) putamen, (6) anterior limb of internal capsule, (7) head of caudate nucleus, (8) septum pellucidum, (9) anterior horn of lateral ventricle, (10) thalamus, (11) fornix, (12) tail of caudate nucleus, (13) choroid plexus, (14) lateral ventricle, (15) splenium of corpus callosum, (16) occipital radiation, (17) occipital pole. (Courtesy of the Yakovlev Collection, NINCDS–AFIP Interagency Agreement N__ Y01–NS–7–0032–04, Armed Forced Institute of Pathology, Washington, D.C. Photo by Paul Reimann, Department of Anatomy, University of Iowa.)

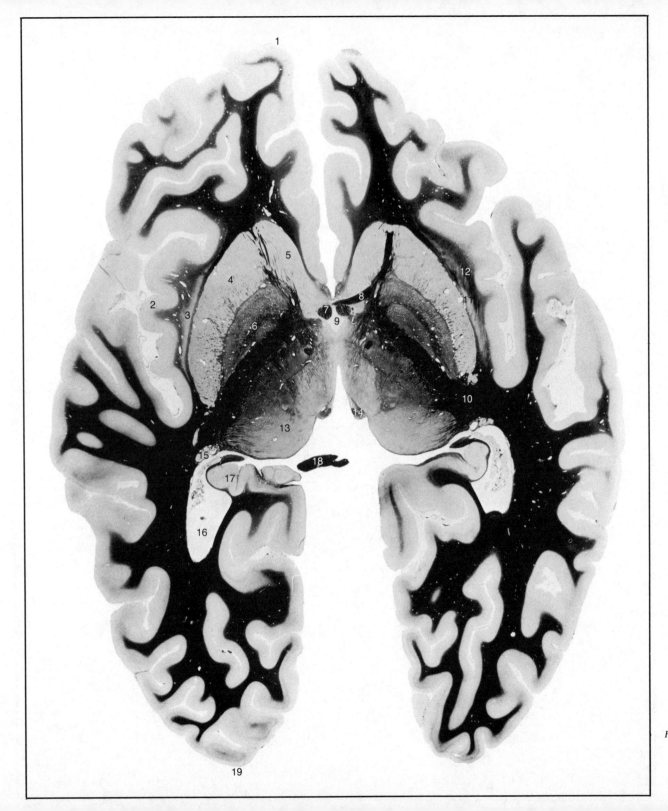

FIGURE 19–15 Photomicrograph of an adult human brain sectioned in the horizontal plane. This figure is the fourth in a series of seven figures progressing from superior to inferior. A myelin stain has been used so that fiber tracts appear dark and cell bodies appear light. (1) frontal pole, (2) insula, (3) claustrum, (4) putamen, (5) caudate nucleus, (6) globus palladus, (7) column of fornix, (8) anterior commissure, (9) third ventricle, (10) internal capsule, (11) external capsule, (12) extreme capsule, (13) thalamus, (14) habenula, (15) tail of caudate nucleus, (16) posterior horn of lateral ventricle, (17) hippocampus, (18) fornix, (19) occipital pole. (Courtesy of the Yakovlev Collection, NINCDS–AFIP Interagency Agreement N__ Y01–NS–7–0032–04, Armed Forces Institute of Pathology, Washington, D.C. Photo by Paul Reimann, Department of Anatomy, University of Iowa.)

CORONAL, SAGITTAL, AND HORIZONTAL SECTIONS OF THE BRAIN

295

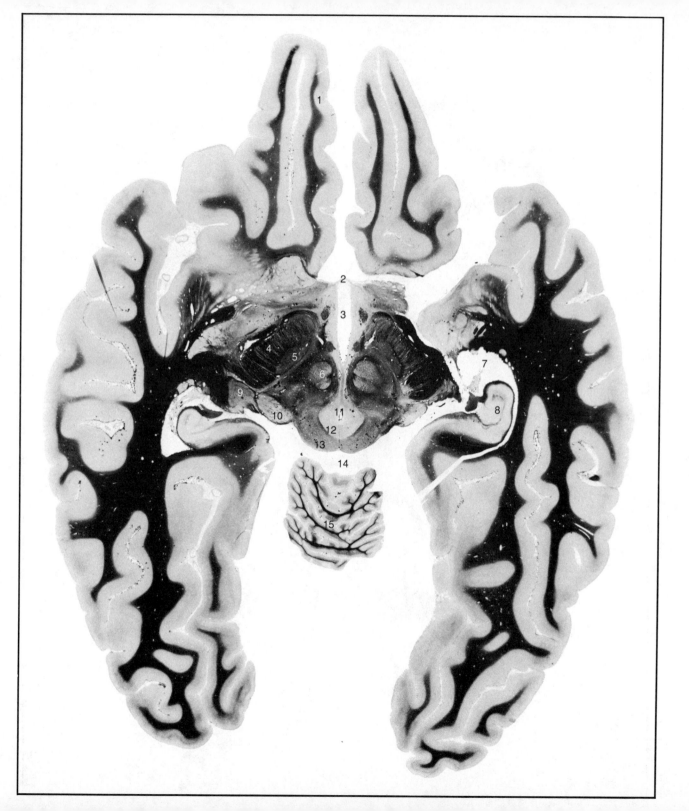

FIGURE 19–16 Photomicrograph of an adult human brain sectioned in the horizontal plane. This figure is the fifth in a series of seven figures progressing from superior to inferior. A myelin stain has been used so that fiber tracts appear dark and cell bodies appear light. (1) straight gyrus, (2) lamina terminalis, (3) third ventricle, (4) cerebral peduncle, (5) substantia nigra, (6) red nucleus, (7) inferior horn of lateral ventricle, (8) hippocampus, (9) lateral geniculate body, (10) medial geniculate body, (11) cerebral aqueduct, (12) periaqueductal gray matter, (13) superior colliculus, (14) quadrigeminal cistern, (15) vermis of cerebellum. (Courtesy of the Yakovlev Collection, NINCDS–AFIP Interagency Agreement N__ Y01–NS–7–0032–04, Armed Forces Institute of Pathology, Washington, D.C. Photo by Paul Reimann, Department of Anatomy, University of Iowa.)

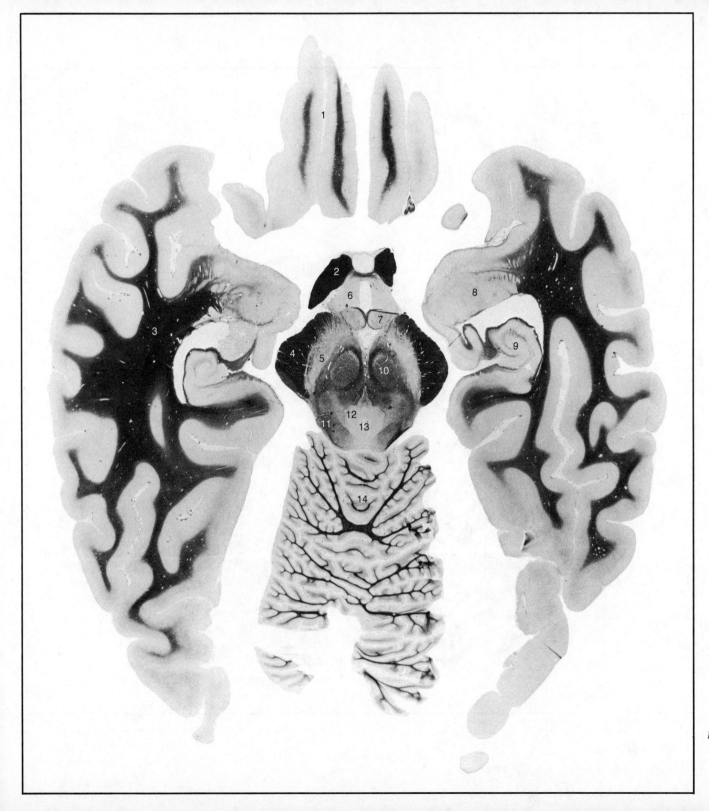

FIGURE 19–17 Photomicrograph of an adult human brain sectioned in the horizontal plane. This figure is the sixth in a series of seven figures progressing from superior to inferior. A myelin stain has been used so that fiber tracts appear dark and cell bodies appear light. (1) olfactory sulcus, (2) optic tract, (3) temporal lobe, (4) cerebral peduncle, (5) substantia nigra, (6) hypothalamus, (7) mammillary body, (8) amygdala, (9) hippocampus, (10) red nucleus, (11) inferior colliculus, (12) periaqueductal gray matter, (13) cerebral aqueduct, (14) vermis of cerebellum. (Courtesy of the Yakovlev Collection, NINCDS–AFIP Interagency Agreement N__ Y01–NS–7–0032–04, Armed Forces Institute of Pathology, Washington, D.C. Photo by Paul Reimann, Department of Anatomy, University of Iowa.)

CORONAL, SAGITTAL, AND
HORIZONTAL SECTIONS OF THE BRAIN

297

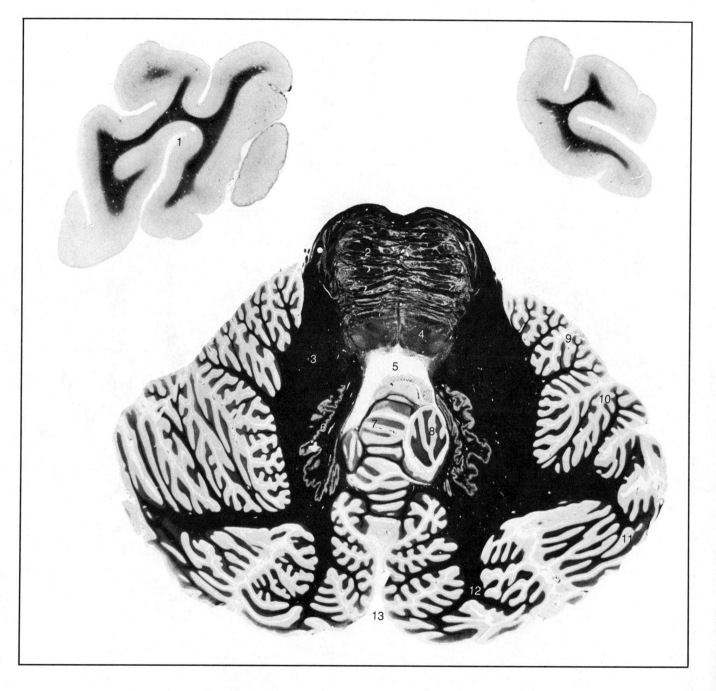

FIGURE 19–18 Photomicrograph of an adult human brain sectioned in the horizontal plane. This figure is the seventh in a series of seven figures progressing from superior to inferior. A myelin stain has been used so that fiber tracts appear dark and cell bodies appear light. (1) inferior tip of temporal lobe, (2) transverse pontine fibers, (3) middle cerebellar peduncle, (4) tegmentum of pons, (5) fourth ventricle, (6) dentate nucleus, (7) vermis, (8) tonsil, (9) quadrangular lobule, (10) simple lobule, (11) superior semilunar lobule, (12) inferior semilunar lobule, (13) posterior incisure. (Courtesy of the Yakovlev Collection, NINCDS–AFIP Interagency Agreement N__ Y01–NS–7–0032–04, Armed Forces Institute of Pathology, Washington, D.C. Photo by Paul Reimann, Department of Anatomy, University of Iowa.)

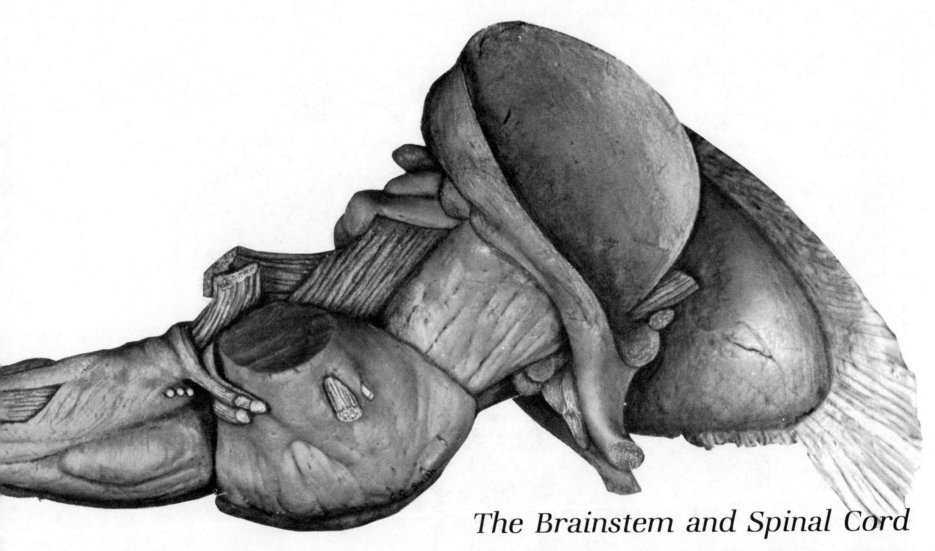

The Brainstem and Spinal Cord

20

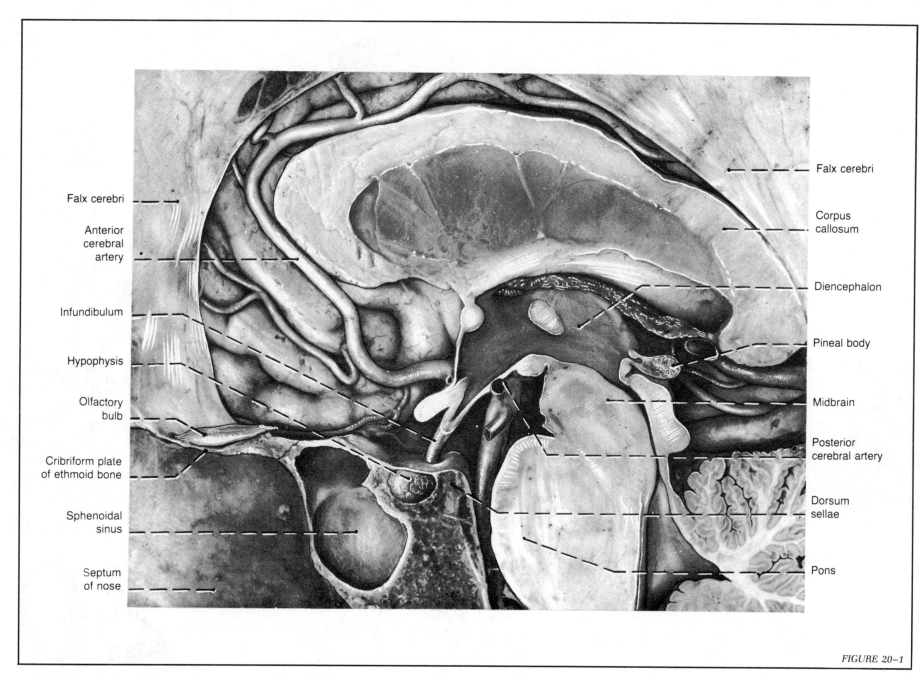

Falx cerebri

Anterior
cerebral
artery

Infundibulum

Hypophysis

Olfactory
bulb

Cribriform plate
of ethmoid bone

Sphenoidal
sinus

Septum
of nose

Falx cerebri

Corpus
callosum

Diencephalon

Pineal body

Midbrain

Posterior
cerebral artery

Dorsum
sellae

Pons

FIGURE 20–1

THE NERVOUS SYSTEM

300

FIGURE 20–1 Midsagittal section of the head to illustrate the corpus collosum, diencephalon, midbrain, pons, and surrounding structures. (Courtesy of Lord Solly Zuckerman, with Deryk Darlington and Peter Lisowski, *A New System of Anatomy*, 2nd Ed. Oxford: Oxford University Press, 1981.)

FIGURE 20–2 Brainstem viewed from the dorsal aspect showing the external morphology. (1) caudate nucleus, (2) right and left fornix anterior to the interventricular foramina, (3) pulvinar, (4) third ventricle, (5) habenular trigone, (6) lateral geniculate body, (7) medial geniculate body, (8) inferior colliculus, (9) superior colliculus, (10) pineal gland, (11) lateral lemniscus, (12) medial lemniscus, (13) cerebral peduncle, (14) middle cerebellar peduncle, (15) inferior cerebellar peduncle, (16) superior cerebellar peduncle, (17) cochlear nucleus, (18) vestibular nuclei, (19) gracilis tubercle, (20) cuneate tubercle, (21) tuberculum cinereum, (22) fasciculus gracilis, (23) fasciculus cuneatus. (From Carlton G. Smith, *Serial Dissections of the Human Brain*. Baltimore: Urban & Schwarzenberg, 1981.)

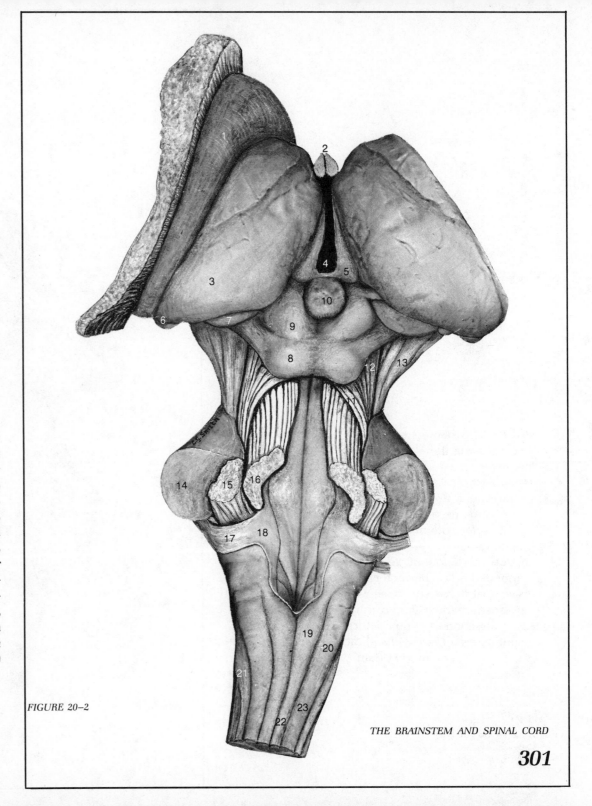

FIGURE 20–2

FIGURE 20–3 Brainstem viewed from the ventral aspect showing the external morphology. (1) right and left fornix, (2) caudate nucleus, (3) lentiform nucleus, (4) striate vessels, (5) lateral surface of diencephalon, (6) lamina terminalis, (7) anterior perforated area, (8) optic nerve, (9) optic chiasma, (10) optic tract, (11) anterior commissure, (12) temporopontine tract, (13) optic radiation, (14) mammillary body, (15) cerebral peduncle, (16) lateral geniculate body, (17) posterior perforated area, (18) motor and sensory branches of trigeminal nerve, (19) facial, vestibular, cochlear, and glossopharyngeal nerves, (20) olive, (21) pyramid, (22) decussation of pyramidal tracts. (From Carlton G. Smith, *Serial Dissections of the Human Brain.* Baltimore: Urban & Swarzenberg, 1981.)

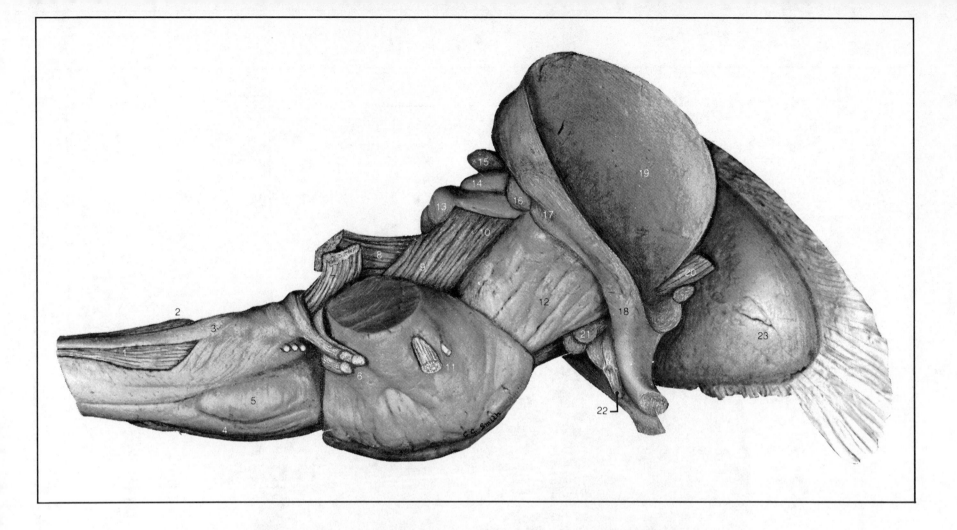

FIGURE 20–4   Brainstem viewed from the lateral aspect showing the external morphology. (1) spinal tract of trigeminal nucleus, (2) gracilis tubercle, (3) cuneate tubercle, (4) pyramid, (5) olive, (6) facial, cochlear, and vestibular nerves, (7) inferior cerebellar peduncle, (8) superior cerebellar peduncle, (9) lateral lemniscus, (10) medial lemniscus, (11) sensory and motor branches of trigeminal nerve, (12) cerebral peduncle, (13) inferior colliculus, (14) superior colliculus, (15) pineal gland, (16) medial geniculate body, (17) lateral geniculate body, (18) optic tract, (19) diencephalon, (20) fornix, (21) mammillary body, (22) infundibulum, (23) caudate nucleus. (From Carlton G. Smith, *Serial Dissections of the Human Brain.* Baltimore: Urban & Schwartzenberg, 1981.)

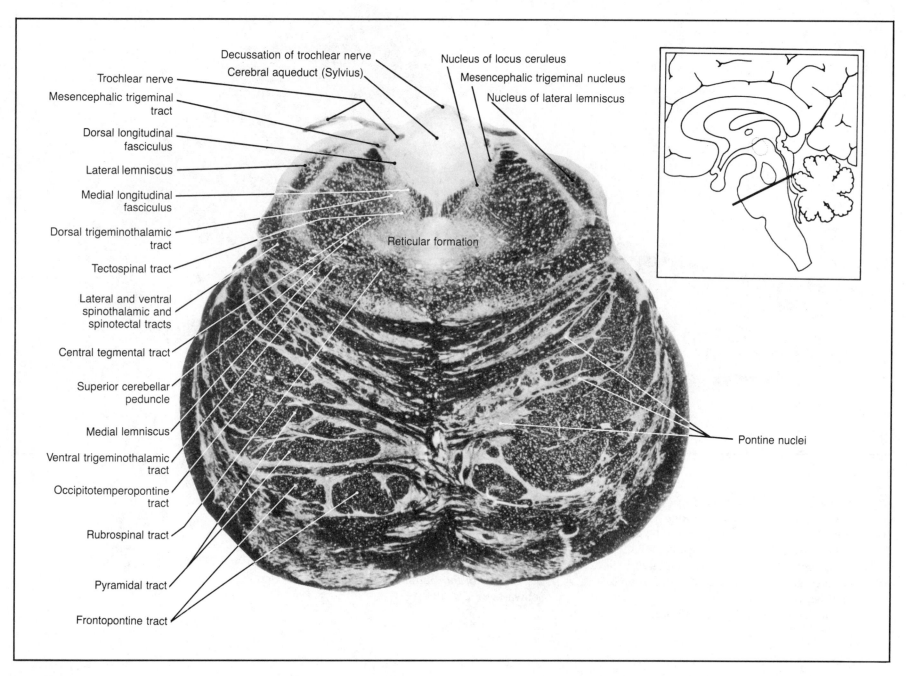

Decussation of trochlear nerve

Trochlear nerve

Cerebral aqueduct (Sylvius)

Nucleus of locus ceruleus

Mesencephalic trigeminal nucleus

Nucleus of lateral lemniscus

Mesencephalic trigeminal tract

Dorsal longitudinal fasciculus

Lateral lemniscus

Medial longitudinal fasciculus

Dorsal trigeminothalamic tract

Tectospinal tract

Reticular formation

Lateral and ventral spinothalamic and spinotectal tracts

Central tegmental tract

Superior cerebellar peduncle

Medial lemniscus

Ventral trigeminothalamic tract

Occipitotemperopontine tract

Rubrospinal tract

Pyramidal tract

Frontopontine tract

Pontine nuclei

FIGURE 20–5 Photomicrograph of transverse section
of human brainstem through pons. (Magnification
× 6.5; Weil stain.) (From *Structure of the Human Brain:
A Photographic Atlas*, Second Edition by Stephen J.
DeArmond, Madeline M. Fusco, Maynard M. Dewey.
Copyright © 1974, 1976 by Oxford University Press,
Inc., New York. Reprinted by permission.)

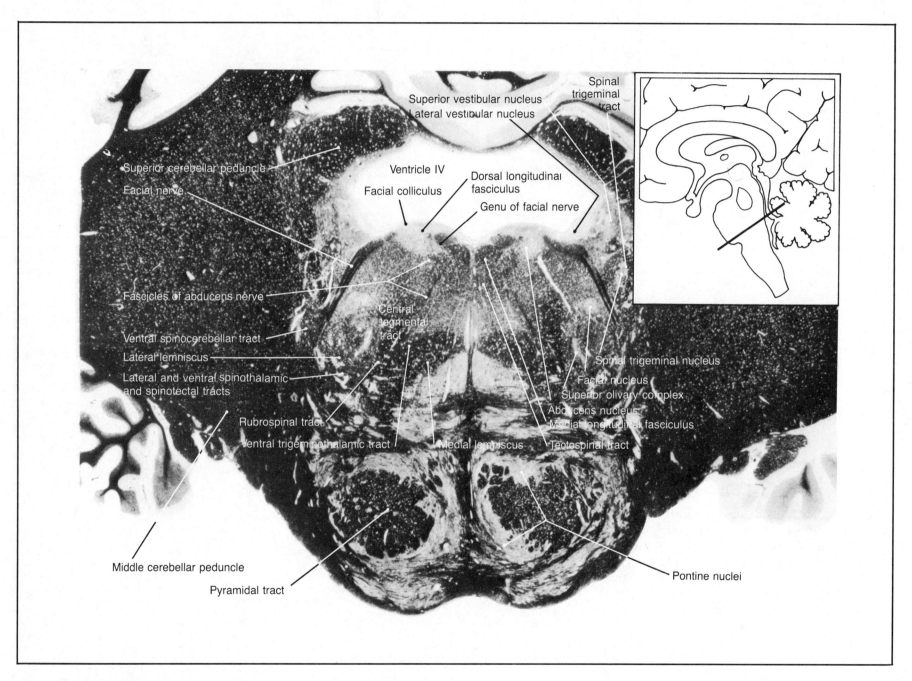

Superior vestibular nucleus

Lateral vestibular nucleus

Spinal trigeminal tract

Superior cerebellar peduncle

Facial nerve

Ventricle IV

Facial colliculus

Dorsal longitudinal fasciculus

Genu of facial nerve

Fascicles of abducens nerve

Central tegmental tract

Ventral spinocerebellar tract

Lateral lemniscus

Lateral and ventral spinothalamic and spinotectal tracts

Spinal trigeminal nucleus

Facial nucleus

Superior olivary complex

Abducens nucleus

Medial longitudinal fasciculus

Rubrospinal tract

Ventral trigeminothalamic tract

Medial lemniscus

Tectospinal tract

Middle cerebellar peduncle

Pyramidal tract

Pontine nuclei

FIGURE 20–6   Photomicrograph of transverse section
of human brainstem through pons at a level slightly
caudal to that of previous figure. (Magnification × 6.5;
Weil stain.) (From *Structure of the Human Brain: A
Photographic Atlas*, Second Edition by Stephen J.
DeArmond, Madeline M. Fusco, Maynard M. Dewey.
Copyright © 1974, 1976 by Oxford University Press,
Inc., New York. Reprinted by permission.)

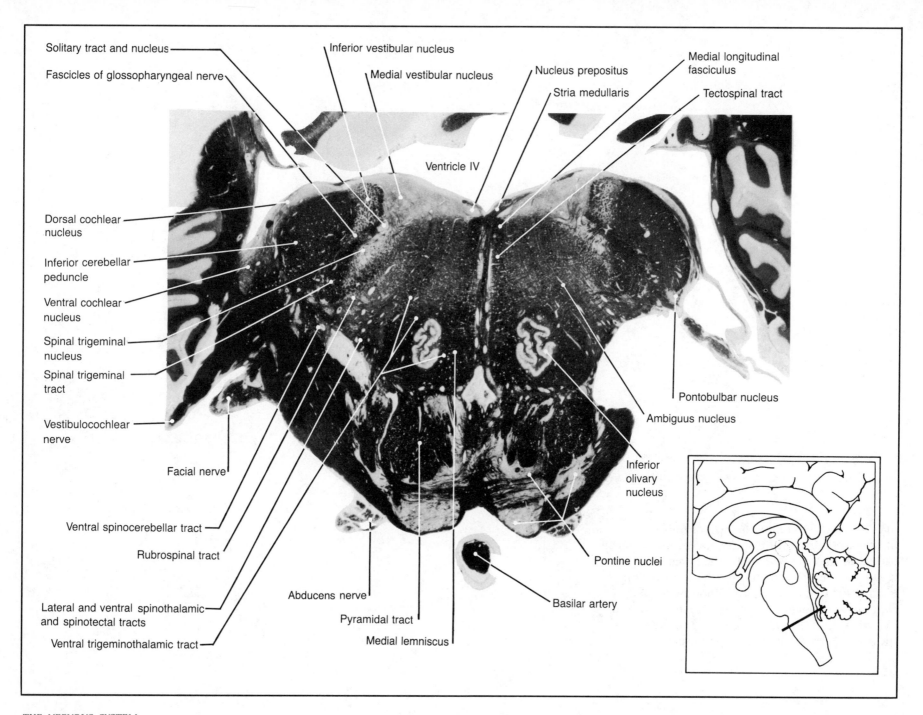

Solitary tract and nucleus

Fascicles of glossopharyngeal nerve

Inferior vestibular nucleus

Medial vestibular nucleus

Nucleus prepositus

Stria medullaris

Medial longitudinal fasciculus

Tectospinal tract

Ventricle IV

Dorsal cochlear nucleus

Inferior cerebellar peduncle

Ventral cochlear nucleus

Spinal trigeminal nucleus

Spinal trigeminal tract

Vestibulocochlear nerve

Facial nerve

Ventral spinocerebellar tract

Rubrospinal tract

Lateral and ventral spinothalamic and spinotectal tracts

Ventral trigeminothalamic tract

Abducens nerve

Pyramidal tract

Medial lemniscus

Basilar artery

Pontine nuclei

Inferior olivary nucleus

Ambiguus nucleus

Pontobulbar nucleus

FIGURE 20–7   Photomicrograph of transverse section
of human brainstem at the level of transition between
pons and medulla oblongata. (Magnification × 6.5;
Weil stain.) (From *Structure of the Human Brain: A
Photographic Atlas*, Second Edition by Stephen J.
DeArmond, Madeline M. Fusco, Maynard M. Dewey.
Copyright © 1974, 1976 by Oxford University Press,
Inc., New York. Reprinted by permission.)

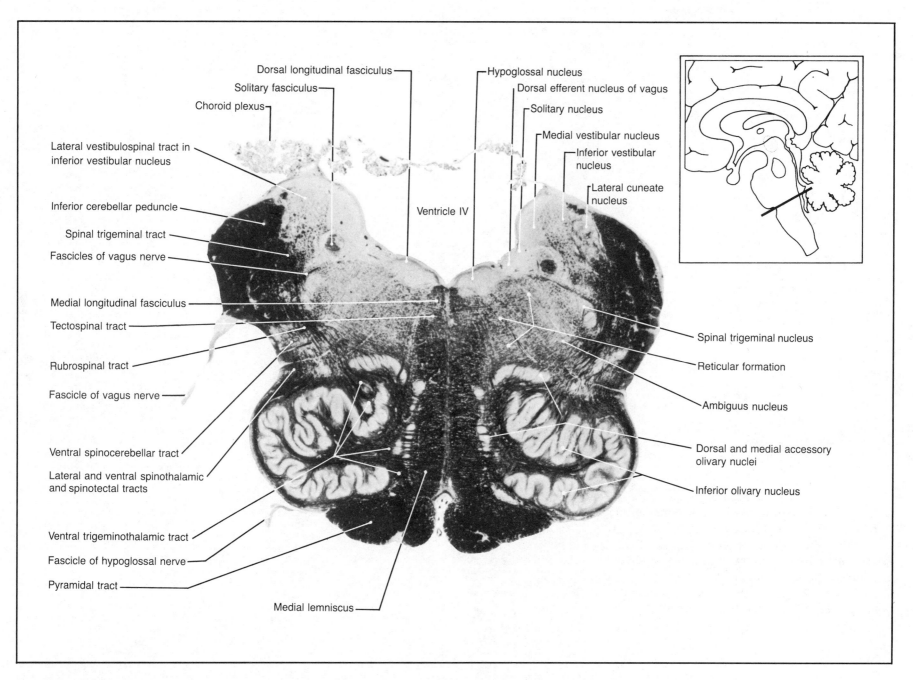

Dorsal longitudinal fasciculus

Solitary fasciculus

Choroid plexus

Lateral vestibulospinal tract in inferior vestibular nucleus

Inferior cerebellar peduncle

Spinal trigeminal tract

Fascicles of vagus nerve

Medial longitudinal fasciculus

Tectospinal tract

Rubrospinal tract

Fascicle of vagus nerve

Ventral spinocerebellar tract

Lateral and ventral spinothalamic and spinotectal tracts

Ventral trigeminothalamic tract

Fascicle of hypoglossal nerve

Pyramidal tract

Medial lemniscus

Hypoglossal nucleus

Dorsal efferent nucleus of vagus

Solitary nucleus

Medial vestibular nucleus

Inferior vestibular nucleus

Lateral cuneate nucleus

Ventricle IV

Spinal trigeminal nucleus

Reticular formation

Ambiguus nucleus

Dorsal and medial accessory olivary nuclei

Inferior olivary nucleus

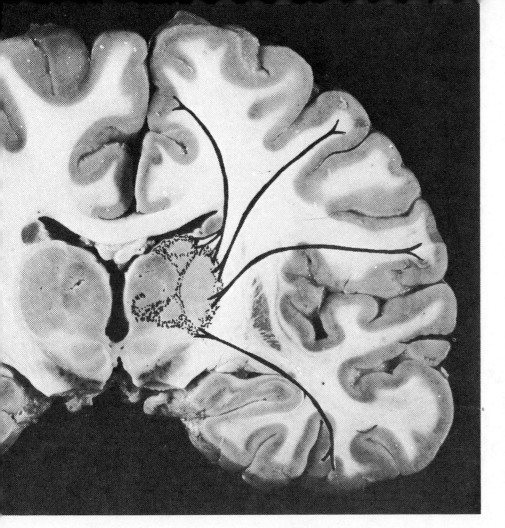

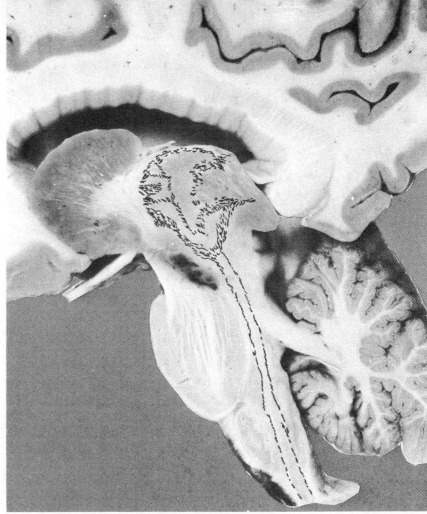

FIGURE 20–9   Cerebrum sectioned coronally with the reticular thalamic nuclei stippled on the photograph. Projections and radiations between reticular thalamic nuclei and "silent" cortical areas have been marked with dark lines. (Courtesy of Jeff Minckler, "Functional Organization and Maintenance," in Jeff Minckler (Ed.), *Introduction to Neuroscience.* St. Louis: The C.V. Mosby Co., 1972.)

FIGURE 20–10   Parasagittal section of the brainstem with the reticular formation stippled and superimposed on the photograph. (Courtesy of Jeff Minckler, "Functional Organization and Maintenance," in Jeff Minckler (Ed.), *Introduction to Neuroscience.* St. Louis: The C.V. Mosby Co., 1972.)

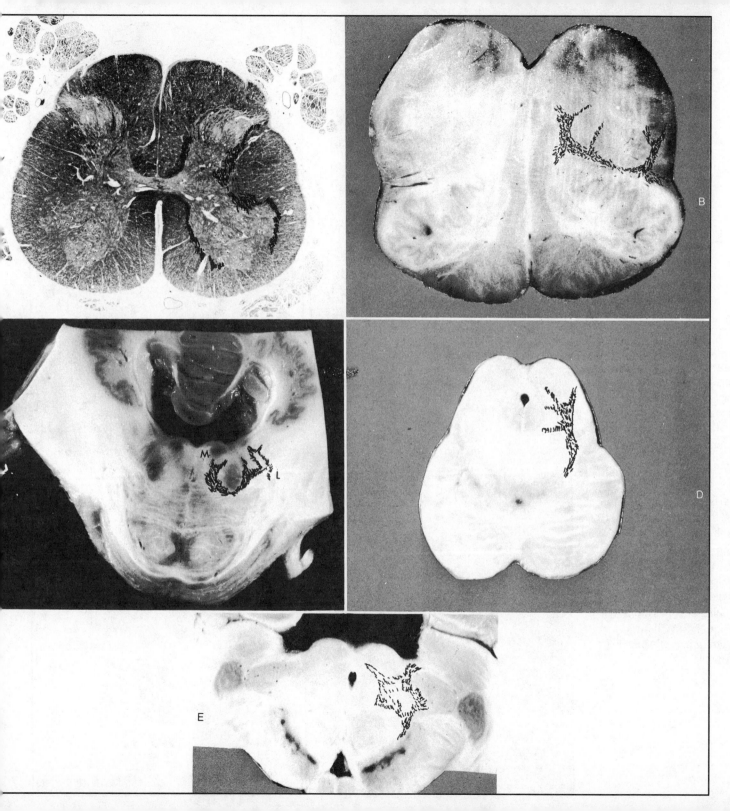

FIGURE 20–11 Position of the reticular formation is illustrated by stippling placed on horizontal sections at various ascending levels. (A) spinal cord; (B) medulla; (C) pons, showing its (L) lateral and (M) medial tegmental paths; (D) lower midbrain; (E) upper midbrain. (Courtesy of Jeff Minckler, "Functional Organization and Maintenance," in Jeff Minckler (Ed.), *Introduction to Neuroscience*. St. Louis: The C.V. Mosby Co., 1972.)

FIGURE 20–12 Brain and spinal cord with attached spinal nerve roots and dorsal root ganglia, viewed from behind. The cauda equina is undisturbed on the right, but has been fanned out on the left to facilitate identification of individual components. The 1st cervical, thoracic, lumbar, and sacral roots are identified with black arrows. (Courtesy of Peter L. Williams and Roger Warwick, *Functional Neuroanatomy of Man.* Edinburgh: Longman Group, Ltd., 1975. Dissection by M.C.E. Hutchinson, Department of Anatomy, Guy's Hospital Medical School.)

FIGURE 20–13 Transverse sections through spinal cord at representative levels. The following regions are evident at all levels, but only labelled at two levels: (1) dorsal funiculus, (2) dorsal grey column, (3) lateral funiculus, (4) ventral grey column, (5) ventral funiculus. Note the changes in overall profile and the relative changes in lightly stained regions of cell bodies and darkly stained regions of myelin-covered fibers. (Magnification × 5.) (Courtesy of Peter L. Williams and Roger Warwick, *Functional Neuroanatomy of Man.* Edinburgh: Longman Group, Ltd., 1975.)

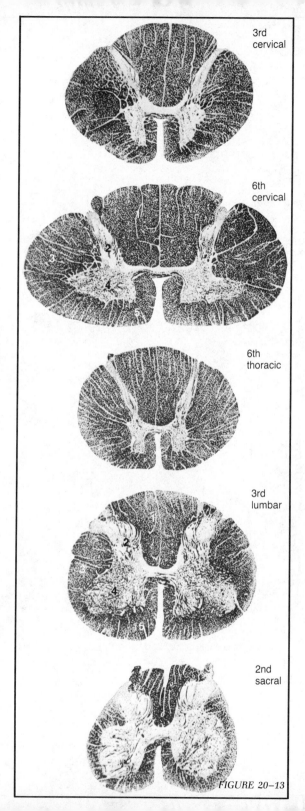

FIGURE 20–12

3rd cervical

6th cervical

6th thoracic

3rd lumbar

2nd sacral

FIGURE 20–13

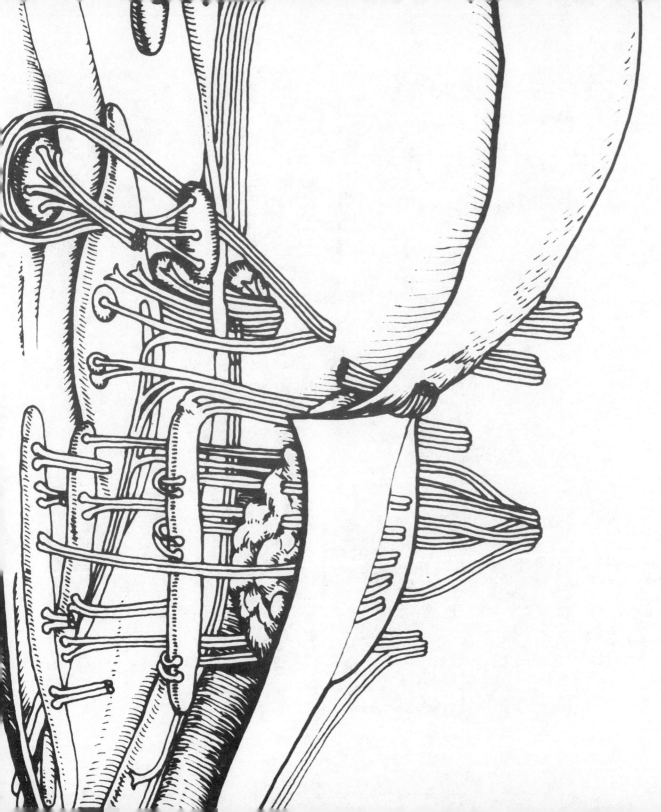

The Cranial Nerves

21

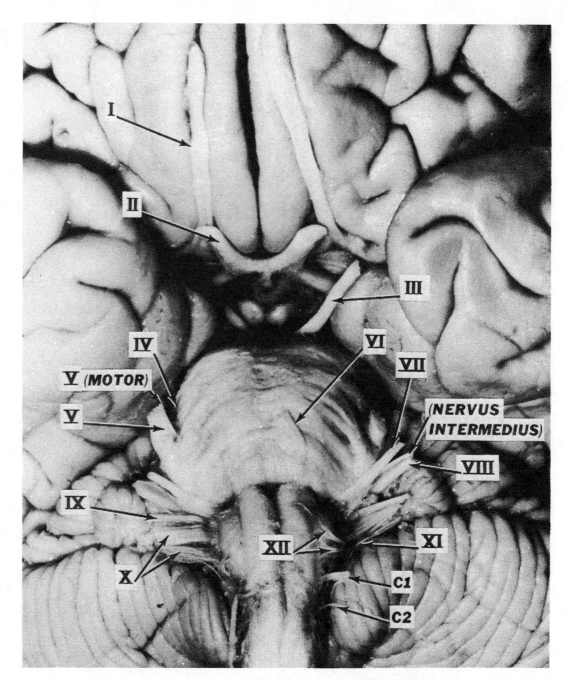

FIGURE 21–1   Ventral view of the brain to demonstrate the location of the cranial nerves as they exit from the central nervous system. The first and second cervical spinal nerves are also labelled. (Courtesy of Jeff Minckler, "Peripheral Nervous System," in Jeff Minckler (Ed.), *Introduction to Neuroscience*. St. Louis: The C.V. Mosby Co., 1972.)

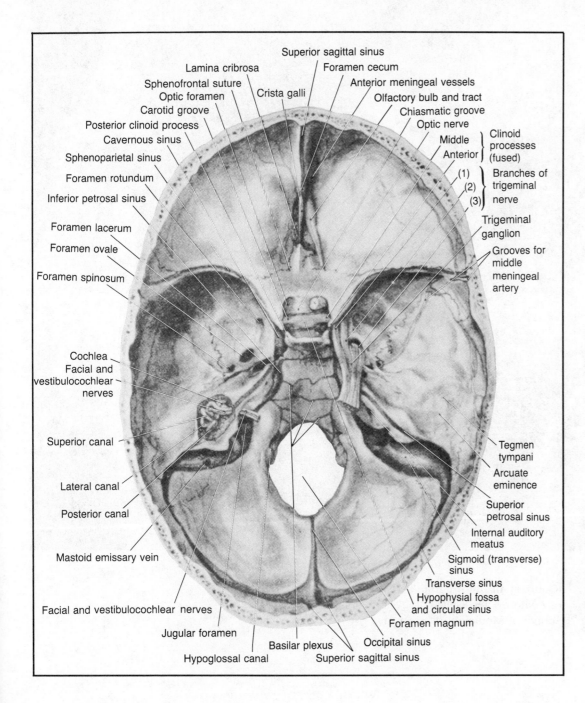

FIGURE 21–2 Drawing of the cranial base showing the trigeminal, facial, vestibulocochlear and hypoglossal nerves exiting through the base of the skull. The cochlea and semicircular canals are exposed on the left. (Courtesy of Fred A. Mettler, *Neuroanatomy*, 2nd Ed. St. Louis: The C.V. Mosby Co., 1948.)

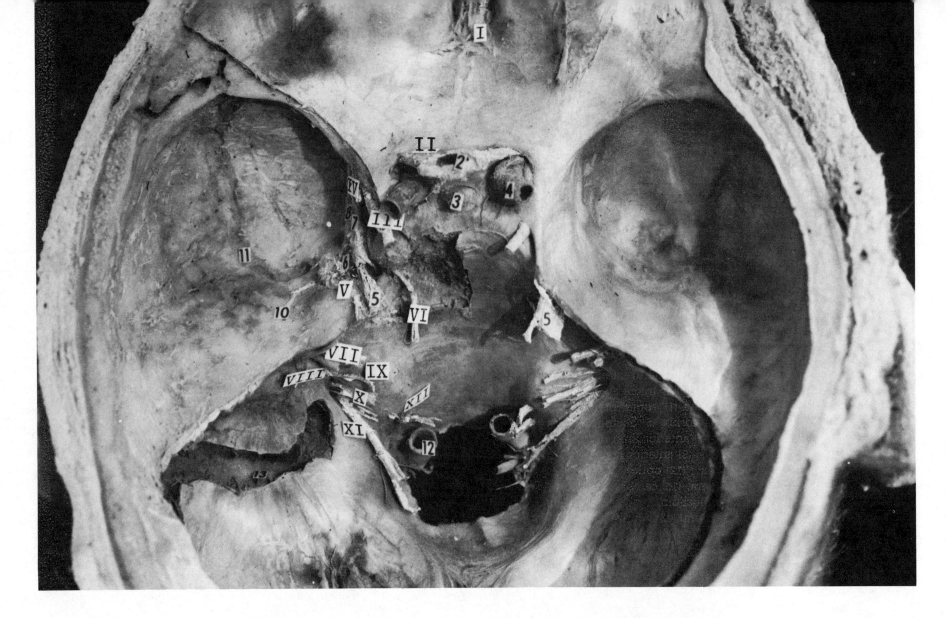

FIGURE 21–3 Cranial base viewed from above, showing cranial nerves exiting through their foramena. This dissection is similar to that shown in Figure 21–2.

(Courtesy of the Anatomy Museum of the Department of Anatomy and Cell Biology, University of Pittsburgh, School of Medicine, Pittsburgh.)

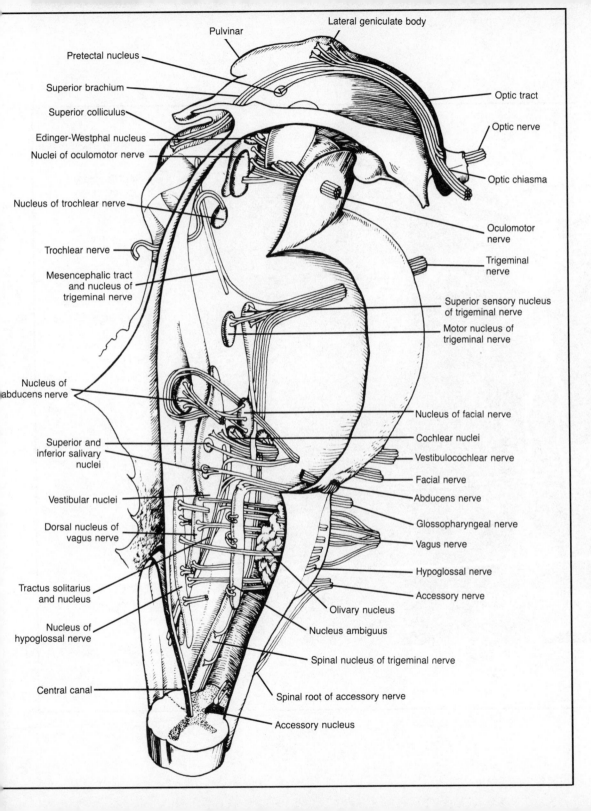

Pulvinar

Lateral geniculate body

Pretectal nucleus

Superior brachium

Superior colliculus

Edinger-Westphal nucleus

Nuclei of oculomotor nerve

Nucleus of trochlear nerve

Trochlear nerve

Mesencephalic tract and nucleus of trigeminal nerve

Nucleus of abducens nerve

Superior and inferior salivary nuclei

Vestibular nuclei

Dorsal nucleus of vagus nerve

Tractus solitarius and nucleus

Nucleus of hypoglossal nerve

Central canal

Accessory nucleus

Optic tract

Optic nerve

Optic chiasma

Oculomotor nerve

Trigeminal nerve

Superior sensory nucleus of trigeminal nerve

Motor nucleus of trigeminal nerve

Nucleus of facial nerve

Cochlear nuclei

Vestibulocochlear nerve

Facial nerve

Abducens nerve

Glossopharyngeal nerve

Vagus nerve

Hypoglossal nerve

Accessory nerve

Olivary nucleus

Nucleus ambiguus

Spinal nucleus of trigeminal nerve

Spinal root of accessory nerve

FIGURE 21–4 Schematic of the cranial nerve nuclei illustrated in a hollow shell of the brainstem. (After Faber and Faber, Ltd., from *Anatomy of the Human Body* by R.D. Lockhart, G.F. Hamilton, and F.W. Fyfe. U.S. publication: Philadelphia: J.B. Lippincott Company, 1959. Reprinted by permission.)

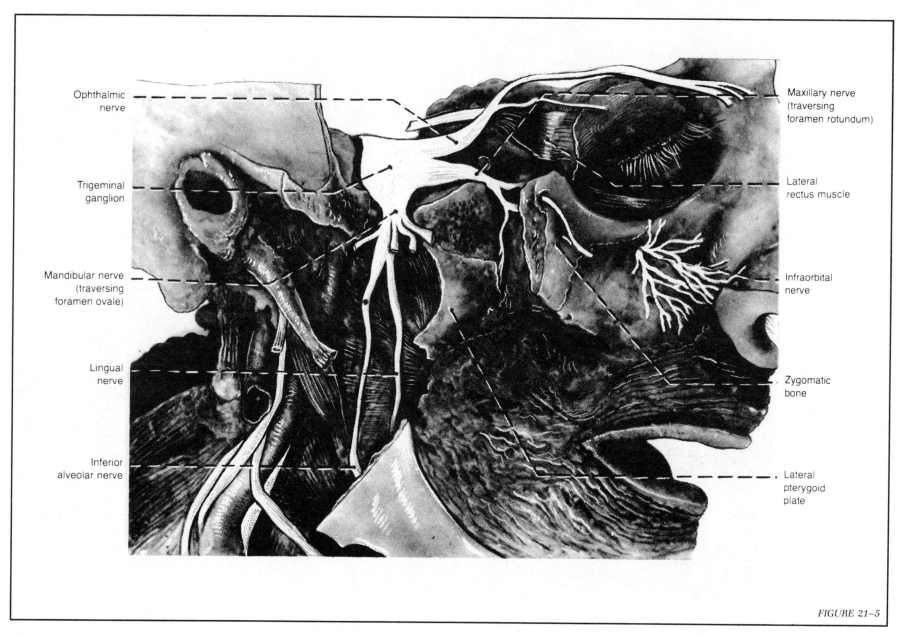

Ophthalmic nerve

Trigeminal ganglion

Mandibular nerve (traversing foramen ovale)

Lingual nerve

Inferior alveolar nerve

Maxillary nerve (traversing foramen rotundum)

Lateral rectus muscle

Infraorbital nerve

Zygomatic bone

Lateral pterygoid plate

FIGURE 21–5

FIGURE 21–5 Dissection to illustrate the three parts of the right trigeminal nerve viewed from an anterolateral angle. Note that many of the facial muscles have been dissected away, and the ramus and parts of the zygomatic and temporal bones have been removed to expose underlying tissue. (Courtesy of Lord Solly Zuckerman, with Deryk Darlington and Peter Lisowski, *A New System of Anatomy*, 2nd Ed. Oxford: Oxford University Press, 1981.)

FIGURE 21–6 Dissection illustrating the primary superficial branches of the right facial nerve. Most of the branches course through the parotid gland, which has been removed. The structure and location of facial nerve branches are not only quite variable among individuals, but also between the two sides of the face. (Courtesy of Lord Solly Zuckerman, with Deryk Darlington and Peter Lisowski, *A New System of Anatomy*, 2nd Ed. Oxford: Oxford University Press, 1981.)

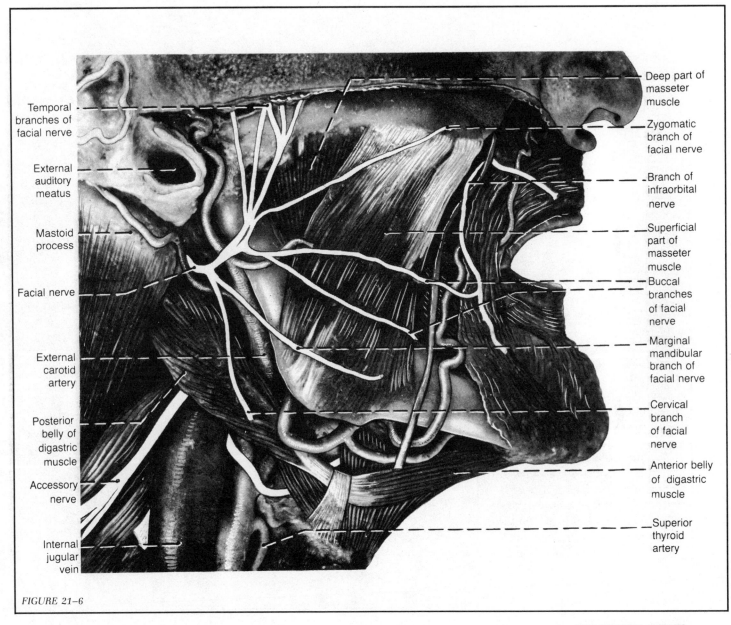

FIGURE 21–6

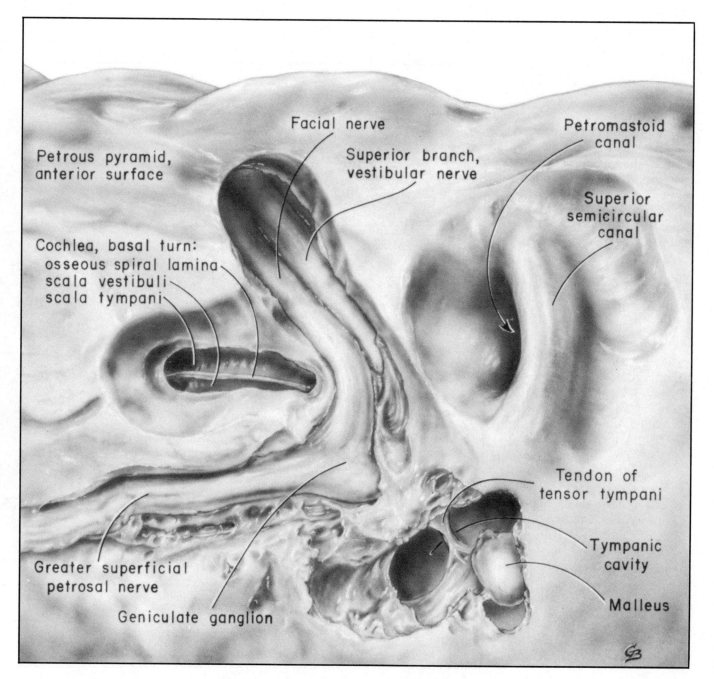

Petrous pyramid, anterior surface

Cochlea, basal turn:
osseous spiral lamina
scala vestibuli
scala tympani

Facial nerve

Superior branch,
vestibular nerve

Petromastoid canal

Superior semicircular canal

Tendon of tensor tympani

Tympanic cavity

Malleus

Greater superficial petrosal nerve

Geniculate ganglion

FIGURE 21–7 Drawing of an unembalmed temporal bone viewed from above and dissected to show the relationship of the facial and vestibular nerves to cochlear, canalicular, and tympanic structures. (Courtesy of Barry J. Anson and James A. Donaldson, *Surgical Anatomy of the Temporal Bone*, 3rd Ed. Philadelphia: W.B. Saunders Company, 1981.)

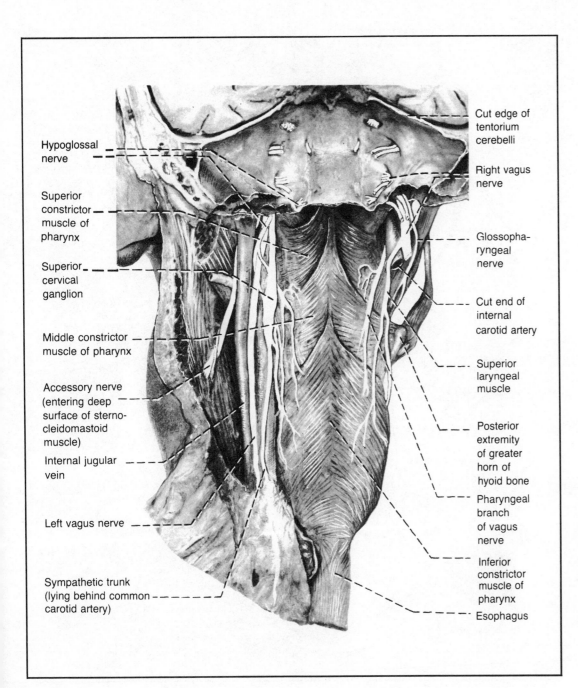

Hypoglossal nerve

Superior constrictor muscle of pharynx

Superior cervical ganglion

Middle constrictor muscle of pharynx

Accessory nerve (entering deep surface of sterno- cleidomastoid muscle)

Internal jugular vein

Left vagus nerve

Sympathetic trunk (lying behind common carotid artery)

Cut edge of tentorium cerebelli

Right vagus nerve

Glossopha- ryngeal nerve

Cut end of internal carotid artery

Superior laryngeal muscle

Posterior extremity of greater horn of hyoid bone

Pharyngeal branch of vagus nerve

Inferior constrictor muscle of pharynx

Esophagus

FIGURE 21–8   Dissection of the posterior aspect of the pharynx illustrating the course of the vagus nerve, hypoglossal nerve, and glossopharyngeal nerve. The right vagus nerve has been cut to provide a better view of the superior laryngeal and pharyngeal branches of the vagus. (Courtesy of Lord Solly Zucker- man, with Deryk Darlington and Peter Lisowski, *A New System of Anatomy,* 2nd Ed. Oxford: Oxford University Press, 1981.)

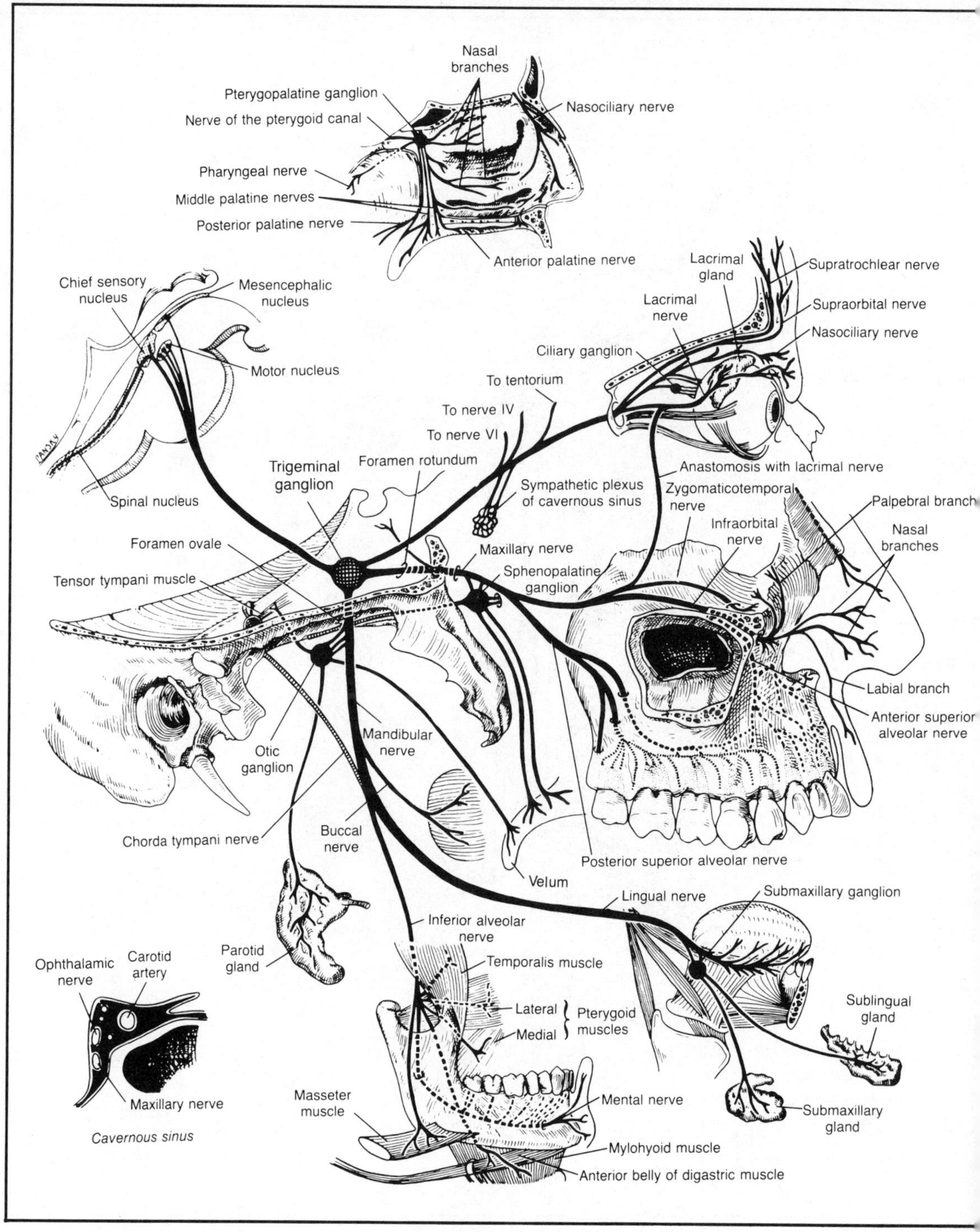

FIGURE 21–9 Schematic showing the course and distribution of the trigeminal (V) nerve. (From E. House and B. Pansky, *A Functional Approach to Neuroanatomy.* New York: McGraw-Hill Book Company, 1960. Used with permission.)

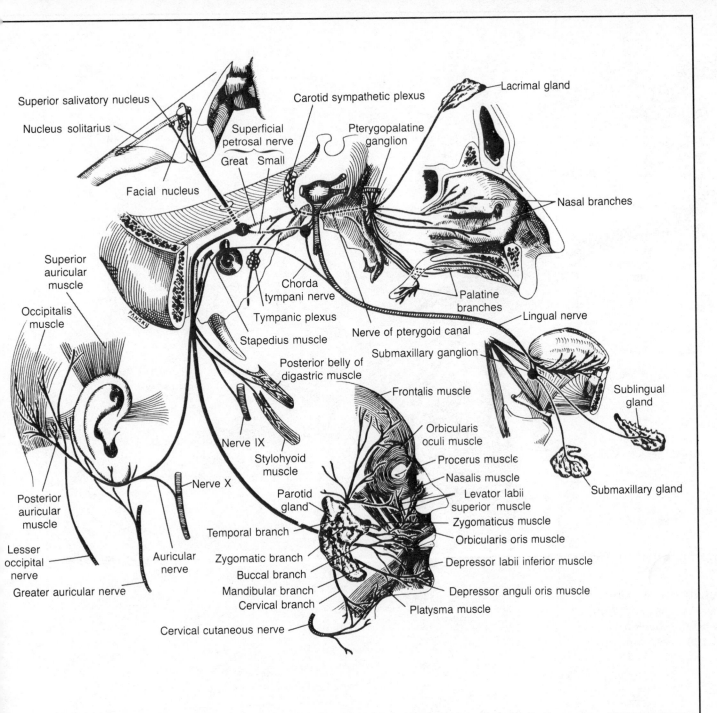

FIGURE 21–10 Schematic showing the course and distribution of the facial (VII) nerve. (From E. House and B. Pansky, *A Functional Approach to Neuroanatomy.* New York: McGraw-Hill Book Company, 1960. Used with permission.)

THE CRANIAL NERVES

325

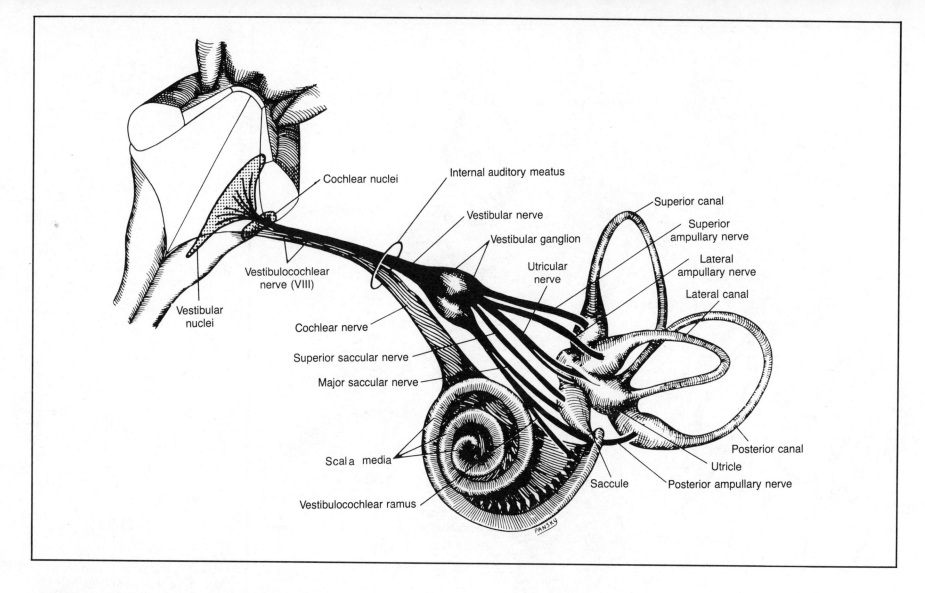

Cochlear nuclei

Internal auditory meatus

Superior canal

Vestibular nerve

Superior ampullary nerve

Vestibular ganglion

Lateral ampullary nerve

Utricular nerve

Lateral canal

Vestibulocochlear nerve (VIII)

Vestibular nuclei

Cochlear nerve

Superior saccular nerve

Major saccular nerve

Posterior canal

Utricle

Scala media

Saccule

Posterior ampullary nerve

Vestibulocochlear ramus

FIGURE 21–11 Schematic showing the course and distribution of the vestibulocochlear (VIII) nerve. (From E. House and B. Pansky, *A Functional Approach to Neuroanatomy.* New York: McGraw-Hill Book Company, 1960. Used with permission.)

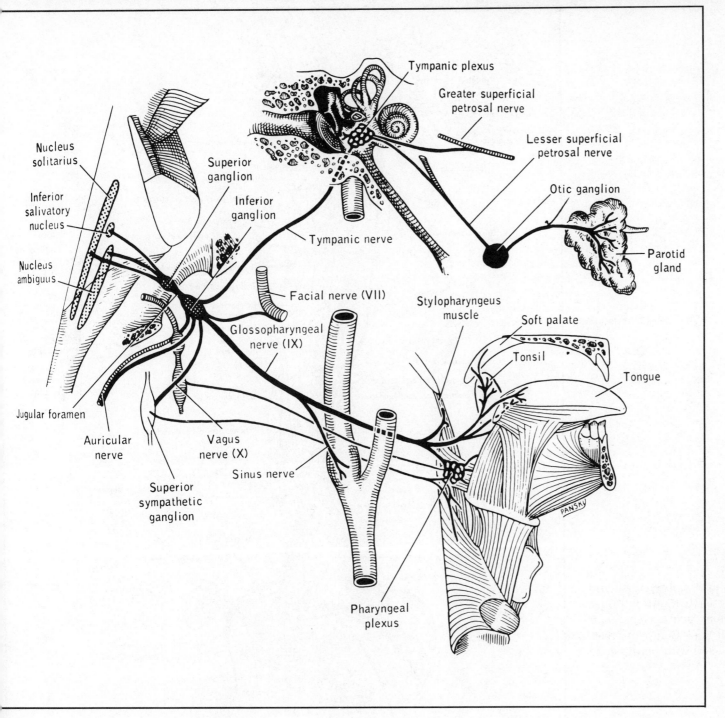

FIGURE 21–12 Schematic showing the course and distribution of the glossopharyngeal (IX) nerve. (From E. House and B. Pansky, *A Functional Approach to Neuroanatomy.* New York: McGraw-Hill Book Company, 1960. Used with permission.)

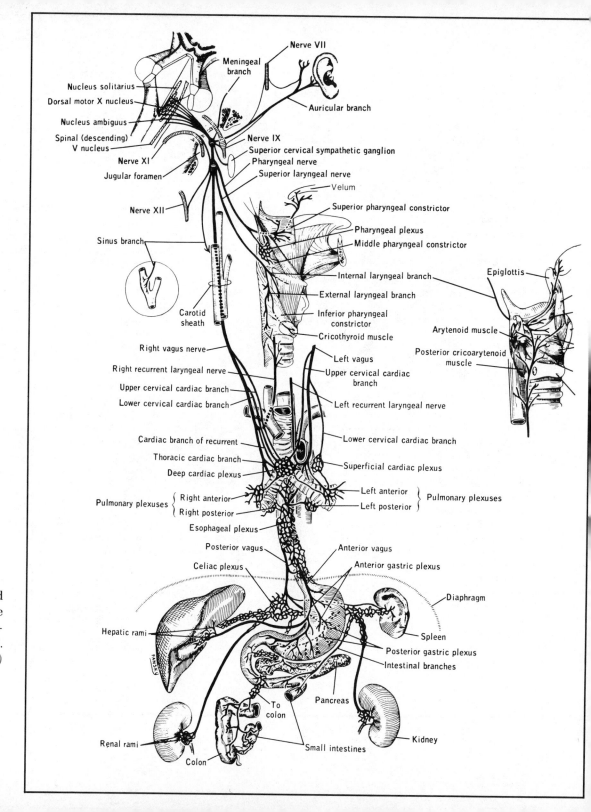

FIGURE 21–13   Schematic showing the course and distribution of the vagus (X) nerve. (From E. House and B. Pansky, *A Functional Approach to Neuroanatomy*. New York: McGraw-Hill Book Company, 1960. Used with permission.)

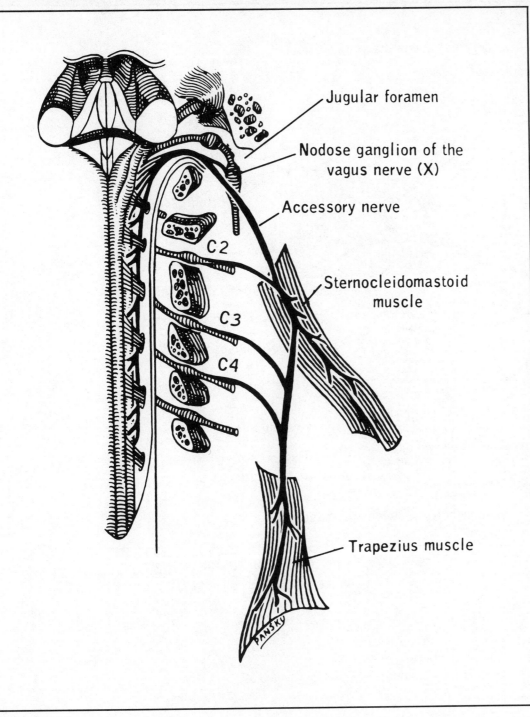

Jugular foramen

Nodose ganglion of the
vagus nerve (X)

Accessory nerve

Sternocleidomastoid
muscle

C 2

C 3

C 4

Trapezius muscle

FIGURE 21–14 Schematic showing the course and
distribution of the (spinal) accessory (XI) nerve. (From
E. House and B. Pansky, *A Functional Approach to
Neuroanatomy*. New York: McGraw-Hill Book Company,
1960. Used with permission.)

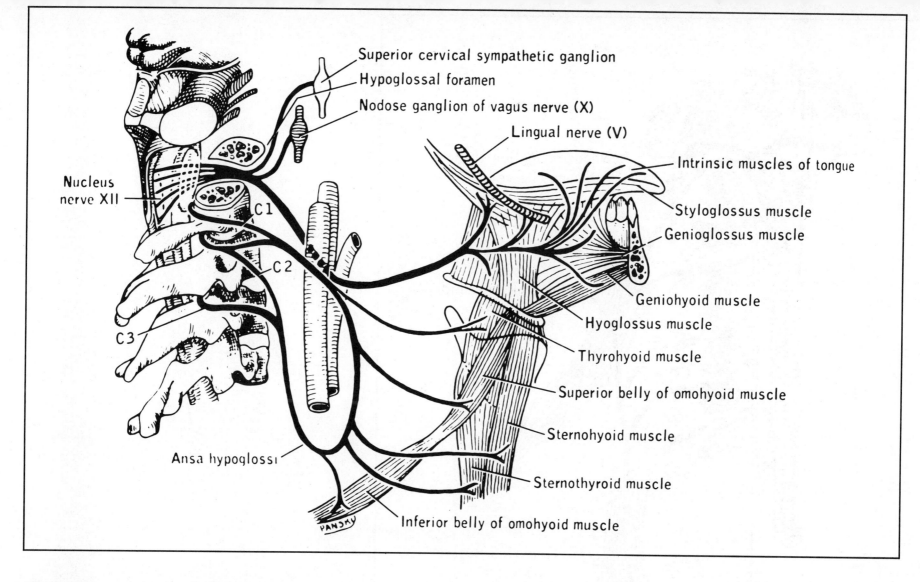

FIGURE 21–15 Schematic showing the course and
distribution of the hypoglossal (XII) nerve. (From
E. House and B. Pansky, *A Functional Approach to
Neuroanatomy.* New York: McGraw-Hill Book Company,
1960. Used with permission.)

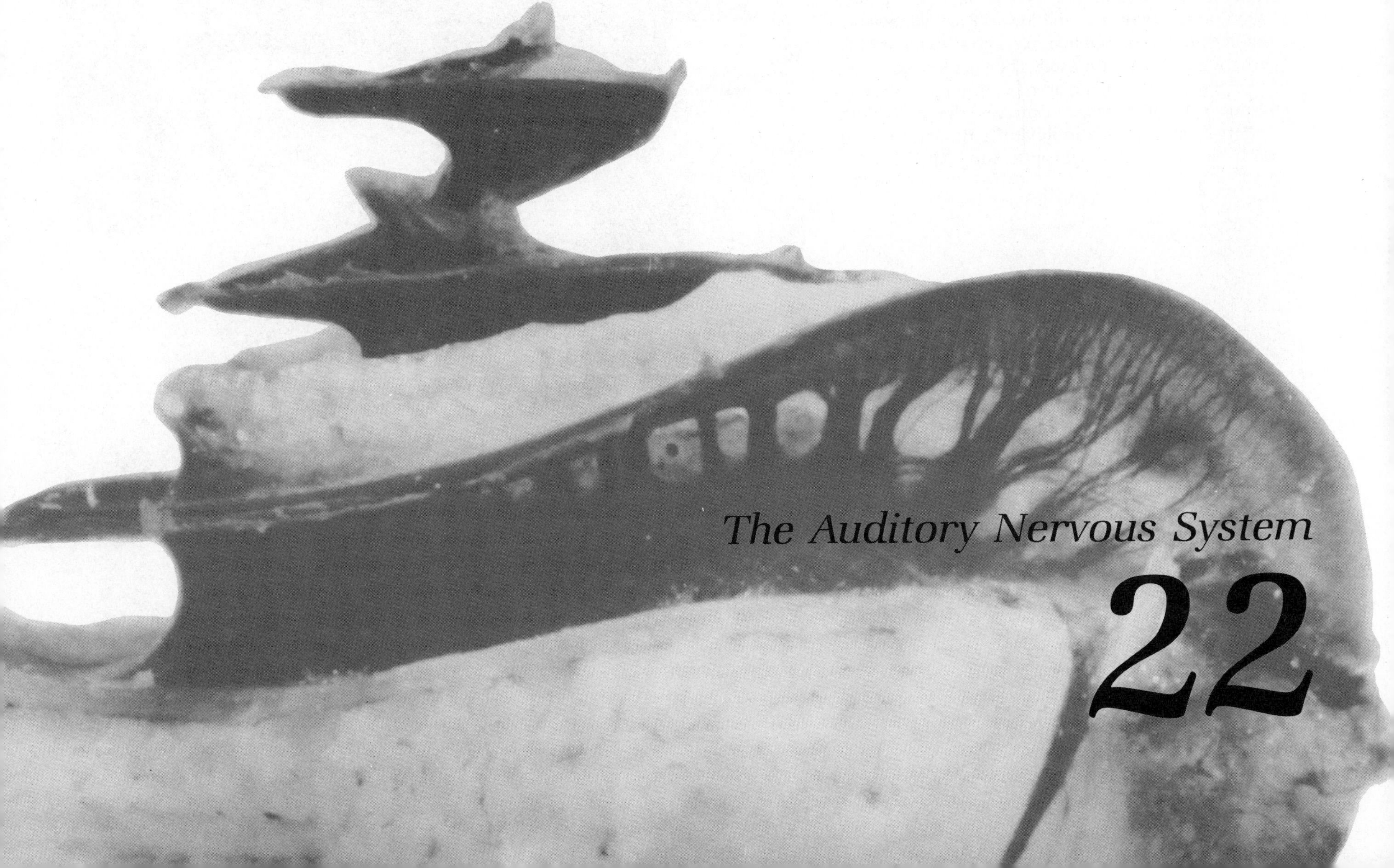

The Auditory Nervous System

22

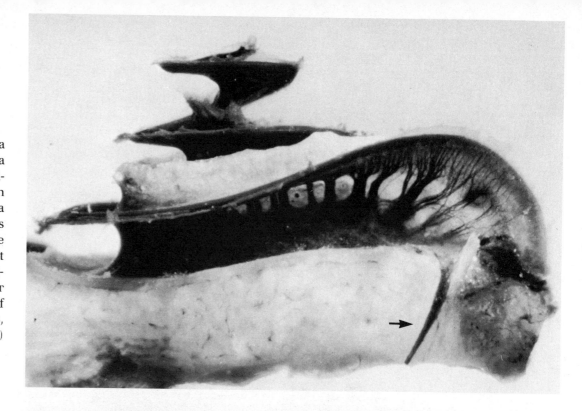

FIGURE 22–1 Dissection of the adult human cochlea showing the modiolus with the osseous spiral lamina and myelinated nerve bundles. The bony capsule, spiral ligament, and Reissner's membrane have been removed. The basal end of the osseous spiral lamina is seen on the right, and the lower basal coil extends to the left side of the photograph. Above it, the middle and apical coils are exposed. The cochlear aqueduct has been opened and is marked with an arrow. (Magnification × 13.) (Courtesy of Goran Bredberg, "Cellular Pattern and Nerve Supply of the Human Organ of Corti," in *Acta Otolaryngologica*, Supplementum 236, 1968, p. 36.)

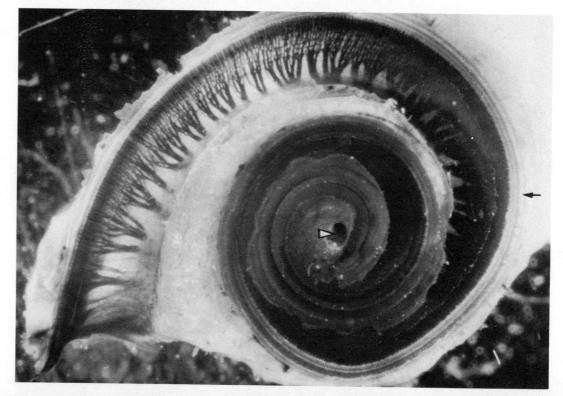

FIGURE 22–2 Dissection of the human cochlea as viewed from above showing myelinated nerve bundles within the osseous spiral lamina. The nerve bundles are seen best in the lower basal coil. The organ of Corti is marked with a black arrow at the peripheral margin of the osseous spiral lamina. The helicotrema is indicated with a white arrow. (Magnification × 13.) (Courtesy of Goran Bredberg, "Cellular Pattern and Nerve Supply of the Human Organ of Corti," in *Acta Otolaryngologica*, Supplementum 236, 1968, p. 37.)

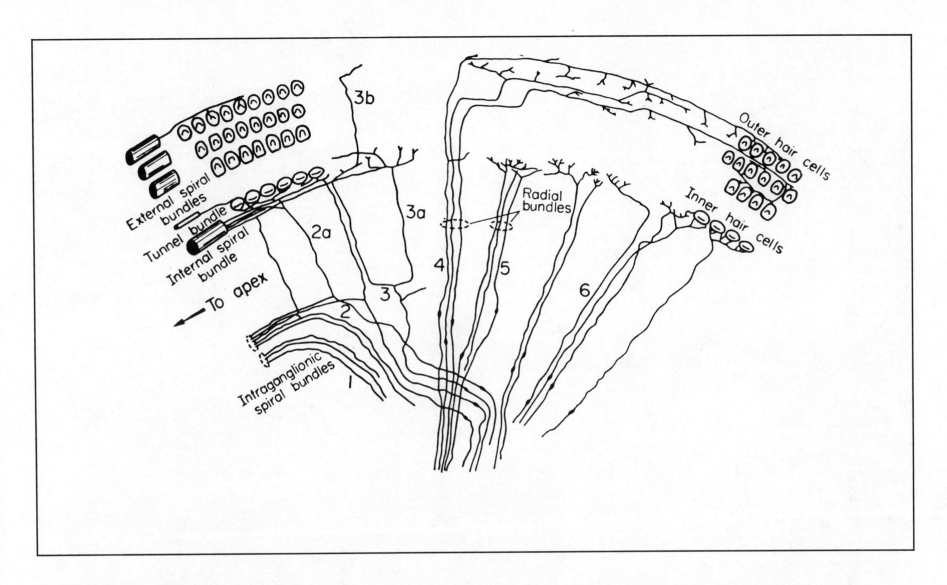

FIGURE 22–3 Innervation of the cochlea. The numbers identify separate bundles of spiral (1, 2, and 3) and radial (4, 5, and 6) fibers from the cochlear nerve.

(Courtesy of T.S. Littler, *The Physics of the Ear*. Elmsford, N.Y.: Pergamon Press, Inc., 1965. Reprinted with permission.)

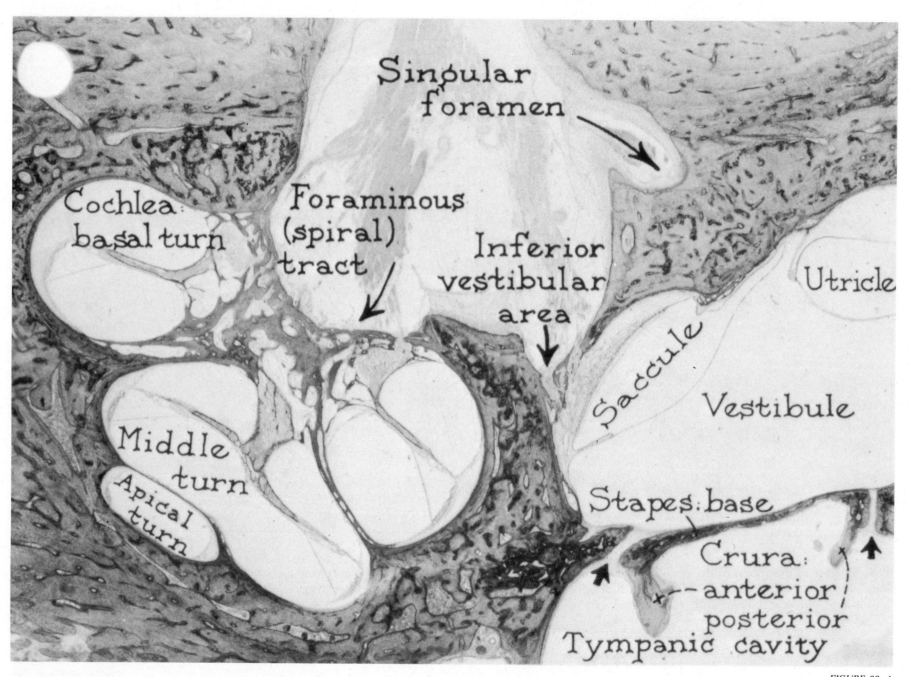

Singular
foramen

Cochlea:
basal turn

Foraminous
(spiral)
tract

Inferior
vestibular
area

Utricle

Saccule

Vestibule

Middle
turn

Apical
turn

Stapes: base

Crura:
anterior
posterior
Tympanic cavity

FIGURE 22–4

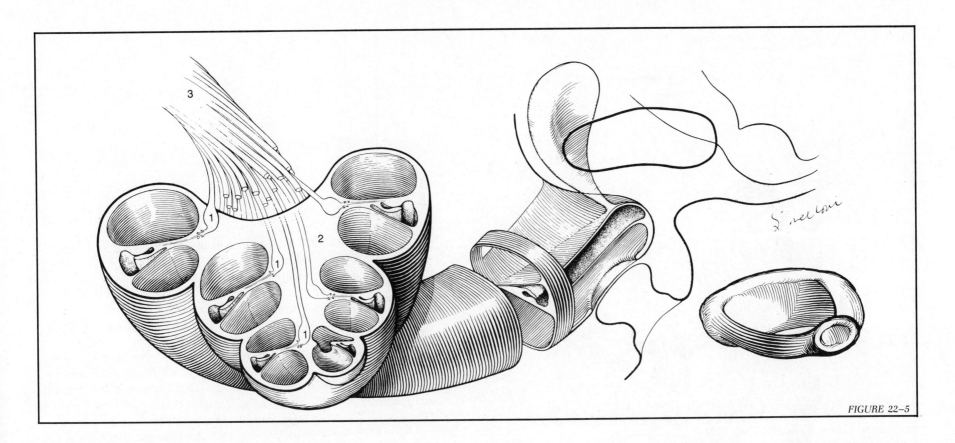

FIGURE 22–5

FIGURE 22–4 Photomicrograph of a horizontal section through the temporal bone showing the cochlear and vestibular divisions of the vestibulocochlear nerve in relation to their channels and foramina. The margins of the oval window are indicated by the unlabelled arrows. The specimen is from a 10-week-old infant. (Magnification × 12; H. & E. stain.) (Courtesy of the Wisconsin Otological Collection, as shown in Barry J. Anson and James A. Donaldson, *Surgical Anatomy of the Temporal Bone*, 3rd Ed. Philadelphia: W.B. Saunders Company, 1981.)

FIGURE 22–5 Cochlea sectioned to illustrate the (1) spiral ganglion in the (2) modiolus, and the course of fibers into the (3) cochlear nerve. (Courtesy of Ida Dox, Biagio John Melloni, and Gilbert M. Eisner, *Melloni's Illustrated Medical Dictionary*. Baltimore: The Williams & Wilkins Co., 1979. Drawing by Biagio John Melloni.)

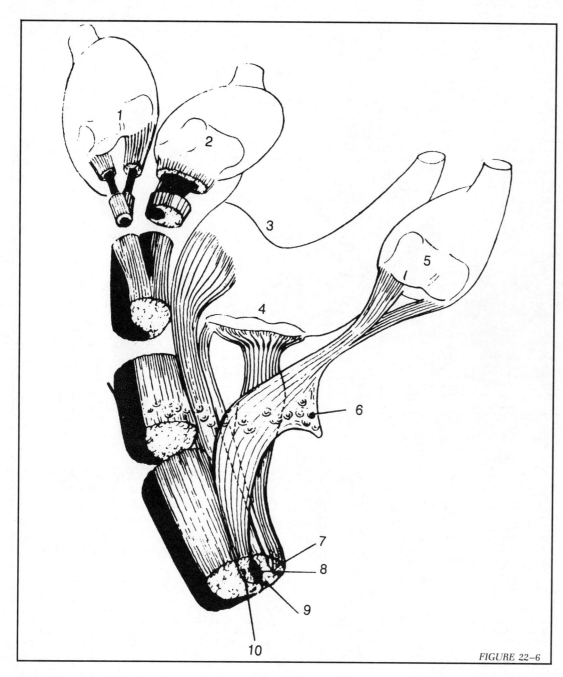

FIGURE 22–6

FIGURE 22–6   Schematic of the innervation of the cristae and macculae. The dark and light areas represent the location of large and small diameter neurons, respectively, to the superior and horizontal cristae. (1) crista ampularis of the superior canal, (2) crista ampularis of the horizontal canal, (3) utricle, (4) saccule, (5) crista ampularis of the posterior canal, (6) Scarpa's ganglion, (7) saccular nerve, (8) efferent fibers, (9) utricular nerve, (10) nerve from crista ampularis of the posterior canal. (Courtesy of R.R. Gacek, "The Course and Central Termination of First Order Neurons Supplying Vestibular Endorgans in the Cat." in *Acta Otolaryngologica*, Supplementum 254, 1969, p. 59.)

FIGURE 22–7   Drawing of the temporal bone as seen from a superior and slightly posterior view to show the relations among the vestibular, cochlear, facial, and greater superficial petrosal nerves. The contents of the undissected temporal bone are shown as if the bone were transparent. (Courtesy of Barry J. Anson and James A. Donaldson, *Surgical Anatomy of the Temporal Bone*, 3rd Ed. Philadelphia: W.B. Saunders Company, 1981.)

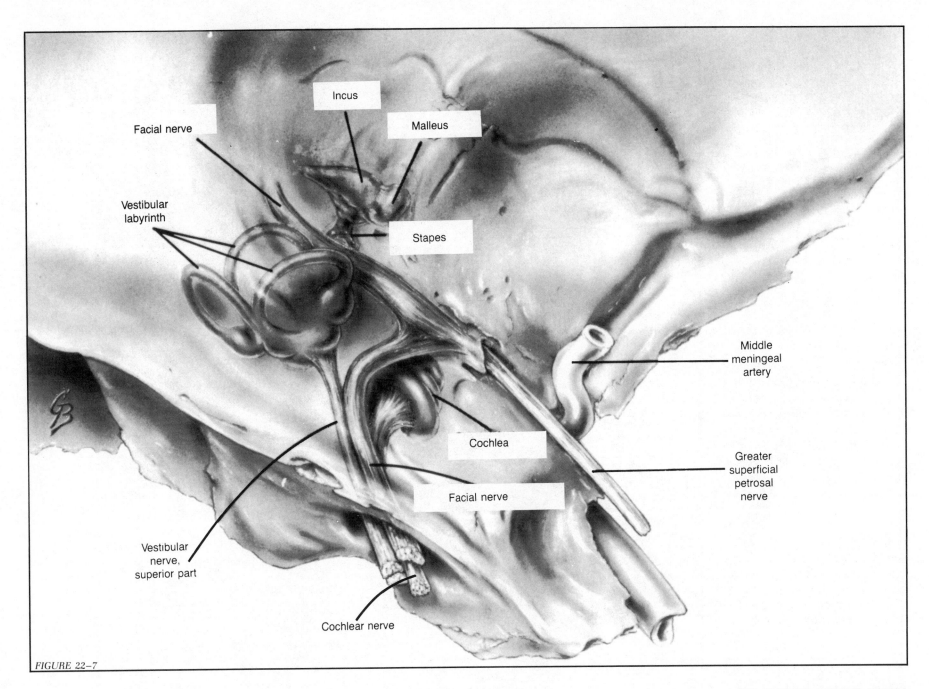

Facial nerve

Incus

Malleus

Stapes

Vestibular
labyrinth

Middle
meningeal
artery

Cochlea

Greater
superficial
petrosal
nerve

Facial nerve

Vestibular
nerve,
superior part

Cochlear nerve

FIGURE 22–7

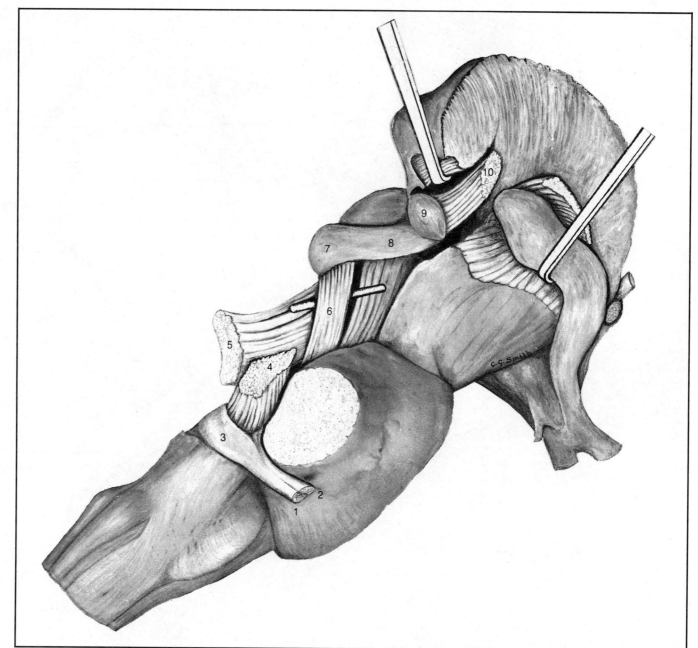

FIGURE 22–8 Dissection of the brainstem to show the auditory pathways. (1) cochlear division of vestibulocochlear nerve, (2) vestibular division of vestibulocochlear nerve, (3) dorsal cochlear nucleus, (4) inferior cerebellar peduncle, (5) superior cerebellar peduncle, (6) lateral lemniscus, (7) inferior colliculus, (8) brachium of inferior colliculus, (9) medial geniculate body, (10) auditory radiation. (From Carlton G. Smith, *Serial Dissections of the Human Brain*. Baltimore: Urban & Schwarzenberg, 1981.)

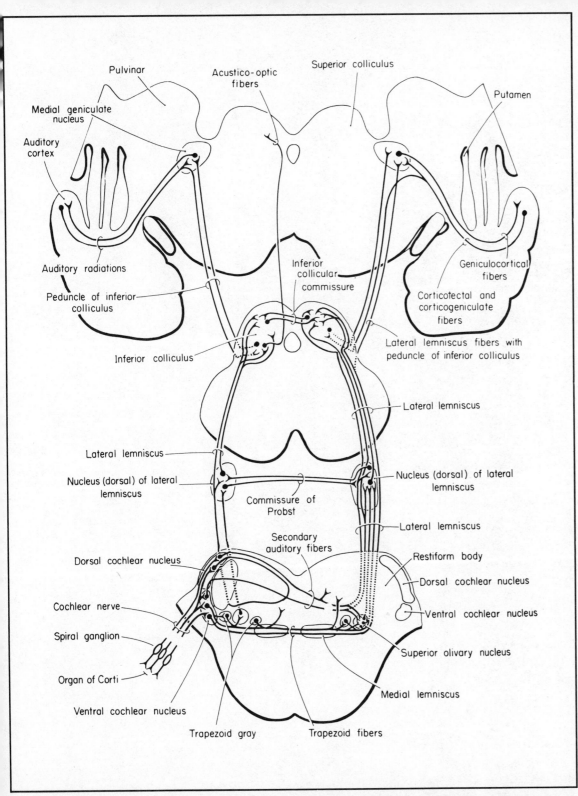

FIGURE 22–9 Diagram illustrating the pathways of the auditory nervous system. (From E. Crosby, T. Humphrey, and E. Lauer, *Correlative Anatomy of the Nervous System*. New York: The Macmillan Co., Inc., 1962.)

Index

muscle, 3–6, 3–7, 3–11, 9–8, 9–12, 9–13, 9–17, 10–11, 21–9

N

naris, 8–2
nasal
  bone, 1–6, 1–15, 8–3, 8–6
  cartilage, 8–3
  cavity, 1–15, 7–2, 8–6, 8–7, 9–13
  choanae, 1–13, 6–2, 8–5
  concha, 1–5, 8–5, 8–7
  crest, 8–6
  septum, 6–2, 6–10, 6–13, 8–5, 20–1
  spine, 6–5, 7–2
nasalis muscle, 11–2, 11–4, 11–5, 11–10, 21–10
nasociliary nerve, 21–9
nasolabial groove, 11–1
nasopharyngeal port, 6–2, 6–14
nasopharynx, 6–2, 6–10, 6–13
nodulus, 18–21, 18–22
nose, 8–1, 8–2, 8–3, 8–4, 8–7
nucleus
  ambiguus, 20–7, 20–8, 21–4, 21–12, 21–13
  gracilis, 19–7
  prepositus, 20–7
  solitarius, 21–10, 21–12, 21–13

O

oblique fissure, 2–24
occipital
  artery, 3–15
  bone, 1–6, 1–7, 1–8, 1–9, 1–10, 1–11
  condyles, 1–9
  forceps, 18–11
  gyri, 18–6, 18–7
  lobe, 19–6
  nerve, 3–15, 21–10
  pole, 18–5, 18–6, 18–7, 18–8, 19–7, 19–8, 19–9, 19–12, 19–13, 19–14, 19–15
  protuberance, 2–3, 3–15
  radiation, 19–14
  sinus, 18–18, 21–2
occipitalis muscle, 21–10
occipitofrontal fascicle, 18–12
occipitotemperopontine tract, 20–5
occipitotemporal gyri, 18–5, 18–8
oculomotor
  nerve (III), 18–17, 21–1, 21–3, 21–4

nucleus, 21–4
olfactory
  area, 8–7
  bulb, 18–4, 20–1, 21–2
  nerve (I), 8–6, 21–1, 21–3
  sulcus, 8–7, 18–5, 19–17
  tract, 18–4, 18–5, 18–17, 21–2
olive, 19–6, 19–7, 20–3, 20–4, 20–6, 20–7, 20–8, 21–4, 22–9
omohyoid muscle, 3–8, 3–9, 3–11, 3–13, 4–31, 4–36, 4–39, 21–15
opthalmic nerve, 21–5, 21–9
optic
  chiasm, 18–6, 18–14, 18–17, 20–3, 21–4
  foramen, 21–2
  nerve (II), 19–7, 20–3, 21–1, 21–2, 21–3, 21–4
  radiation, 19–10, 20–3
  tract, 18–13, 19–3, 19–8, 19–17, 20–3, 20–4, 21–4
oral cavity, 6–2, 6–10, 7–2, 7–3, 7–8, 7–9, 7–10, 7–14, 7–15
orbicularis oculi muscle, 11–3, 11–4, 11–5, 11–11, 11–12, 21–10
  pars lacrimalis (Horner) muscle, 11–2
orbicularis oris
  inferior muscle, 10–9, 11–2, 11–3, 11–4, 11–7, 11–11, 11–12, 21–10
  superior muscle, 10–9, 11–3, 11–4, 11–7, 11–10, 11–11, 11–12, 21–10
orbital
  cavity, 1–5, 1–6
  gyri, 18–5, 19–1
  surface, 18–4
organ of Corti, 16–3, 16–6, 17–1, 17–2, 17–3, 17–5, 17–6, 17–7, 17–8, 17–9, 17–10, 17–11, 17–12, 22–2, 22–9
oropharynx, 6–2, 9–20
osseous labyrinth, 12–8, 16–1
osseous spiral lamina, 21–7, 22–1, 22–2
otic
  capsule, 16–5
  ganglion, 21–9, 21–12
otolithic membrane, 16–13, 16–14
otoliths, 16–14
oval window, 12–8, 15–11, 16–1, 16–3, 22–4

P

palatal
  aponeurosis, 6–5, 6–7, 7–2
  periosteum, 6–3

palate
  hard, 1–12, 5–1, 6–9, 7–2, 7–3, 7–6, 7–7, 7–8, 8–6, 9–8, 9–11, 9–16, 21–13
  soft (see velum)
palatine
  bone, 1–9, 1–12, 1–14, 1–15
  foramina, 1–12
  glands, 9–13
  nerve, 21–9,
  process, 1–9,
  raphe, 7–6, 7–7
  suture, 1–12
  tonsils, 9–2
palatoglossus muscle, 6–3, 6–4, 9–2
palatopharyngeus muscle, 5–3, 6–4, 6–7, 6–12, 6–13, 9–8
pancreas, 21–13
papilla
  circumvallate, 9–2, 9–3, 9–4
  filiform, 7–12, 9–4, 9–8
  foliate, 7–12, 9–4, 9–8
  fungiform, 7–12, 9–4
  vallate, 9–8
paracentral lobule, 18–8
paraflocculus, 18–22
parahippocampal gyrus, 18–5, 18–8
parathyroid gland, 5–4
parietal
  bone, 1–6, 1–7, 1–8, 1–10
  lobe, 18–7
  peritoneum, 2–16, 2–17
  pleura, 2–19, 2–20
parieto-occipital sulcus, 18–8, 19–7
parolfactory gyrus, 18–8
parotid
  duct, 7–11, 10–9, 11–2, 11–3
  gland, 10–24, 21–9, 21–10
patella, 1–3
pectoralis
  major muscle, 2–1, 2–2, 2–4, 2–5, 2–6, 2–20
  minor muscle, 2–1, 2–2, 2–5, 2–6, 2–20
pelvis, 1–3
periacqueductal gray, 19–5, 19–16, 19–17
pericardial cavity, 2–11
pericardium, 2–19, 2–21, 2–24
petromastoid canal, 21–7
petrosal
  nerve
    greater superficial, 21–7, 21–10, 21–12, 22–7
    lesser superficial, 21–12

vertebral
    artery, 18–17, 18–18
    column, 6–10
vertical tongue muscle, 9–3, 9–7, 9–11, 9–12, 9–13, 9–15
vestibular aqueduct, 12–4
vestibular artery, 16–8
vestibular cecum, 16–1
vestibular fold, 4–4, 4–32, 4–34, 4–35, 4–45
vestibular ganglion, 21–11
vestibular nuclei, 20–2, 20–6, 20–7, 20–8, 21–4, 21–11
vestibular vein, 16–8
vestibulocochlear

    artery, 16–6
    nerve (VIII), 15–11, 16–1, 16–5, 16–6, 16–7, 18–17, 20–3, 20–4, 20–7, 20–8, 21–1, 21–2, 21–3, 21–4, 21–7, 21–11, 22–3., 22–4, 22–7, 22–8, 22–9
    ramus, 16–1, 21–11
vestibulospinal tract, 20–8
visceral pleura, 2–20
visual auditory association area, 18–9
vocal
    fold, 4–4, 4–34, 4–35, 4–47, 4–48, 4–49, 9–2
    ligament, 4–47, 4–49
vomer bone, 1–9, 1–13, 1–14, 8–6
vomeronasal cartilage, 8–6

Z

zygomatic
    arch, 10–20
    bone, 1–5, 1–6, 1–9, 10–9, 21–5
    nerve, 21–10
    process, 1–9, 10–17, 12–3, 12–4, 12–5, 12–6, 21–2
zygomaticotemporal nerve, 21–9
zygomaticus
    major muscle, 11–2, 11–3, 11–4, 11–5, 11–11, 11–12, 21–10
    minor muscle, 11–2, 11–3, 11–4, 11–5, 21–10